Infective Endocarditis

Gilbert Habib

Editor

Infective Endocarditis

Epidemiology, Diagnosis, Imaging, Therapy, and Prevention

Springer

Editor
Gilbert Habib
Cardiology Department
Hôpital La Timone
Marseille
France

ISBN 978-3-319-32430-2   ISBN 978-3-319-32432-6   (eBook)
DOI 10.1007/978-3-319-32432-6

Library of Congress Control Number: 2016947177

Printed on acid-free paper

This Springer imprint is published by Springer Nature
The registered company is Springer International Publishing AG Switzerland

Preface

Infective Endocarditis: A Changing Disease

An up-to-date textbook on infective endocarditis is missing and sorely needed. With this book, we hope to have supplied precisely this.

Although infective endocarditis is a cardiac disease that has been known to us for a very long time, it also is an ever-changing disease, with completely varying epidemiology, more and more nosocomial cases, more atypical clinical presentations, new microorganisms, new diagnostic techniques, and, finally, a persistent, severe prognosis.

During the previous 2 years, three international guidelines have been published (two American, one European) summarizing our knowledge of this disease and presenting clear recommendations about the best ways to diagnose and treat patients with suspected or confirmed endocarditis.

Challenges remain, however, mainly:

- How to manage infective endocarditis patients who have intracardiac devices and prostheses, which will probably be the most frequent types of patients in the years to come, due to the radical increase in the number of percutaneous procedures.
- When and how to implement the new diagnostic techniques: With which patients should they be used? PET/CT is an example of a new technology recently brought on board for diagnosing endocarditis.
- When surgery should be considered. If endocarditis is clearly "a surgical disease," nonetheless uncertainties still persist concerning the best indications and timing for surgical intervention.
- How endocarditis can be prevented: This was probably the most hotly debated topic of the past year in this field.

To answer all these questions, the top endocarditis specialists in the world agreed to share their unique knowledge and experience on all the aspects of this disease by contributing chapters to this project. I would like to thank the chapter authors for their kind participation in this textbook.

Finally, this book represents the present. We hope readers will find herein all the most relevant and up-to-date information on this fascinating and challenging disease in which the patient is at the center, surrounded by numerous specialists: cardiologists, cardiac surgeons, infectiologists, microbiologists, radiologists, nuclear medicine specialists, internal medicine specialists, anesthesiologists, neurologists, neurosurgeons, and other specialists who constitute the multidisciplinary "Endocarditis Team."

Marseille, France   Gilbert Habib, MD, FESC, FASE

Contents

Part VIII   Prevention and Prophylaxis

Part IX   Conclusion

Contributors

Sana Arif, MB, BS Department of Internal Medicine, Duke University Medical Center, Durham, NC, USA

Larry M. Baddour, MD Department of Infectious Diseases and Cardiovascular Diseases, Mayo Clinic College of Medicine, Rochester, MN, USA

Aref A. Bin Abdulhak, MD Department of Internal Medicine, University of Iowa Hospitals and Clinics, Iowa City, IA, USA

Roberto Boni, MD Department of Nuclear Medicine, Department of Translational Research and New Technology in Medicine, University of Pisa, Azienda Ospedaliero Universitaria Pisana, Pisa, Italy

Berto J. Bouma, MD, PhD Department of Cardiology, Academic Medical Center, Amsterdam, The Netherlands

Jean-Paul Casalta, MD Unité de Recherche sur les Maladies Infectieuses et Tropicales Emergentes, UMR CNRS 7278, IRD 198, Institut National de la Santé et de la Recherche Médicale (INSERM) 1095, Faculté de Médecine, Aix-Marseille Université, Marseille, France

Fréderic Collart, MD Department of Cardiac Surgery, La Timone Hospital, Marseille, France

Xavier Duval, MD, PhD Department of Infectious Diseases, Bichat Claude Bernard University Hospital, Paris, France

Sophie Edouard, PharmD, PhD Microbiological Laboratory, Hospital La Timone, APHM Marseille, Marseille, France

Paola Anna Erba, MD, PhD Department of Translational Research and New Technology in Medicine, University of Pisa, Azienda Ospedaliero Universitaria Pisana, Pisa, Italy

Artur Evangelista Masip, PhD Servei de Cardiologia, Hospital Universitari Vall d'Hebron, Barcelona, Spain

Carlos Ferrera Durán, MD Department of Cardiology, Hospital Clínico San Carlos, Madrid, Spain

Pierre-Edouard Fournier, MD, PhD Microbiology Laboratory, Institut Hospitalo-Universitaire Méditerranée-Infection, Hospital La Timone, Marseille, France

Luc Frimat, MD, PhD Department of Nephrology, University Hospital of Nancy, Vandoeuvre les Nancy, France

François Goehringer, MD Department of Infectious and Tropical Diseases, University Hospital of Nancy, Vandoeuvre les Nancy, France

Maria Teresa Gonzàlez-Alujas, PhD Servei de Cardiologia, Hospital Universitari Vall d'Hebron, Barcelona, Spain

Frederique Gouriet, MD, PhD Pôle de Maladies Infectieuses, Hôpital de la Timone, Marseille, France

Unité de Recherche sur les Maladies Infectieuses et Tropicales Emergentes, Aix-Marseille Université, Faculté de Médecine, Marseille, France

Gilbert Habib, MD, FESC Cardiology Department, Hôpital La Timone, Marseille, France

Bradley Hayley, MD Division of Cardiology, The Health Sciences Centre, Memorial University, St. John's, Newfoundland and Labrador, Canada

Olivier Huttin, MD Department of Cardiology, University Hospital of Nancy, Vandoeuvre les Nancy, France

Bernard Iung, MD Department of Cardiology, Hôpital Bichat, DHU Fire and Paris Diderot University, Paris, France

Duk-Hyun Kang, MD, PhD Department of Cardiology, University of Ulsan, Asan Medical Center, Seoul, South Korea

Joey Mike Kuijpers, MD, MSc Department of Cardiology, Academic Medical Center, Amsterdam, The Netherlands

Cristiane C. Lamas, MD, PhD, MRCP Department of Valvular Heart Disease, Instituto Nacional de Cardiologia, Rio de Janeiro, Brazil

Patrizio Lancellotti, MD, PhD Department of Cardiology, University of Liège, Liège, Belgium

Elena Lazzeri, MD, PhD Department of Nuclear Medicine, Azienda Ospedaliero Universitaria Pisana, Pisa, Italy

Hubert Lepidi, MD, PhD Department of Pathology, Hôpital de la Timone, Marseille, France

Kwan Leung Chan, MD, FRCPC, FAHA, FACC Department of Cardiology, University of Ottawa Heart Institute, Ottawa, ON, Canada

Javier López Díaz, MD, PhD Instituto de Ciencias Del Corazón (ICICOR), Hospital Clínico Universitario de Valladolid, Valladolid, Spain

Sylvestre Marechaux, MD, PhD Département de Cardiologie, Groupement des Hôpitaux de l'Institut Catholique de Lille, Hôpital Saint Philibert, Lomme, France

Luis Maroto Castellanos, MD, PhD Department of Cardiac Surgery, Hospital Clínico San Carlos, Madrid, Spain

Barbara J.M. Mulder, MD, PhD Department of Cardiology, Academic Medical Center, Amsterdam, The Netherlands

Paul N. Newton, BM, BCh, DPhil, MRCP, DTM&H Microbiology Laboratory, Mahosot Hospital, Vientiane, Lao PDR, Laos

Carmen Olmos Blanco, MD, PhD Department of Cardiology, Hospital Clínico San Carlos, Madrid, Spain

Didier Raoult, PUPH, MD Unité de Recherche sur les Maladies Infectieuses et Tropicales Emergentes, UMR CNRS 7278, IRD 198, Institut National de la Santé et de la Recherche Médicale (INSERM) 1095, Faculté de Médecine, Aix-Marseille Université, Hospital La Timone, Marseille, France

Alberto Riberi, MD Department of Cardiac Surgery, La Timone Hospital, Marseille, France

José Alberto San Román Calvar, MD, PhD Instituto de Ciencias Del Corazón (ICICOR), Hospital Clínico Universitario de Valladolid, Valladolid, Spain

Cristina Sarriá Cepeda, MD, PhD Department of Internal Medicine and Infectious Diseases, Hospital Universitario de la Princesa, Madrid, Spain

Christine Selton-Suty, MD Department of Cardiology, University Hospital of Nancy, Institut Lorrain du Coeur et des Vaisseaux, Vandoeuvre les Nancy, France

Ulrika Snygg-Martin, MD, PhD Department of Infectious Diseases, Sahlgrenska University Hospital, Gothenburg, Sweden

M. Rizwan Sohail, MD Department of Infectious Diseases and Cardiovascular Diseases, Mayo Clinic College of Medicine, Rochester, MN, USA

Martina Sollini, MD Department of Nuclear Medicine, IRCCS MultiMedica, Sesto San Giovanni, Italy

Pierre Tattevin, MD, PhD Intensive Care Unit and Department of Infectious Diseases, Pontchaillou University Hospital, Rennes, France

Franck Thuny, MD, PhD Unit of Heart Failure and Valve Heart Disease, Nord Hospital, Marseille, France

Imad M. Tleyjeh, MD, MSc College of Medicine, Al Faisal University, Riyadh, Saudi Arabia

Department of Medicine, Infectious Diseases Section, King Fahad Medical City, Riyadh, Saudi Arabia

Division of Infectious Diseases, Division of Epidemiology, Mayo Clinic, Rochester, MN, USA

Pilar Tornos, MD, FESC Department of Cardiology, Hospital General Universitario Vall d'Hebron, Barcelona, Spain

Christophe Tribouilloy, MD, PhD Service de Cardiologie, Centre Hospitalier Universitaire d'Amiens, Hôpital Sud, Amiens, France

Isidre Vilacosta, MD, PhD Department of Cardiology, Hospital Clínico San Carlos, Madrid, Spain

David Vivas Balcones, MD, PhD Department of Cardiology, Hospital Clínico San Carlos, Madrid, Spain

George Watt, MD, PhD Department of Internal Medicine, John A. Burns School of Medicine, University of Hawaii at Manoa, Honolulu, HI, USA

Part I
Definition and Epidemiology

Chapter 1
Definition and Epidemiology of Infective Endocarditis

Imad M. Tleyjeh and Aref A. Bin Abdulhak

Historical Aspects and Definition of Infective Endocarditis

William Osler (1849–1919) of Canada loaned his name to the skin manifestations of infective endocarditis early in the last century; however, the history of this infection started more than 350 years ago [1–4]. The history of the evolving understanding of endocarditis beautifully illustrates how human knowledge of a disease develops over time, and certain important milestones warrant mention (Fig. 1.1a, b) [1–5]. A detailed account of historical events that led to the understanding of endocarditis is well presented by Contrepois [1, 2] and other authors [3, 4].

Inflammation of the inner layer of the heart was probably first recognized in 1646 in France by Lazare Riviere (1589–1655) who described the cardiac autopsy of a patient who presented with palpitations and died after a relatively short course. He described "round carbuncles" that resemble "clusters of hazelnuts" in the left ventricle outflow track. His observation was followed by the description of excrescences on valve tissues, which were assumed to be of valvular tissue origin, by Giovanni Maria Lancisi in Italy (1654–1720). The term "vegetation" was first used by Jean Nicholas Corvisart in France (1755–1821), who described it as a cauliflower, and attributed it to syphilis due to its resemblance to syphilitic nodules [1–4].

I.M. Tleyjeh, MD, MSc (✉)
College of Medicine, Al Faisal University, Riyadh, Saudi Arabia

Department of Medicine, Infectious Diseases Section, King Fahad Medical City, Riyadh, Saudi Arabia

Division of Infectious Diseases, Division of Epidemiology, Mayo Clinic, Rochester, MN, USA
e-mail: itlaygeh@gmail.com

A.A. Bin Abdulhak, MD
Department of Internal Medicine, University of Iowa Hospitals and Clinics, Iowa City, IA, USA
e-mail: Aref146@gmail.com

© Springer International Publishing Switzerland 2016
G. Habib (ed.), *Infective Endocarditis*, DOI 10.1007/978-3-319-32432-6_1

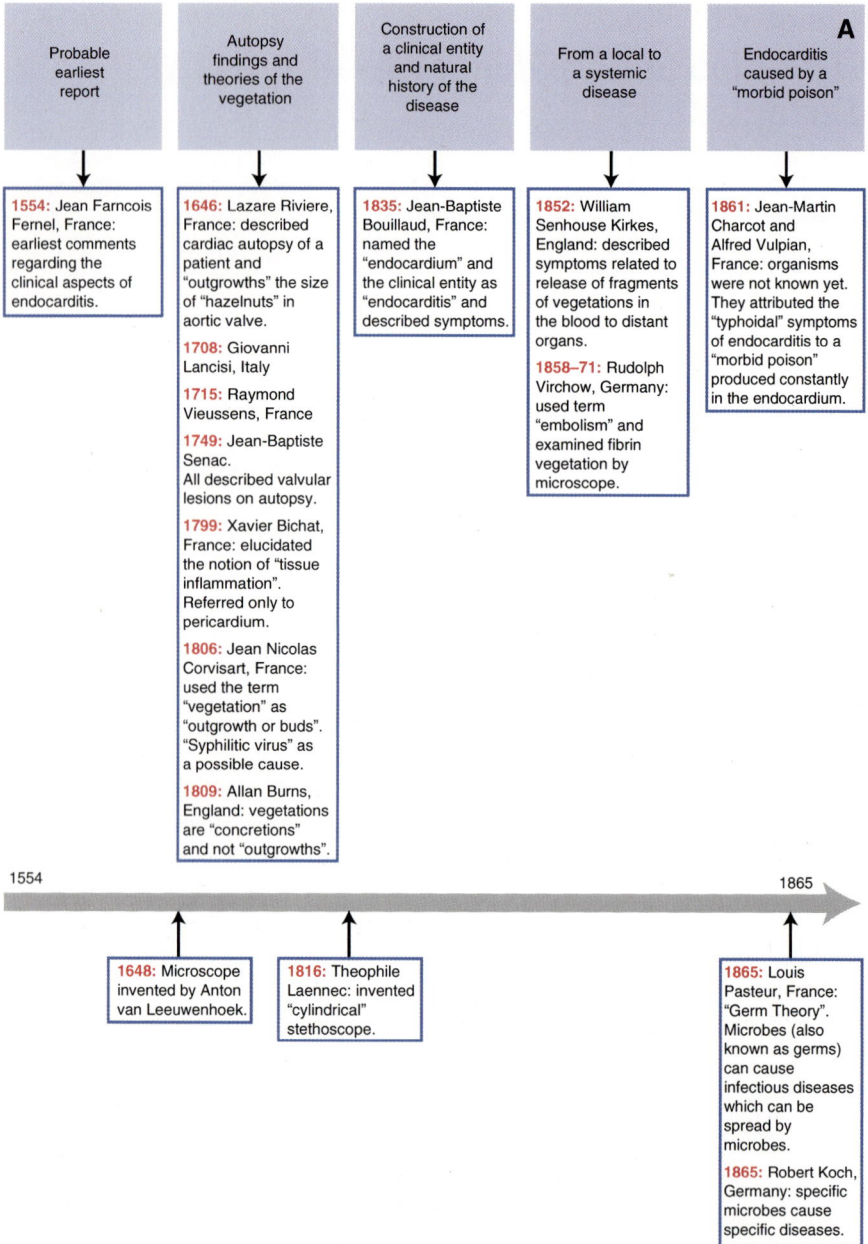

Probable earliest report	Autopsy findings and theories of the vegetation	Construction of a clinical entity and natural history of the disease	From a local to a systemic disease	**A** Endocarditis caused by a "morbid poison"

1554: Jean Farncois Fernel, France: earliest comments regarding the clinical aspects of endocarditis.

1646: Lazare Riviere, France: described cardiac autopsy of a patient and "outgrowths" the size of "hazelnuts" in aortic valve.

1708: Giovanni Lancisi, Italy

1715: Raymond Vieussens, France

1749: Jean-Baptiste Senac. All described valvular lesions on autopsy.

1799: Xavier Bichat, France: elucidated the notion of "tissue inflammation". Referred only to pericardium.

1806: Jean Nicolas Corvisart, France: used the term "vegetation" as "outgrowth or buds". "Syphilitic virus" as a possible cause.

1809: Allan Burns, England: vegetations are "concretions" and not "outgrowths".

1835: Jean-Baptiste Bouillaud, France: named the "endocardium" and the clinical entity as "endocarditis" and described symptoms.

1852: William Senhouse Kirkes, England: described symptoms related to release of fragments of vegetations in the blood to distant organs.

1858–71: Rudolph Virchow, Germany: used term "embolism" and examined fibrin vegetation by microscope.

1861: Jean-Martin Charcot and Alfred Vulpian, France: organisms were not known yet. They attributed the "typhoidal" symptoms of endocarditis to a "morbid poison" produced constantly in the endocardium.

1554   1865

1648: Microscope invented by Anton van Leeuwenhoek.

1816: Theophile Laennec: invented "cylindrical" stethoscope.

1865: Louis Pasteur, France: "Germ Theory". Microbes (also known as germs) can cause infectious diseases which can be spread by microbes.

1865: Robert Koch, Germany: specific microbes cause specific diseases.

Fig. 1.1 AB Although it is difficult to give an accurate account for all historical details that led to the understanding of endocarditis, these two figures highlight important milestones up to the beginning of the twentieth century: (**a**) 1554 through 1865; (**b**) 1869 through 1909

"Parasitic" disease; Point of entry; Circulation via blood	Valvular lesion as a predisposing factor	Experimental Endocarditis	Blood culture for Endocarditis	A unified view of Endocarditis **B**
1869: Emmanuel Winge, Norway: "parasitic organisms" entered skin and transported to heart via blood. **1872:** Hjalmar Heiberg, Norway: puerperal endocarditis. Uterine as port of entry for "vibrions". **1878:** Edwin Klebs, Germany: all cases of endocarditis were of infectious origin.	**1878:** Karl Koester, Germany: if the valves were exposed over a long period to abnormal mechanical attacks, this would create a favourable terrain for bacteria.	**1878:** Ottomar Rosenbach, Poland: first endocarditis animal model. **1886:** Vladimir Wyssokowitsch and Johannes Orth, Germany: various bacteria introduced in the bloodstream can cause endocarditis in animals with injured valves.	**1881–1886:** Arnold Netter and Joseph Grancher, France: aseptic blood sampling and culture. Same microorganisms in blood cultures and vegetations from autopsy. Grancher named disease: "infective endocarditis."	**1885–1908:** William Osler, Canada: the eponym of endocarditis. He synthesized the work of previous scientists to create a unified view of endocarditis. Used discriminative terms. Described substrate of non bacterial thrombotic nucleus of vegetation. Postulated a diversity of causative organisms. Described cardiac and systemic clinical symptoms. **1909:** Thomas Horder, England: pre-exisiting valvulopathy, oral and intestinal port of entry, mycotic aneurysms, predominance of streptococcal etiology.

1869 ——————————————————————→ 1909

1882: Hans Christian Gram, Denmark: gram staining method.

1890: Louis Malasez, France: invented a glass syringe.

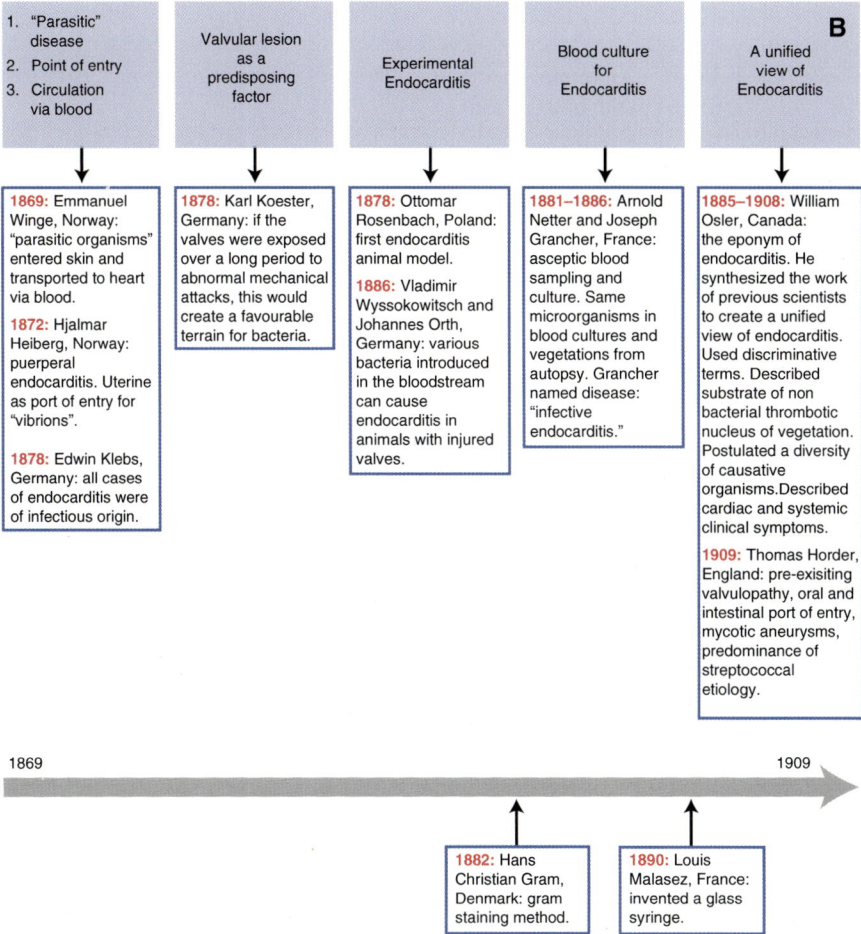

Fig. 1.1 (continued)

Knowledge of the disease further evolved when scientists started to propose new theories, such as the association between "typhoid endocarditis" and "acute rheumatoid arthritis" suggested by Jean-Baptiste Bouillaud (1796–1881) in France, who introduced the term "endocardium" and called "endocarditis" as a clinical entity in 1835. This was followed by the discovery that endocarditis was a systemic disease and not only confined to the endocardium. The concept of embolic events was proposed by William Senhouse Kirkes (1822–1864) in England, who discovered fragments of valve vegetations in distant foci such as the brain, kidney and spleen. The pathology of the disease was regularly reformulated and its definition varied from period to period and from country to country.

Before the proof of the germ theory by Louis Pasteur and Robert Koch in the middle of the nineteenth century, Emmanuel Winge (1817–1894) in Norway described "parasitic microorganisms" in aortic valve vegetation in a patient who suffered from endocarditis 1 month after having a skin infection. This led to the theory by Edwin Klebs (1834–1913) in Germany that there is a point of entry for microorganisms that are later transported in the bloodstream [1–4].

A theory that valvular impairment is a predisposing factor for endocarditis was later proposed by Ottomar Rosenbach (1851–1907) in Poland, who conducted the first animal experiments. In 1886, Vladimir Wyssokowitsch and Johannes Orth of Germany discovered, using animal endocarditis models, that various bacteria introduced in the bloodstream can cause endocarditis in animals with injured valves [1–4].

The germ theory, and the use of microscopes and experimental animal models, changed the view and concept of the disease at the end of the century. William Osler built on earlier findings to give a more comprehensive understanding of this infection. He differentiated between ulcerative, malignant, septic, and pyemic endocarditis. He also described the symptoms of endocarditis and the deposition of fibrin and platelets on damaged endocardium, which constituted the nucleus of the vegetation. He proposed that a diversity of microorganisms can cause endocarditis. Years later, Lord Thomas Horder (1871–1955) in England published 150 cases of IE and described their pathological lesions. He classified IE in five categories: latent, fulminant, acute, chronic, and subacute [1–4].

Despite these discoveries provided by the synthesis of clinical medicine, pathology and microbiology, IE was without effective treatment and carried a dismal prognosis until the discovery of sulfonamides in the 1940s. Even then, the cure rate improved only to 5–16 % [3]. The use of penicillin starting in 1944 resulted in a 70 % cure rate, and provided significant optimism that endocarditis is a curable disease [3, 4]. In 1963, Andrew G. Wallace from Duke University in USA performed the first valve excision and aortic valve replacement in a patient with endocarditis who failed to respond to antibiotic therapy [5].

Today, IE has been clearly established as an infection of the endocardial lining of the heart that includes heart valves, mural endocardium, and endocardial covering of the implanted material such as prosthetic valves and intracardiac devices [6]. The infection is mostly caused by bacteria, with *Staphylococcus* and *Streptococcus* species causing 80 % of cases; however, it [7] may occasionally be due to fungal pathogens.

Incidence, Sequelae, and Global Burden of Infective Endocarditis

The incidence of IE varies widely based on the geographic region and population at risk. There is also significant heterogeneity between published incidence studies due to referral and case ascertainment biases, disease misclassification, use of different study designs and case definitions, and the change of IE definition over time [8].

IE continues to be an uncommon infectious disease, with an annual incidence ranging from 3 to 7 cases per 100,000 person-years in the most contemporary population surveys [9, 10]. The Global Burden of Diseases Project-GBD 2010 IE expert group conducted a comprehensive systematic review of IE epidemiology literature between 1980 and 2008 [11]. Several medical and science databases were searched, yielding 115 studies published in ten languages. Eligible studies were population-based (17%), multicenter hospital-based (11%), and single-center hospital-based (71%). Population-based studies were reported from only ten countries: Australia, Denmark, France, Greece, Italy, the Netherlands, Sweden, Tunisia, the United States, and the United Kingdom. The crude incidence of IE ranged between 1.5 and 11.6 cases per 100,000 people. The overall mean proportion of IE patients that developed stroke was $15.8 \pm 9.1\%$, and the mean proportion of patients that underwent valve surgery was $32.4 \pm 18.8\%$ and the mean case fatality risk was $21.1 \pm 10.4\%$.

Data were missing or sparse from the majority of other countries. Accordingly, IE incidence remains largely unknown from many parts of the world as the available data were mostly reported from developed countries (Fig. 1.2).

The mean age of persons with IE was reported as 57.2 years [12], with incidence increasing with age. The male to female case ratio is over 2:1 [7].

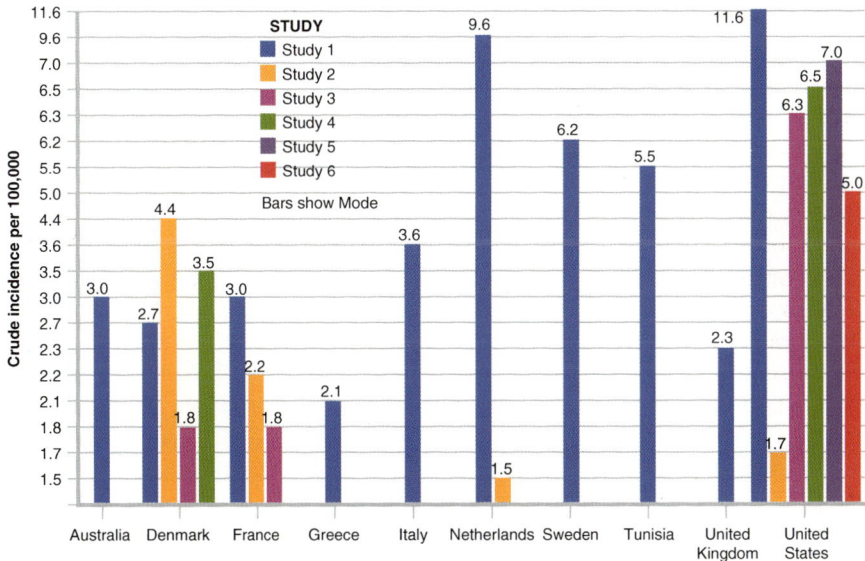

Fig. 1.2 Infective endocarditis incidence among different countries (From Bin Abdulhak et al. [11]. Reprinted with permission from Elsevier Limited)

Risk Factors of Infective Endocarditis

IE has been traditionally linked to the presence of rheumatic heart disease, congenital heart disease, prosthetic valves, and previous episodes of IE. However, many other risk factors have been identified that predispose to the development of IE [7, 13], including intracardiac devices, intravenous drug use, advanced age, degenerative valvular heart disease, hemodialysis, HIV infection, diabetes mellitus, cardiac transplant with development of valvulopathy, and poor dentition or dental infection.

Some of these more recently identified risk factors may have taken predominance over the traditional risk factors as predisposing to IE, especially in developed countries. Nonetheless, about 50 % of IE cases have no predisposing condition identified [7].

Temporal Trends in the Epidemiology of Infective Endocarditis

The earlier description of infective endocarditis as a disease of pre-existing valvular heart conditions that is mostly caused by *S. viridans* has undergone significant epidemiological changes during the recent decades, particularly in developed countries. However, there are certain degrees of heterogeneity with regard to the changing epidemiology of IE among different nations [8, 14].

Temporal trends in the epidemiology of IE have been examined using different study designs. The first approach used longitudinal follow-up data from the small population of Olmsted County, MN, USA [10, 15, 16], which provides a unique opportunity to conduct population-based studies because its population is stable and medical care is limited to a few local facilities. The long-established Rochester Epidemiology Project [17] facilitates data collection and ensures detection of virtually all cases. In 2000, the population of Olmsted County was 90,000 adults. Between 1970 and 2006, there were 150 cases with IE with 3 % intravenous drug (IVD) use. The age- and sex-adjusted incidence rates of IE ranged between 5.0 and 7.9 cases per 100,000 person-years. IE incidence among men was relatively stable across the study period and ranged from 8.6 to 12.7 cases per 100,000 person-years (P = .79). In contrast, there was a significant increase in incidence among women, from 1.4 cases per 100,000 person-years at the beginning of the study period to 6.7 at the end of the period (P = .006) (Fig. 1.3a). Among incident cases, there was a temporal trend of increasing age on presentation (Spearman correlation coefficient, 0.17; P = .04), with median age increasing from 46.5 years in 1980–1984 to 70.5 years in 2001–2006. From 1975 to 1979 to 2001–2006, the proportion of cases with rheumatic heart disease as a predisposing factor declined from 31 to 5 % (P = .02), while the proportion of patients undergoing surgery increased from 0 to 30 % (p = 0.09). There was no significant temporal trend in the incidence of either *S aureus* or viridans group streptococcal IE (Fig. 1.3b).

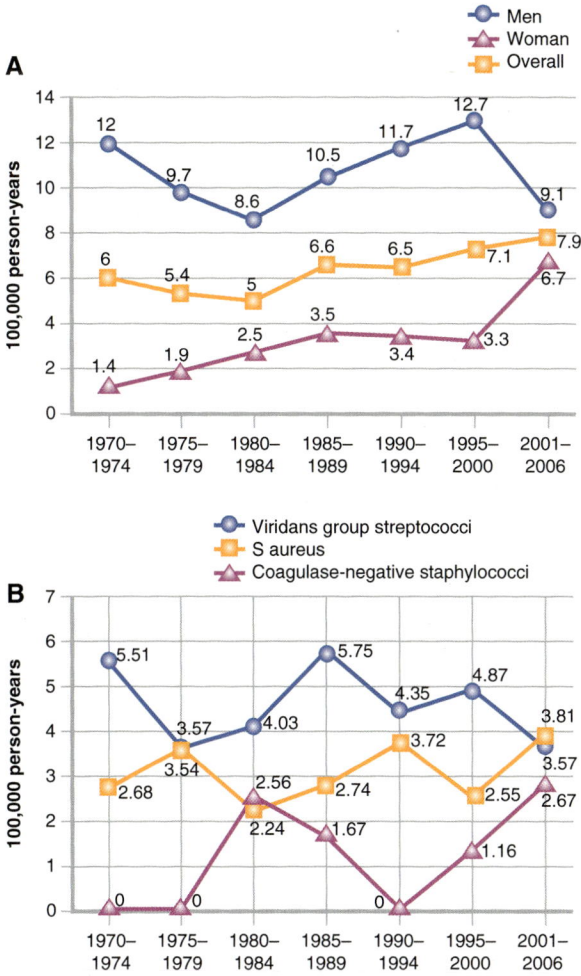

Fig. 1.3 Epidemiological trends of infective endocarditis in Olmsted County, Minnesota. (**a**) Age-adjusted incidence of infective endocarditis over time; for trend in women, P = .006; for trend in men, P = .79. (**b**) Age-adjusted incidence of infective endocarditis by causative organisms over time (Both from Correa de Sa et al. [10]. Reprinted with permission from Elsevier Limited)

The second study design compared repeated temporal cross-sectional surveys of a large population in France [9, 18–20]. These studies included three French regions (Greater Paris, Lorraine and Rhone-Alpes) with 11 million inhabitants (24 % of the French population). Three 1-year population-based surveys were conducted in 1991, 1999, and 2008 by prospectively collecting IE cases from all medical centers using a survey design. Overall, 993 expert-validated IE cases were analyzed (323 in 1991; 331 in 1999; and 339 in 2008). The age- and sex-standardized annual IE incidence did not change significantly across the 3 surveys (Fig. 1.3a, b), but it decreased significantly in patients with previously known native heart

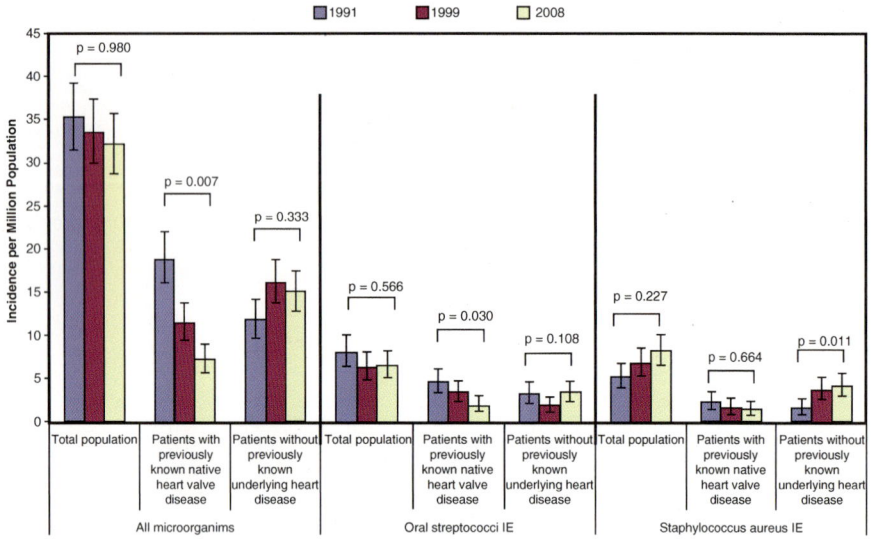

Fig. 1.4 Temporal trends in IE age- and sex-standardized incidence for all micro-organisms and according to underlying heart disease and micro-organisms in France (From Duval et al. [9]. Reprinted with permission from Elsevier Limited)

valve disease. The incidence of oral streptococcal IE did not increase in the overall population or in the population of patients with previously known native heart valve disease, in whom it significantly decreased. The incidence of both *S. aureus* and coagulase-negative staphylococcal IE increased significantly in patients without previously known native heart valve disease (Fig. 1.4). Mean age increased over time from 58 to 62 years (P=0.013). IE predominated in males in all 3 surveys. The rate of patients with no previously known heart valve disease increased from 34 % in 1991 to 49 % in 1999 and remained stable in 2008 (47 %) (P<0.001).

Microorganisms responsible for IE were identified in 87, 93, and 93 % from 1991 to 2008. *Streptococcal sp.* were the most frequent microorganisms across the 3 surveys. The proportion of *Staphylococcus aureus* increased regularly and significantly (16, 21, and 26 %; P=0.011). The rate of cardiac surgery performed during the acute phase of the disease increased from 1991 to 1999 (31–50 %) and then remained stable (50 %) (P<0.001). In-hospital death rates were not significantly different among the three periods (21 %, 15 %, and 21 %, respectively).

The third approach used pooled analyses of temporal trends across different population studies [8]. Fifteen population-based investigations from seven countries (Denmark, France, Italy, the Netherlands, Sweden, United Kingdom, and United States) from 1969 to 2005 were eligible. Using meta-regression analyses, the authors observed a decline in the proportion of IE cases with underlying rheumatic heart disease (−12 %/decade), an increase in the proportion of IE patients undergoing surgery (+9 %/decade), and no temporal trends in causative organisms.

Controversy surrounds the dominant pathogens and temporal trends of pathogenic organisms of IE. A large-scale review of data from hospital-based studies

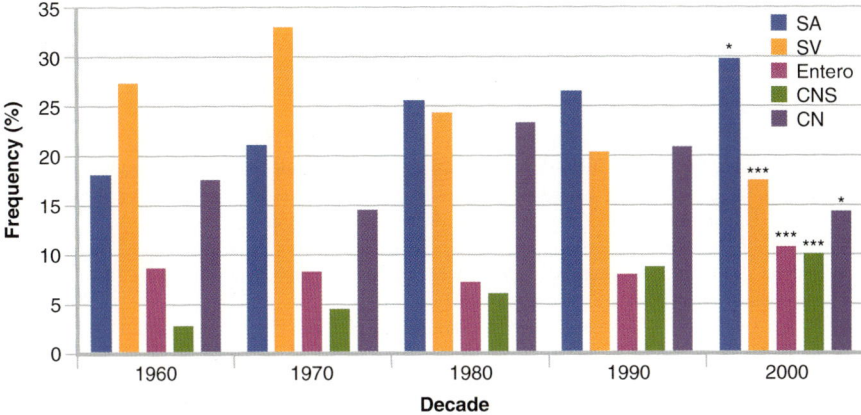

Fig. 1.5 Worldwide frequency distribution and trends of infective endocarditis pathogens over five decades. *SA* Staphylococcus aureus, *SV* streptococcus viridans, *Entero* enterococcus, *CNS* coagulase negative staphylococcus, *CN* culture negative endocarditis. *=p<0.05; **=p<0.01; ***=p<0.001 (Reproduced with permission from Slipczuk et al. [12]. Open access)

demonstrated that staphylococcal and enterococcal infection rates have increased over the last five decades, whereas *S. viridians* and culture negative endocarditis rates have declined over the same period of time [12]. Figure 1.5 illustrates worldwide distribution and trends of endocarditis pathogens [12]. *S. aureus* was the most commonly identified pathogen over the last decade followed by *S. viridians*, culture negative endocarditis, enterococcus group, and coagulase negative staphylococcus [12]. The overall worldwide increase in the frequency of *S aureus* endocarditis was driven by an increase in North America [12]. The increase in *S aureus* endocarditis in North American was paralleled by an increase in intravenous drug use-associated endocarditis in the last decade, which may partially explain its higher frequency [12].

Outcome in Infective Endocarditis

IE continues to be characterized by increased morbidity and mortality, and is now the fourth most common life-threatening infection syndrome, after sepsis, pneumonia, and intra-abdominal abscess. Globally, in 2010, IE was associated with 1.58 million disability-adjusted life years (DALYs) or years of healthy life lost due to death and non-fatal illness or impairment [21].

Despite advances in medical knowledge, technology, and antimicrobial therapy, IE is still associated with devastating outcomes. Almost one in every four cases will not survive the disease [11]. IE is associated with up to 22 % in-hospital mortality and 45 % 5 -year mortality rates [20, 22]. Globally, IE was estimated to be associated with 35,900 thousands deaths (95 % uncertainty interval [UI]: 30.0, 44.5) in 1990, increasing to 48,300 thousand deaths (95 % UI: 39.3, 55.5) in 2010 [23].

References

1. Contrepois A. Notes on the early history of infective endocarditis and the development of an experimental model. Clin Infect Dis. 1995;20(2):461–6.
2. Contrepois A. Towards a history of infective endocarditis. Med Hist. 1996;40(1):25–54.
3. Grinberg M, Solimene M. Historical aspects of infective endocarditis. Rev Assoc Med Bras. 2011;57(2):228–33.
4. Millar B, Moore J. Emerging issues in infective endocarditis. Emerg Infect Dis. 2004; 10(6):1110–6.
5. Wallace A, Young W, Osterhout S. treatment of acute bacterial endocarditis by valve excision and replacement. Circulation. 1965;31:450–3.
6. Thuny F, Grisoli D, Cautela J, Riberi A, Raoult D, Habib G. Infective endocarditis: prevention, diagnosis, and management. Can J Cardiol. 2014;30(9):1046–57.
7. Hoen B, Duval X. Infective endocarditis. N Engl J Med. 2013;369(8):785.
8. Tleyjeh IM, Abdel-Latif A, Rahbi H, Scott CG, Bailey KR, Steckelberg JM, et al. A systematic review of population-based studies of infective endocarditis. Chest. 2007;132(3): 1025–35.
9. Duval X, Delahaye F, Alla F, Tattevin P, Obadia JF, Le Moing V, et al. Temporal trends in infective endocarditis in the context of prophylaxis guideline modifications: three successive population-based surveys. J Am Coll Cardiol. 2012;59(22):1968–76.
10. Correa de Sa DD, Tleyjeh IM, Anavekar NS, Schultz JC, Thomas JM, Lahr BD, et al. Epidemiological trends of infective endocarditis: a population-based study in Olmsted County, Minnesota. Mayo Clin Proc. 2010;85(5):422–6.
11. Bin Abdulhak A, Baddour L, Erwin P, Hoen B, Chu V, Mensah G, et al. Global and regional burden of infective endocarditis, 1990–2010: a systematic review of the literature. Glob Heart. 2014;9(1):131–43.
12. Slipczuk L, Codolosa JN, Davila CD, Romero-Corral A, Yun J, Pressman GS, et al. Infective endocarditis epidemiology over five decades: a systematic review. PLoS One. 2013; 8(12):e82665. doi:10.1371/journal.pone.0082665.
13. Lockhart PB, Brennan MT, Thornhill M, Michalowicz BS, Noll J, Bahrani-Mougeot FK, et al. Poor oral hygiene as a risk factor for infective endocarditis-related bacteremia. J Am Dent Assoc. 2009;140(10):1238–44.
14. Tleyjeh IM, Steckelberg JM. Changing epidemiology of infective endocarditis. Curr Infect Dis Rep. 2006;8(4):265–70.
15. Tleyjeh IM, Steckelberg JM, Murad HS, Anavekar NS, Ghomrawi HM, Mirzoyev Z, et al. Temporal trends in infective endocarditis: a population-based study in Olmsted County, Minnesota. JAMA. 2005;293(24):3022–8.
16. Desimone D, Tleyjeh I, Correa de Sa DD, Anavekar N, Lahr B, Sohail M, Mayo Cardiovascular Infections Study Group, et al. Incidence of infective endocarditis caused by viridans group streptococci before and after publication of the 2007 American Heart Association's endocarditis prevention guidelines. Circulation. 2012;126(1):60–4.
17. Melton L. History of the Rochester epidemiology project. Mayo Clin Proc. 1996;71(3): 266–74.
18. Delahaye F, Goulet V, Lacassin F, Ecochard R, Selton-Suty C, Hoen B, et al. Characteristics of infective endocarditis in France in 1991. A 1-year survey. Eur Heart J. 1995;16(3): 394–401.
19. Hoen B, Alla F, Selton-Suty C, Béguinot I, Bouvet A, Briançon S, et al. Changing profile of infective endocarditis: results of a 1-year survey in France. JAMA. 2002;288(1):75–81.
20. Selton-Suty C, Celard M, Le Moing V, Doco-Lecompte T, Chirouze C, Iung B, et al. Preeminence of Staphylococcus aureus in infective endocarditis: a 1-year population-based survey. Clin Infect Dis. 2012;54(9):1230–9.

21. Murray CJ, Vos T, Lozano R, Naghavi M, Flaxman AD, Michaud C, et al. Disability-adjusted life years (DALYs) for 291 diseases and injuries in 21 regions, 1990–2010: a systematic analysis for the Global Burden of Disease Study 2010. Lancet. 2012;380(9859):2197–223.
22. Sy RW, Kritharides L. Health care exposure and age in infective endocarditis: results of a contemporary population-based profile of 1536 patients in Australia. Eur Heart J. 2010;31(15): 1890–7.
23. Lozano R, Naghavi M, Foreman K, Lim S, Shibuya K, Aboyans V, et al. Global and regional mortality from 235 causes of death for 20 age groups in 1990 and 2010: a systematic analysis for the Global Burden of Disease Study 2010. Lancet. 2012;380(9859):2095–128.

Part II
Pathophysiology

Chapter 2
Pathophysiology of Infective Endocarditis

Franck Thuny

Introduction

Infective endocarditis usually occurs on an endocardium with pre-existing lesions or on intracardiac foreign materials. From various portals of entry (oral, digestive, cutaneous, etc.) and subsequent bacteraemia, pathogens can adhere and colonize the previously damaged endocardium thanks to numerous complex processes based on a unique host-pathogen interaction [1, 2]. Then, severe life-threatening complications can occur such as acute heart failure or embolic events.

The Host's Underlying Lesions

Under normal conditions, the endocardium is resistant to infection. However, degenerative processes (fibrosis, calcifications), turbulent blood flows created by valvular or congenital heart diseases and mechanical lesions secondary to material implantation can provoke endocardial damage, resulting in the exposure of the extracellular matrix, apoptosis, production of tissue factor and then thrombus formation (non-bacterial vegetation). Moreover, the presence of underlying endocardial damage may induce an exposure of altered phospholipids (cardiolipin) on the outer membrane of endothelial cells, resulting in the production of antiphospholipid antibodies by the immune cells. The implication of antiphospholipid antibodies in this thrombotic step of the endocarditis pathogenesis has been suggested even in the absence of autoimmune disease [3]. Indeed, the antiphospholipid antibodies react with negatively charged phospholipids. They require beta-$_2$-glycoprotein 1 as a cofactor to bind to phospholipids. This beta-$_2$-glycoprotein 1 inhibits factor Xa

F. Thuny, MD, PhD
Unit of Heart Failure and Valve Heart Disease, Nord Hospital, Marseille, France
e-mail: Franck.thuny@gmail.com

© Springer International Publishing Switzerland 2016
G. Habib (ed.), *Infective Endocarditis*, DOI 10.1007/978-3-319-32432-6_2

synthesis on activated platelets. Thus, antiphospholipid antibodies may interfere with this inhibition leading to factor Xa generation and thrombin formation [3]. Immunoglobulin fractions from patients with antiphospholipid antibodies can bind to endothelial cells, resulting in endothelial cell activation and phenotypic changes, with induction of a pro-adhesive, pro-thrombotic surface causing a subsequent perturbation of the endothelium-platelet axis, thrombin generation and reduced fibrinolysis. The formation of such non-bacterial thrombotic endocarditis is the key event that will facilitate the pathogens adherence and infection.

Alternatively, an endocardium free of previous mechanical lesions, but with inflammation, can also form, by itself, an adhesive surface for circulating virulent pathogens, such as *S. aureus*, thanks to expression of integrins by the endothelial cells [4].

The Bacteraemia

The role of bacteraemia has been studied in animals with catheter-induced non-bacterial thrombotic endocarditis. Both the magnitude of bacteraemia and the ability of the pathogen to attach to damaged valves are important. Of note, bacteraemia does not occur only after invasive procedures, but also as a consequence of the daily routine activities such as chewing, flossing and tooth brushing. The cumulating numbers of circulating bacteria are even greater after these activities than after an invasive procedure. Such spontaneous, low grade, short duration but repeated bacteraemia may explain why most cases of IE are not preceded by invasive procedures, questioning the efficiency of the one-dose prescription of antibioprophylaxis. Also of increasing concern are health-care-associated bacteremias, such as in chronic hemodialysis patients who represent a new at-risk group for IE [5–8].

The Host-Pathogen Interaction

During bacteraemia, some pathogens can adhere to the components of the non-bacterial thrombotic vegetation or the enflamed endocardium. Molecules such as fibrinogen, fibronectin or platelets proteins are recognized by adhesins located on the surface of pathogens [1, 9]. The predominance of gram-positive pathogens as the leading cause of most IE can be explained by the fact that they are the most equipped with these surface adhesins that mediate attachment to the extracellular host matrix proteins. These adhesins are collectively referred to as Microbial Surface Component Reacting with Adhesive Matrix Molecules [1]. After adhesion, the subsequent colonization and invasion of the endocardium maintain both the inflammation and the coagulation processes, resulting in a vicious circle with

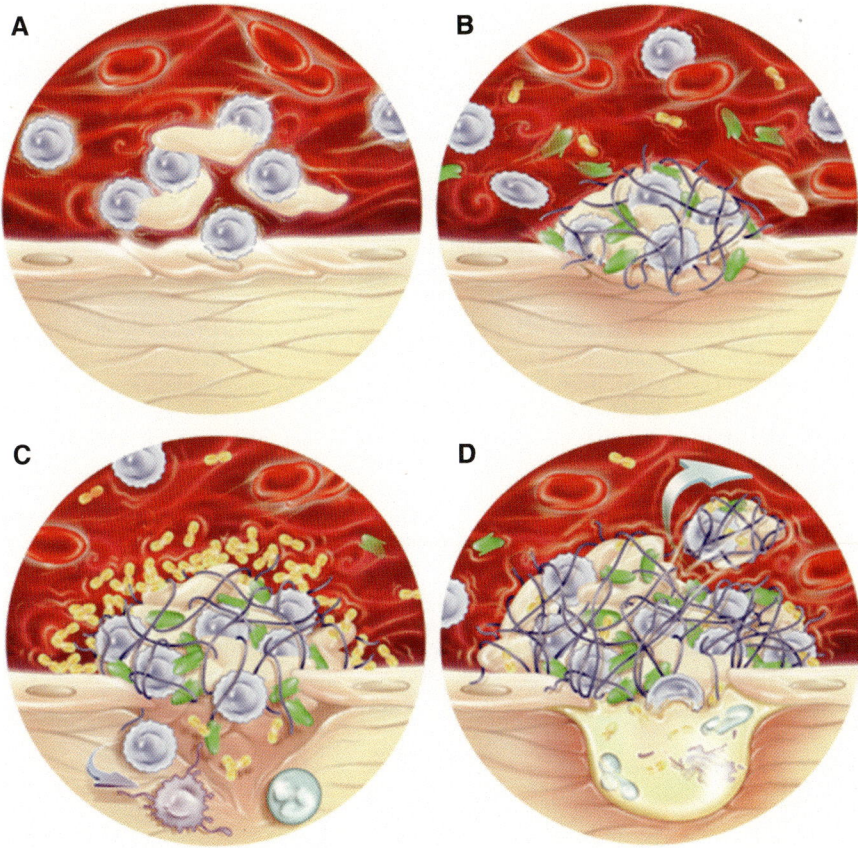

Fig. 2.1 Illustration of the infective endocarditis (IE) pathophysiology. The natural history of IE may be demonstrated in successive steps including cell apoptosis that may be promoted by blood turbulence in the vicinity of valve lesion (**a**), procoagulant activity that results in fibrin and platelet deposition (**b**), bacterial colonization and chemoattraction of neutrophils increasing vegetation size (**c**), and tissue remodelling and neoangiogenesis leading to the functional destruction of the valve (**d**). At this stage, the situation is irreversible and cardiac surgery is necessary (All from Benoit et al. [2]. Open access)

the formation of infective vegetation in which the pathogens persist, multiply and escape from the host defenses. Consequently, the vegetation will grow, a neoangiogenesis process will occur, and the valve tissue will be destroyed, resulting ultimately in embolic events, abscess formation, and valve dysfunction [2]. Moreover, the excessive host response can be responsible for the aggravation of the lesions by secondary autoimmune effects, such as immune complex glomerulonephritis and vasculitis, but also an increasing risk of embolic events due to hypersecretion and activation of the matrix metalloproteinases [10] and the increased production of antiphospholipid antibodies [3] (Fig. 2.1a–d).

References

1. Que YA, Moreillon P. Infective endocarditis. Nat Rev Cardiol. 2011;8:322–36.
2. Benoit M, Thuny F, Le Priol Y, et al. The transcriptional programme of human heart valves reveals the natural history of infective endocarditis. PLoS One. 2010;5:e8939.
3. Kupferwasser LI, Hafner G, Mohr-Kahaly S, et al. The presence of infection-related antiphospholipid antibodies in infective endocarditis determines a major risk factor for embolic events. J Am Coll Cardiol. 1999;33:1365–71.
4. Que YA, Haefliger JA, Piroth L, et al. Fibrinogen and fibronectin binding cooperate for valve infection and invasion in staphylococcus aureus experimental endocarditis. J Exp Med. 2005; 201:1627–35.
5. Cabell CH, Jollis JG, Peterson GE, et al. Changing patient characteristics and the effect on mortality in endocarditis. Arch Intern Med. 2002;162:90–4.
6. Fowler Jr VG, Miro JM, Hoen B, et al. Staphylococcus aureus endocarditis: a consequence of medical progress. JAMA. 2005;293:3012–21.
7. Sy RW, Kritharides L. Health care exposure and age in infective endocarditis: results of a contemporary population-based profile of 1536 patients in Australia. Eur Heart J. 2010;31: 1890–7.
8. Thuny F, Avierinos JF, Habib G. Changing patterns in epidemiological profiles and prevention strategies in infective endocarditis: from teeth to healthcare-related infection. Eur Heart J. 2010;31:1826–7.
9. Moreillon P, Que YA. Infective endocarditis. Lancet. 2004;363:139–49.
10. Thuny F, Habib G, Le Dolley Y, et al. Circulating matrix metalloproteinases in infective endocarditis: a possible marker of the embolic risk. PLoS One. 2011;6:e18830. 2007;154:923–8.

Part III
Diagnosis

Chapter 3
Clinical Features of Infective Endocarditis

Pilar Tornos

Introduction

The diagnosis of infective endocarditis (IE) is based on a combination of clinical symptoms, microbiologic findings and imaging techniques, in particular echocardiography, but with an increasing role for computed tomography and nuclear techniques. The diagnosis of IE is usually straightforward when the symptoms are recognized: blood cultures and echocardiography will confirm or rule out the diagnosis in most cases. A number of difficult cases will remain that will need further microbiologic investigations or additional imaging techniques.

However, the most important challenge in the diagnosis of IE is that the clinical suspicion is very often delayed because the early clinical symptoms are not properly evaluated. There are several reasons to explain this. Besides the fact that IE is a rather uncommon and complex disease, important changes in epidemiology have recently occurred and consequently the clinical picture has been modified.

The classical IE occurring in young patients with valve disease is nowadays uncommon [1]; IE is now diagnosed in older people [2], in patients with no previous history of valvular disease [3], in patients with comorbidities who suffer from nosocomial IE [4], and in patients with pacemakers, defibrillators and valvular prostheses [5].

IE can present as a subacute disease. In those cases the initial symptoms consisting of fever and malaise do not seem to correspond to a serious disease, and IE is only suspected after the appearance of complications.

On the other hand, IE can present acutely, with fever, sepsis and major emboli. In those cases, extra cardiac symptoms may predominate and patients present to a

P. Tornos, MD, FESC
Department of Cardiology, Hospital General Universitario Vall d'Hebron, Barcelona, Spain
e-mail: ptornos@vhebron.net

© Springer International Publishing Switzerland 2016
G. Habib (ed.), *Infective Endocarditis*, DOI 10.1007/978-3-319-32432-6_3

Table 3.1 Clinical data considered as minor diagnostic criteria in the modified Duke criteria for the diagnosis of infective endocarditis

Predisposition
Fever
Vascular phenomena:
Major arterial emboli
Septic pulmonary infarcts
Mycotic aneurysm
Intracranial haemorrhages
Janeway lesions
Immunologic phenomena:
Glomerulonephritis
Osler's nodes
Roth's spots

variety of specialists. Very often, alternative diagnoses are considered before the suspicion of endocarditis arises.

According to the Duke criteria [6], clinical symptoms are considered minor criteria (Table 3.1).

However, as Li et al. point out [6], Duke criteria are useful for research purposes in order to compare series of patients but their use in clinical decision making is not clear. Although the use of Duke's clinical criteria are very useful clinical judgement remains crucial in the evaluation and diagnosis of IE.

In the present chapter, the clinical situations and signs and symptoms of IE are discussed.

Clinical Data

Predisposition

Patients at increased risk of infective endocarditis are patients with valvular heart disease, patients with previous episodes of endocarditis, patients with congenital heart diseases, and patients with valvular prostheses. In recent years, IE is being diagnosed frequently in patients with pacemakers and other intracardiac devices.

On the other hand, patients at risk are intravenous drug addicts and patients with comorbidities that require frequent medical instrumentation or that result in immunosuppression, for example renal patients on haemodialysis or cancer patients. In those patients, even low grade fever should indicate the practice of blood cultures, and the diagnosis of IE should be considered.

Nevertheless, IE occurs often in patients who were unaware of having any heart problem. This makes the clinical diagnosis more difficult.

Fever

Fever is present in almost 90 % of all cases of IE. The diagnosis of IE should be always considered in patients with longstanding fever, especially when this causes chills and when there are signs consistent with bacteraemia.

In patients with low virulent organisms, fever can be low grade and well tolerated. Valvular patients and patients with congenital heart disease should know about the risk of IE and should be educated to report cases of fever lasting for several days. Blood cultures then will allow for an early diagnosis. Unfortunately, many patients with IE are unaware of having any cardiac disease, and the diagnosis of IE is only considered after the development of heart failure or embolic episodes.

Patients with IE caused by virulent organisms such as *staphylococci* can present within hours or within a few days with high fever and in a severe septic status. In those very acute cases, the diagnosis of IE can also be missed, in particular if there is a lack of previous history of valve disease. In these very septic patients, it is difficult to hear murmurs and non cardiac symptoms, such as neurologic symptoms, or respiratory insufficiency can predominate. Nevertheless, when blood cultures are positive per *staphylococci,* or other microorganisms common in endocarditis the diagnosis of IE should be considered and investigations performed.

Fever is a common finding in the early postoperative period after valve surgery. In this clinical setting, there are many causes for fever, but when an obvious cause is not present, the diagnosis of IE should be on the list and blood cultures and other investigations performed.

In patients with pacemakers and defibrillators, endocarditis can occur in combination with an infection of the pocket of the device, and patients present with fever and clear signs of pocket infection. However, other patients can have infections of the leads causing IE with no apparent signs of pocket infection. Those patients usually present with several episodes of well tolerated low grade fever, sometimes with respiratory symptoms due to lung embolism that can be viewed as pulmonary infections. A high index of suspicion is needed to consider the possibility of IE.

Fever in hospitalized patients with intravenous lines, haemodialysis, or exposed to chemotherapy or other medical instrumentations should be carefully studied, blood cultures performed and close follow up of patients with positive blood cultures performed, in particular when blood cultures are positive for microorganisms that are common in IE.

The absence of fever makes the diagnosis of IE unlikely, although fever can be absent in patients with renal failure or in cases where there are very low virulent infections.

Cardiac Murmur

The presence of a cardiac murmur in a patient presenting with fever can raise the suspicion of IE. However, a systolic murmur caused by the increased cardiac output can occur in the absence of any cardiac problem. Nevertheless, the presence of a murmur, in particular a diastolic murmur of aortic regurgitation or a murmur of mitral regurgitation, should encourage investigations to rule out IE. All textbooks on IE state that any change in a previous murmur or an increase in a previous murmur is very specific to IE, although this finding is very uncommon. Rarely, a change in a previous murmur can occur during the course of IE. For example, a continuous murmur can appear when a fistula occurs between left and right cardiac cavities.

In patients with valvular prostheses, any murmur consistent with a prosthetic leak should also raise the possibility of IE, in particular in the presence of fever. Also, when a new prosthetic leak is discovered, the possibility of endocarditis should be considered, even in the absence of fever.

Cardiac Symptoms

Patients with IE can develop heart failure. Therefore, this diagnosis should be suspected in any patient with heart failure and fever. Heart failure can be secondary to the febrile status, anemia, and tachycardia, but more often heart failure is due to the acute valvular insufficiency caused by the infectious process. In patients with acute heart failure, the diagnosis of severe acute aortic or mitral regurgitation can be difficult because the murmur is usually faint, the heart is not enlarged, and pulmonary edema can be erroneously diagnosed as a pulmonary infection in patients with fever and septic shock.

Patients can present with pericardial signs such as a pericardial rub. In those cases, periannular or myocardial abscesses are likely to be present causing pyopericardium. In patients with periannular abscesses, new conduction defects can appear (Fig. 3.1a, b), and therefore IE has to be ruled out in any patient with fever and heart block.

Myocardial infarction can occur as a result of coronary embolism. Rarely can mycotic coronary aneurysm be found [7].

Neurological Symptoms

Clinical neurological events occur in 20–40 % of patients with IE, and occult cerebral lesions in asymptomatic patients occur in almost 70 % of patients [8]. Neurological symptoms are sometimes present at the time of diagnosis. Patients may present with encephalopathy that can be secondary to sepsis or to underlying central nervous system complications. The most common include ischemic or hemorrhagic stroke as a consequence of embolism [9]. Therefore, the diagnosis of endocarditis should always be suspected in patients with stroke and fever. Ischemic strokes most commonly occur in the middle cerebral artery; however, multifocal infarction is also common

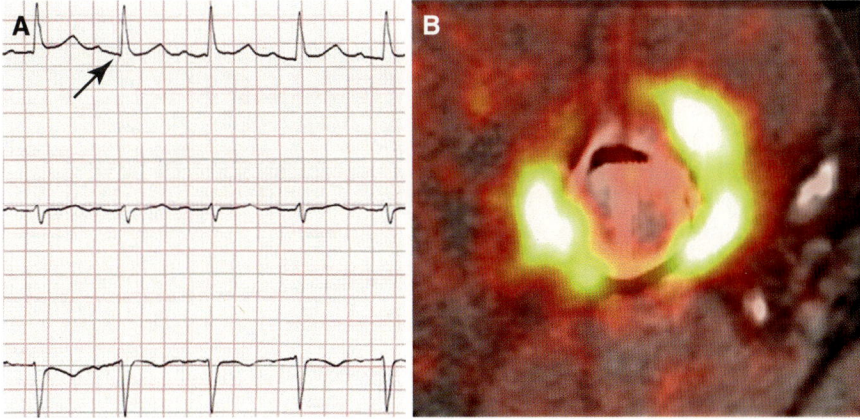

Fig. 3.1 (**a**) ECG showing prolonged PR (*arrow*) in a patient with prosthetic valve endocarditis with perianular extension. (**b**) 18 FDG PET/CT showing the periprosthetic abscess

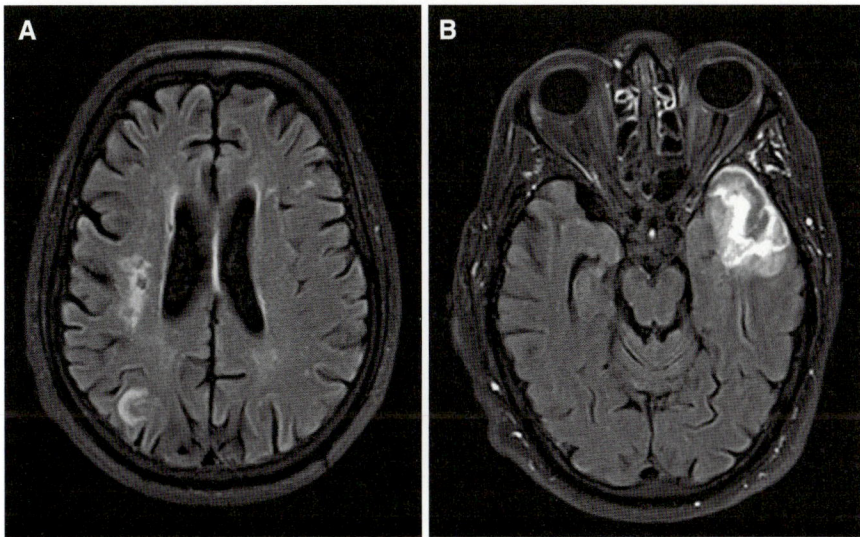

Fig. 3.2 (**a**) MRI showing multiple embolic infarcts in a patient with IE caused by *S aureus* who presented with fever and encephalopathy. (**b**) MRI of the same patient with a large infarct in the anterior temporal lobe

(Fig. 3.2a, b). Hemorrhage in the brain can be subarachnoid or parenchymal as a result of hemorrhagic conversion of a prior ischemic infarct or rupture of an infectious aneurysm. Other neurological complications include meningitis, brain abscess, and infectious intracranial aneurysms. In those cases, headache and seizures in a febrile patient can be the initial symptomatology.

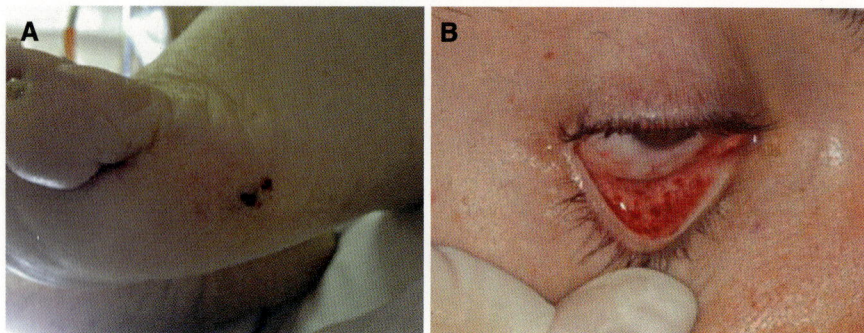

Fig. 3.3 (**a**) Peripheral emboli in a patient with prosthetic infective endocarditis caused by *Enterococcus faecalis*. (**b**) Conjunctival petechiae in a patient with *S mitis* IE

Musculoskeletal Symptoms

Patients with IE can present with nonspecific arthralgia or myalgia. Sometimes, patients are erroneously diagnosed of polymyalgia rheumatica or giant cell arteritis [10]. Back pain is also a common manifestation of IE, but in patients with fever and severe back pain spondylodiscitis should be suspected and blood cultures performed. In patients presenting with pyogenic vertebral osteomyelitis, the incidence of infective endocarditis is high [11].

Peripheral Signs

Petechiae or purpura and splinter haemorrhages are nonspecific findings that occur in up to 20 % of patients with IE (Fig. 3.3a, b). In a recent study [12], specific skin manifestations occurred in 12 % of cases, purpura being the most common. Osler nodes, Janeway lesions, and conjunctival haemorrhages occurred more infrequently. Roth spots are also rare but, when present the diagnosis of IE, should be suspected

Renal Symptoms

Renal impairment can occur in IE as a result of the infection or in relation to antibiotic toxicity. Glomerulonephritis is rather uncommon, but can present as acute kidney injury, and the most common biopsy pattern is necrotizing and crescentic glomerulonephritis [13]. Patients can also present with haematuria and back pain as a result of embolism to the kidney.

Other

Systemic embolisms in the spleen or kidney causing abdominal pain or silent and discovered at the time of a radiological examination should also arouse suspicion of

IE. In patients with right sided IE, pulmonary embolisms presenting as pulmonary infections can be the clue for establishing the diagnosis of IE. Mycotic aneurysms are rarely diagnosed before rupture, but in rare cases peripheral aneurysms can be seen.

References

1. Hill EE, Herijgers P, Claus P, Vanderschuren S, Herreods MC, Peetermans WE. Infective endocarditis: changing epidemiology and predictors of 6 month mortality. A prospective cohort. Eur Heart J. 2007;28:196–203.
2. Hoen B, Alla F, Selton-Suty C, Beguinot I, Bouvet A, Briancon S, Casalta JP, Danchin N, Delahaye F, Etienne J, Le Moing V, Leport C, Mainardi JL, Ruimy R, Vandernesch F. Changing profile of infectve endocarditis: results of a 1 year survey in France. JAMA. 2002;288:5–81.
3. Tornos P, Iung B, Permanyer-Miralda G, Baron G, Delhaye F, Gohlke-Barwolf CH, Butchart EG, Ravaud P, Vahanian A. Infective endocarditis in Europe:lessons from the Euro Heart Survey. Heart. 2005;91:571–5.
4. Fernandez-Hidalgo N, Almirante B, Tornos P, Pigrau C, Sambola A, Iual A, Pahissa A. Contemporary epidemiology and prognosis of health care-associated infective endocardits. Clin Infect Dis. 2008;47:1287–97.
5. Murdoch DR, Corey GR, Hoen B, Miro JM, Fowler Jr VG, Bayer AS, Karchmer AW, Olaison L, Pappas PA, Moreillon P, Chambers ST, Chu VH, Falco V, Holland DJ, Jones P, Klein JL, Raymond NJ, Read KM, Tripodi MF, Utili R, Wang A, Woods CW, Cabell CH. Clinical presentation, etiology and outcome of infective endocarditis of the 21st century: the International Collaboration on Endocarditis-Prospective Cohort study. Arch Intern Med. 2009;169:463–73.
6. Li JS, Sexton DJ, Mick N, Netles R, Fowler Jr VG, Ryan T, Bashore T, Corey GR. Proposed modifications to the Duke criteria for the diagnosis of infective endocarditis. Clin Infect Dis. 2000;30:633–63.
7. Pfahl KW, Osinelli DA, Raman S, Fistenberg M. The diagnosis and treatment of a mycotic coronary artery aneurysm: a case report. Echocardiography. 2013;30:E304–6.
8. Hess A, Klein I, Iung B, Lavallee P, Ilic-Habernaus E, Domic Q, Arnoult F, Mimoun L, Wolff M, Duval X, Laissy JP. Brain MRI findings in neurologically asymptomatic patients with infective endocarditis. Am J Neuroradil. 2013;4:1579–84.
9. Garcia-Cabrera E, Fernandez-Hidalgo N, Almirante B, Ivanova-Giorgieva R, Noureddine M, Plata A, Lomas JM, Galvez-Acebal J, Hidalgo-Tenorio C, Ruiz-Morales J, Martinez-Marcos FJ, Reguera JM, de la Torre-Lima J, de Alarcon Gonzalez A. Neurolgical complications of infective endocarditis: risk factors, outcome and impact in cardiac surgery: a multicenter observational study. Circulation. 2013;127:2272–84.
10. Auzary C, Le Thi Huong D, Delabre X, Sbai A, Lhote F, Papo T, Wechsler B, Cacoub P, Martin-Hundayi C, Piette JC. Subacute bacterial endocarditis presenting as polymialgia rheumatica or giant cell arteritis. Clin Exp Rheumatol. 2006;24:S38–40.
11. Pigrau C, Almirante B, Flores X, Falco V, Rodrguez D, Gasser I, Villanueva C, Pahissa A. Spontaneous pyogenic vertebral osteomyelitis and endocarditis: incidencerisk factors and outcome. Am J Med. 2005;118:1287.
12. Servy A, Valeyrie-Allanore L, Alla F, Leriche C, Nazeyrollas P, Chidiac C, Hoen B, Chosidow O, Dual X. Prognostic value of skin manifestations of infective endocarditis. JAMA Dermatol. 2014;150:494–500.
13. Boils CL, Nasr SH, Walker PD, Couser WG, Larsen CP. Update on endocarditis-associated glomerulonephritis. Kidney Int. 2015;87(6):1241–9.

Chapter 4
Microbiological Diagnosis in Infective Endocarditis

Jean-Paul Casalta, Frederique Gouriet, Sophie Edouard,
Pierre-Edouard Fournier, Hubert Lepidi, and Didier Raoult

Blood Culture-Positive Endocarditis (BCPE)

Currently, blood culture is the most significant assay for the diagnosis of bacterial infections, especially for bloodstream infections and endocarditis. Positive blood cultures remain the cornerstone of diagnosis and provide live bacteria for both identification and susceptibility testing. Three sets are taken at 30 min interval including in the first one aerobic and one anaerobic, in the second and third one anaerobic, each containing 10 mL of blood for a total of 40 ml obtained from a peripheral vein using meticulous sterile technique, is virtually always sufficient to identify usual causative microorganisms. Automates perform continuous monitoring of bacterial growth,

J.-P. Casalta, MD (✉) • D. Raoult, PUPH, MD
Unité de Recherche sur les Maladies Infectieuses et Tropicales Emergentes, UMR CNRS
7278, IRD 198, Institut National de la Santé et de la Recherche Médicale (INSERM) 1095,
Faculté de Médecine, Aix-Marseille Université, Marseille, France
e-mail: Jean-paul.casalta@wanadoo.fr; Didier.raoult@gmail.com

F. Gouriet, MD, PhD
Pôle de Maladies Infectieuses, Hôpital de la Timone, Marseille, France

Unité de Recherche sur les Maladies Infectieuses et Tropicales Emergentes, Faculté de
Médecine, Aix-Marseille Université, Marseille, France
e-mail: Frederique.gouriet@ap-hm.fr

S. Edouard, PharmD, PhD
Microbiological Laboratory, Hospital La Timone, APHM Marseille, Marseille, France
e-mail: Soph.edouard@gmail.com

P.-E. Fournier, MD, PhD
Microbiology Laboratory, Institute Hospitalo-Universitaire Méditerranée-Infection,
Hospital La Timone, Marseille, France
e-mail: Pierre-edouard.fournier@univ-amu.fr

H. Lepidi, MD, PhD
Department of Pathology, Hôpital de la Timone, Marseille, France
e-mail: Hubert.lepidi@ap-hm.fr

© Springer International Publishing Switzerland 2016
G. Habib (ed.), *Infective Endocarditis*, DOI 10.1007/978-3-319-32432-6_4

which ensures quick reports to the physicians. When a blood culture bottle is identified as growing bacteria by the automate, presumptive identification is based on Gram staining, which allows classification of bacteria as either cocci or bacilli and as Gram-positive or Gram-negative. This information is immediately given to clinicians in order to adapt presumptive antibiotic therapy. The positive blood culture suspension is then subcultured on agar plates in order to obtain bacterial colonies that will be subjected to identification. Routine bacterial identification is based on phenotypic tests, including Gram staining, culture and growth characteristics and biochemical patterns. Complete identification is routinely achieved within 2 days, but may require longer time for fastidious or atypical organisms [1–3]. As the delay between blood culture sampling and definitive identification of the organism responsible for the bacteremia and antibiotic susceptibility testing is long, many improvements have been proposed to speed up the process of detection and identification. These systems are based on a quick identification of bacteria that have grown in blood culture bottles. First of all, improvements in culture media and detection of growth procedures have reduced these delays. The most recent generation of automates can detect even weak bacterial growth. When growth is detected by the automate, it is possible to perform direct identification of bacteria by molecular biology, such as universal amplification and sequencing, nucleic acid-based fluorescence hybridization probes, such as FISH, DNA microarrays or molecular detection amplification and specific probes. The latter systems are usually not open and only allow detection of one or a few specific targets; however, they may provide no information about presumptive antibiotic susceptibility (i.e., detection of MRSA). These procedures are efficient but are expensive and/or require highly qualified bacteriology technicians. Among the most recent procedures for rapid identification, bacterial identification based on peptide spectra obtained by matrix-assisted laser desorption ionization time-of-flight mass spectrometry (MALDI-TOF MS) has recently demonstrated its usefulness in clinical microbiology. Not only may this method replace routine identification of bacterial colonies as it enables identification of bacterial isolates grown in agar for a few cents and within minutes, but it may also be applied to bacterial suspensions, as it has also recently been used successfully for the routine identification of bacterial colonies directly in the blood culture bottle supernatant [4, 5].

Blood Culture-Negative Endocarditis (BCNE)

Blood culture-negative endocarditis (BCNE) refers to endocarditis in which no causative microorganism can be grown using usual blood culture methods. BCNE occurs in 2.5–31 % of all cases of endocarditis (BCNE) and often causes considerable diagnostic and therapeutic dilemmas. First, BCNE are often caused by fungi or fastidious bacteria, notably obligatory intracellular bacteria. Isolation of these microorganisms requires culturing them on specialized media, and their growth is relatively slow, when possible, on axenic culture media. Second, the initiation of antibiotic therapy is often delayed, with profound impact on clinical outcome. Third, the usual empirical antibiotic therapy used for BCNE, i.e., an association of a β-lactam and an aminoglycoside, may not appropriate for several causative agents of BCNE that require a specific treatment, such as *Coxiella burnetii, Tropheryma whipplei* or fungi, potentially affecting the outcome of the disease. Four, BCNE may be caused by a manifestation of non-infectious diseases such as anti-phospholipid syndrome or systemic lupus erythematosus (Libmann-Sacks endocarditis), cancer (marantic or non-bacterial thrombotic endocarditis) [6] or allergy to pork in patients with porcine valvular bioprostheses. In these diseases, antibiotics are totally inefficient.

The variation in incidence of BCNE among series may be explained by several factors, including (i) differences in the diagnostic criteria used; (ii) specific epidemiological factors, as may be the case for fastidious zoonotic agents; (iii) variations in the early use of antibiotics prior to blood sampling; (iv) differences in sampling strategies; or (v) involvement of unknown pathogens. It's important to highlight the major role of zoonotic agents and the underestimated role of non-infective diseases in BCNE. Therefore, according to local epidemiology, systematic serological testing for *Coxiella burnetii, Bartonella spp., Aspergillus spp., Mycoplasma pneumonia, Brucella spp., Legionella pneumophila, Brucella spp.* should be proposed [7], followed by specific PCR assays for *T. whipplei, Bartonella species*, and fungi *(Candida spp, Aspergillus spp)* from blood [1]. Most studies using blood PCR for the diagnosis of BCNE have highlighted the importance of *Streptococcus gallolyticus* and *mitis, Enterococci, Staphylococcus aureus, Escherichia coli* and fastidious bacteria, the respective prevalence of which vary according to the status and condition of the patient [2, 8, 9].

Two other major diagnostic methods for BCNE are histological examination and broad-spectrum 16S and 18S ribosomal RNA PCR applied to valvular biopsies.

When all microbiological assays are negative, the diagnosis of non-infectious endocarditis should systematically be considered, and assays for antinuclear antibodies as well as antiphospholipid syndrome [anti –cardiolipine (IgG) and anti Beta2 glycoprotein 1 (IgG and IgM)] be performed [5]. When all other tests are negative and the patient has a porcine bioprosthesis and markers of allergy, anti-pork antibodies should be searched [10].

Histologic Diagnosis of Infective Endocarditis

Pathological examination of resected valve tissue or embolic fragments remains the gold standard for the diagnosis of IE [11]. All tissue samples that are excised during the course of the surgical removal of cardiac valves must be collected in a sterile container without fixative or culture medium. The entire sample is taken without delay to the diagnostic microbiology laboratory for optimal recovery and identification of microorganisms. After the selection of valve tissue samples for bacteriologic procedures such as valve tissue culture and polymerase chain reaction amplification, the remaining tissue samples are fixed in neutral buffered formalin, decalcified if necessary, and embedded in paraffin. Tissue specimens are cut to 3-mm thickness and stained with hematoxylin-eosin by use of routine methods. During the histo- logic examination, valve lesions are classified as (i) consistent with IE, (ii) showing no histologic features of IE, (iii) intermediate status according to criteria defined elsewhere. Non-specific special stains, including Giemsa, Grocott-Gomori methe- namine silver, Warthin-Starry, periodic acid Schiff, Brown-Brenn and Brown-Hopps tissue Gram stains, are used when necessary to better visualize bacterial colonies or fungal hyphae. Moreover, immunohistological detection, as specific method of detection, can be used to detect bacteria, particularly in case of bacteria with an intracellular growth [12–15]. Detection and specific identification of bacteria in tis- sue samples can be also achieve by fluorescence in situ hybridization (FISH), a recent molecular method [16].

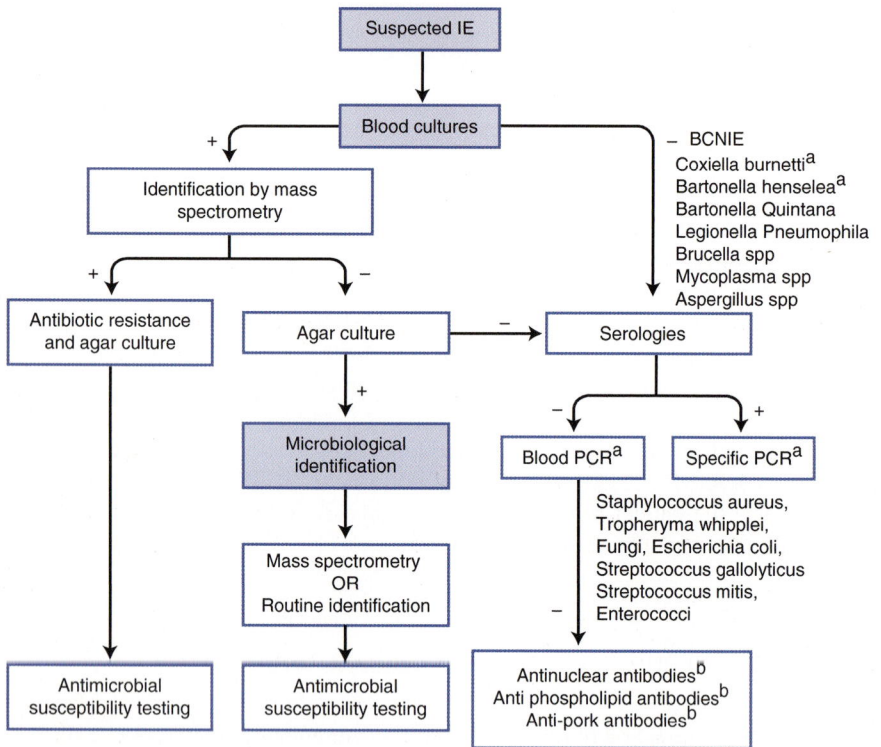

BCNIE: Blood culture-negative endocarditis
a: Qualified microbiological laboratory
b: Immunological laboratory

Fig. 4.1 Microbiologic decision algorithm (From Habib et al. [17]. Used with permission of Oxford University Press)

Strategy for the Standard Diagnostic of Culture-Positive and Culture-Negative IE

In recent decades, standard diagnostic schemes have been developed to improve the sensitivity and specificity of the diagnosis of endocarditis. Despite progress with diagnostic criteria, the type and timing of laboratory tests used to diagnose infective and non-infective endocarditis have not been standardized. One of solutions is the realization of diagnostic kit taken in 1 h and including four blood bottles, systematic serological testing for *Coxiella burnetii, Bartonella spp., Aspergillus spp., Legionella pneumophila, brucella spp., Mycoplasma pneumonia*, rheumatoid factor for the positive diagnosis, serological tests for antiphospholipid syndrome [anti –cardio-lipine (IgG) and anti Beta2 glycoprotein 1 (IgG and IgM)], antinuclear antibodies and anti-pork antibodies. The kit is used to indicate to the microbiological laboratory the patient suspected of IE. At 24 h, when the results of blood cultures are negatives (most bacteria are growing within 24 h) the laboratory can perform the other tests of the kit (serologies and PCRs). These investigations performed in accordance with a decision algorithm proposed by the European Society of Cardiology [17] (Fig. 4.1) can be a complete solution with cost- effectiveness [4]. In addition, cardiac valvular materials obtained at surgery were subjected systematical culture, histologic examination and included PCR aimed at documenting the presence of fastidious organisms.

References

1. Fenollar F, Raoult D. Molecular diagnosis of bloodstream infections caused by non-cultivable bacteria. Int J Antimicrob Agents. 2007;30 Suppl 1:S7–15.
2. Fournier PE, Thuny F, Richet H, Lepidi H, Casalta JP, Arzouni JP, Maurin M, Célard M, Mainardi JL, Caus T, Collart F, Habib G, Raoult D. Comprehensive diagnostic strategy for blood culture-negative endocarditis: a prospective study of 819 new cases. Clin Infect Dis. 2010;51(2):131–40.
3. Lagacé-Wiens PR, Adam HJ, Karlowsky JA, Nichol KA, Pang PF, Guenther J, Webb AA, Miller C, Alfaa MJ. Identification of blood culture isolates directly from positive blood cultures by use of matrix-assisted laser desorption ionization–time of flight mass spectrometry and a commercial extraction system: analysis of performance, cost, and turnaround time. J Clin Microbiol. 2012;50(10):3324–8.
4. La Scola B, Raoult D. Direct identification of bacteria in positive blood culture bottles by matrix-assisted laser desorption ionisation time-of-flight mass spectrometry. PLoS One. 2009;4(11):e8041.
5. Lee L, Naguwa SM, Cheema GS, Gershwin ME. Revisiting libman-sacks endocarditis: a historical review and update. J Clin Rev Allergy Immunol. 2009;36(2–3):126–30.
6. Mazokopakis EE, Syros PK, Starakis IK. Nonbacterial thrombotic endocarditis (marantic endocarditis) in cancer patients. Cardiovasc Hematol Disord Drug Targets. 2010;10(2):84–6.
7. Raoult D, Casalta JP, Richet H, Khan M, Bernit E, Rovery C, Branger S, Gouriet F, Imbert G, Bothello E, Collart F, Habib G. Contribution of systematic serological testing in diagnosis of infective endocarditis. J Clin Microbiol. 2005;43(10):5238–42.

8. Leli C, Moretti A, Pasticci MB, Cenci E, Bistoni F, Mencacci A. A commercially available multiplex real-time PCR for detection of pathogens in cardiac valves from patients with infective endocarditis. Diagn Microbiol Infect Dis. 2014;79(1):98–101.
9. Rovery C, Greub G, Lepidi H, Casalta JP, Habib G, Collart F, Raoult D. PCR detection of bacteria on cardiac valves of patients with treated bacterial endocarditis. J Clin Microbiol. 2005;43(1):163–7.
10. Loyens M, Thuny F, Grisoli D, Fournier PE, Casalta JP, Vitte J, Habib G, Raoult D. Link between endocarditis on porcine bioprosthetic valves and allergy to pork. Int J Cardiol. 2013;167(2):600–2.
11. Lepidi H, Durack DT, Raoult D. Diagnostic methods: current best practices and guidelines for histologic evaluation in Infective endocarditis. Infect Dis Clin N Am. 2002;16:339–61.
12. Lepidi H, Fournier PE, Raoult D. Quantitative analysis of valvular lesions during Bartonella endocarditis. Am J Clin Pathol. 2000;114:880–9.
13. Lepidi H, Houpikian P, Liang Z, Raoult D. Cardiac valves in patients with Q fever endocarditis: microbiological, molecular and histologic studies. J Infect Dis. 2003;187:1097–106.
14. Lepidi H, Fenollar F, Dumler JS, Gauduchon V, Chalabreysse L, Bammert A, Bonzi MF, Thivolet-Béjui F, Vandenesch F, Raoult D. Cardiac valves in patients with Whipple endocarditis: microbiological, molecular, quantitative histologic, and immunohistochemical studies of 5 patients. J Infect Dis. 2004;190:935–45.
15. Lepidi H, Coulibaly B, Casalta JP, Raoult D. Auto-immunohistochemistry, a new method for histologic diagnosis of infective endocarditis. J Infect Dis. 2006;193:1711–7.
16. Mallmann C, Siemoneit S, Schmiedel D, Petrich A, Gescher DM, Halle E, Musci M, Hetzer R, Göbel UB, Moter A. Fluorescence hybridization to improve the diagnosis of endocarditis: a pilot study. Clin Microbiol Infect. 2010;16:767–73.
17. Habib G, et al. 2015 ESC guidelines for the management of infective endocarditis. The task force for the management of infective endocarditis of the European Society of Cardiology (ESC). Eur Heart J. 2015;36(44):3075–128.

Chapter 5
Echocardiography in Infective Endocarditis Diagnosis

Maria Teresa Gonzàlez-Alujas and Artur Evangelista Masip

Introduction

Early and reliable diagnostic and risk stratification strategies are critical to reduce delays in the initiation of appropriate antimicrobial therapy and identify patients who require urgent valve surgery. The development of two-dimensional and later transoesophageal echocardiography (TOE) has significantly improved the non-invasive detection of vegetations. Moreover, Doppler echocardiography provides clinically important information on the presence and degree of valvular destruction and their haemodynamic consequences, as well as on the existence of perivalvular infection. The diagnostic strategy proposed by Durack et al. [1] (the Duke criteria) combined echocardiographic findings with clinical and microbiological data. Three echocardiographic findings were considered to be major criteria for the diagnosis of endocarditis: (a) presence of vegetations defined as mobile echodense masses implanted in a valve or mural endocardium in the trajectory of a regurgitant jet or implanted in prosthetic material with no alternative anatomical explanation; (b) presence of abscesses; or (c) presence of a new dehiscence of a valvular prosthesis. Abnormal echocardiographic findings not fulfilling these definitions were considered minor criteria. More recently, the use of TOE has resulted in better imaging and therefore doubtful findings are no longer considered minor criteria [2]. Since the definitive diagnosis of endocarditis requires the presence of two major criteria or one major and three minor criteria, it is clear that echocardiography has assumed a crucial role in the diagnosis of the disease, particularly when blood cultures are negative.

Electronic supplementary material The online version of this chapter (doi:10.1007/978-3-319-32432-6_5) contains supplementary material, which is available to authorized users.

M.T. Gonzàlez-Alujas, PhD (✉) • A. Evangelista Masip, PhD
Servei de Cardiologia, Hospital Universitari Vall d'Hebron, Barcelona, Spain
e-mail: teresagonzalu@gmail.com; arturevangelistamasip@gmail.com

© Springer International Publishing Switzerland 2016
G. Habib (ed.), *Infective Endocarditis*, DOI 10.1007/978-3-319-32432-6_5

Table 5.1 Anatomic and echocardiographic definitions of IE findings

	Echocardiography	Surgery/Necropsy
Vegetation	Echo-dense mass on valve or other endocardial structures or in implanted intracardiac material	Infected mass attached to an endocardial structure, or on implanted intracardiac material
Abscess	Thickened, non-homogeneus perivalvular area with echo dense or echolucent appearance	Perivalvular cavity with necrosis and purulent material not communicating with the cardiovascular lumen
Pseudoaneurysm	Pulsatile perivalvular echo-free cavity with colour-Doppler flow detected	Perivalvular cavity communicating with the cardiovascular lumen
Valvular aneurysm	Saccular dilatation of valvular tissue in "jet" impact areas	Saccular outpouching of valvular tissue
Perforation	Solution of continuity in the valve leaflets with evidence of flow passage through it	Interruption of endocardial valve continuity
Fistula	Non anatomic connection between two cardiac chambers, with flow passage through it	Communication between two neighbouring cardiac cavities through a perforation
Prosthesis dehiscence	Perivalvular regurgitation identified by TTE or TEE, with or without "rocking" motion of the prosthesis	Dehiscence of the prosthesis

Detection of Vegetations

There is no better technique for the non-invasive visualisation of vegetations than echocardiography. Typically, a vegetation presents as an oscillating mass attached to a valvular structure, with a movement independent of that of this valve (Table 5.1). Overall, the detection rate for vegetations by transthoracic echocardiography (TTE) in patients with clinically suspected endocarditis [3] is around 75 % (Fig. 5.1, Video 5.1). However, the sensitivity of TTE may be reduced by several factors: (a) image quality, (b) echogenicity and vegetation size, (c) vegetation location, (d) presence of previous valvular disease or valvular prosthesis, (e) experience and skill of the examiner, and (f) pre-test probability of endocarditis.

A vegetation may also present as a non-oscillating mass and with an atypical location. Vegetations are usually located on the atrial side of the atrio-ventricular valves and on the ventricular side of the aortic and pulmonary valves. Less frequently, vegetations are located on papillary muscles or mural endocardium. Over time, vegetations tend to decrease in size with therapy, although they may persist indefinitely as less mobile and more echogenic masses. Vegetations persisting after effective treatment must not be interpreted as a clinical recurrence of the disease unless supported by clinical features and bacteriological evidence.

Not all intracardiac mass lesions are vegetations from IE. For instance, in systemic lupus erythematosus inflammatory mass lesions (Libman-Sacks) related to

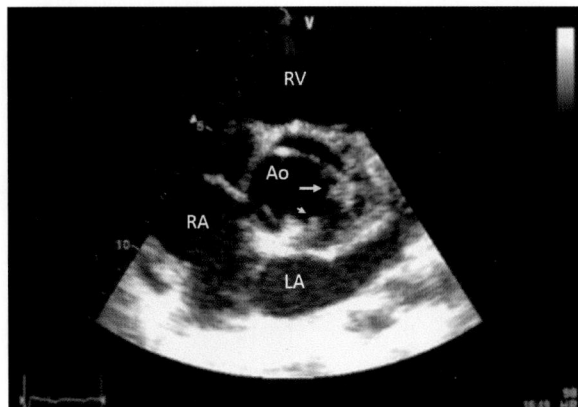

Fig. 5.1 Transthoracic echocardiography showing a large vegetation on the sigmoid of bicuspid aortic valve (*arrow*) and another small vegetation at the posterior commissure (*small arrow*). *RV* right ventricle, *RA* right atrial, *Ao* aortic valve, *LA* left atrial

the disease usually have broad bases and are small. Other sterile vegetations, such as in marantic endocarditis, may also be present in patients with advanced malignancies. A mass effect may be seen in patients with myxomatous valves, ruptured chordae unrelated to infection or heart tumours. Moreover, normal variants, such a Lambl excrescences (small filiform processes on the medial tip of the aortic valve), a Chiari network, and a Eustachian valve in the right atrium, may mimic IE vegetations on the echocardiogram [4, 5]. Echocardiography must be performed rapidly, as soon as IE is suspected. However, the sensitivity and specificity of TTE and TOE are diminished when applied indiscriminately, particularly in patients with a low likelihood of IE. Appropriate use of echocardiography using simple clinical criteria improves the diagnostic yield [6]. An exception is in patients with *staphylococcus aureus* bacteraemia when routine echo is warranted owing to the aggressiveness of this infection. The list of clinical situations in which IE must be suspected has been clearly established in the ESC guidelines [7].

Native Valve Infective Endocarditis

TTE is the initial technique of choice for study. However, vegetation size affects TTE sensitivity [8] since only 25 % of vegetations less than 5 mm and 70 % of those between 6 and 10 mm are identified [9]. Underlying valve disease may influence the diagnostic accuracy of TTE when a myxomatous mitral valve or sclerotic or calcified valves are present. These limitations have been overcome by TOE owing to its better resolution and multiple study planes (Fig. 5.2, Video 5.2). Many studies have compared the sensitivity and specificity of TTE and TOE in the diagnosis of vegetations. In the majority of these studies TTE sensitivity varies between 40 and 63 % and that of TOE between 90 and 100 % [4, 5, 8, 9]. TOE is mandatory in cases of doubtful TTE. in prosthetic and pacemaker IE.

A negative TOE has a major clinical impact on the diagnosis of endocarditis with a high negative predictive value ranging from 86 to 97 %. In patients with native

Fig. 5.2 Large vegetation visualised by 3D-TOE at the atrial side of the posterior mitral valve (P2), with a mobile component in the upper part (*arrow*)

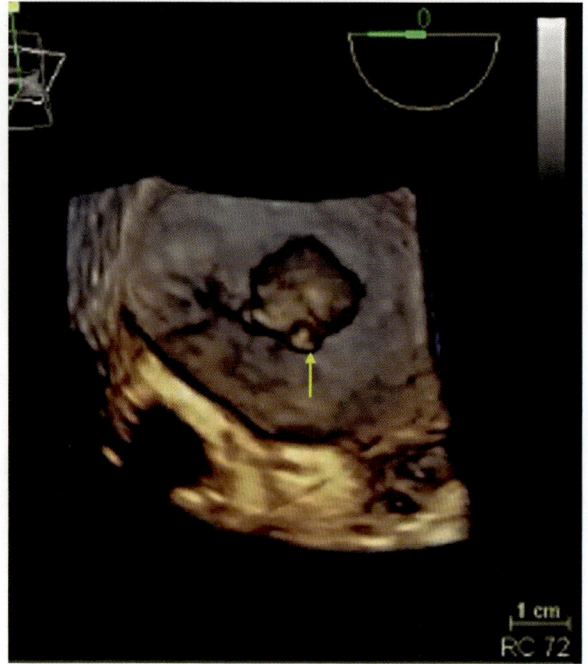

heart valves, a negative TOE virtually rules out the diagnosis of infective endocarditis. However, in the study of Sochowski et al. [10], 5 out of 65 patients (7.6 %) with an initially negative TOE were finally diagnosed of endocarditis: In 3 of these, TOE performed in 1–2 weeks after the initial examination showed the presence of vegetations. This study underlines the importance of recognising the phase of the disease in which the study is performed since vegetations may not be large enough to be visualised when endocarditis is suspected very early on. The usefulness of TOE in patients with suspected endocarditis on a native valve depends on the TTE results. TOE is useful when TTE is negative or inconclusive.

Prosthetic Valve Endocarditis

Vegetations on prosthetic valves are more difficult to detect by TTE than those involving native valves; thus, TOE should always be used if the diagnosis of prosthetic endocarditis is suspected (Fig. 5.3, Video 5.3). The sewing ring and support structures of mechanical and bioprosthetic valves are strongly echogenic and may prevent vegetations detection within the valve apparatus or its shadow. The vegetative growth appears as thickening and irregularity of the normally smooth contour of the sewing ring. Both thrombus and pannus have a similar appearance and cannot be distinguished from vegetative material. It is also important to recognise strands to avoid false-positive diagnosis. Strands are commonly

Fig. 5.3 TOE showing a large vegetation on the annulus of mitral valve bileaflet prosthesis (*arrows*). *LA* left atrial, *LV* left ventricle

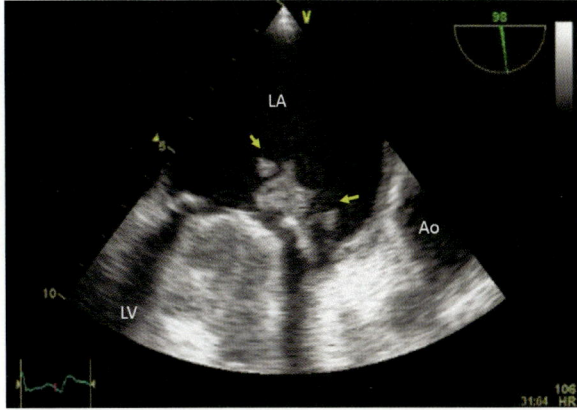

Fig. 5.4 TTE shows a large, mobile vegetation in tricuspid valve (*arrows*). *RV* right ventricle, *Ao* aortic valve, *RA* right atrial

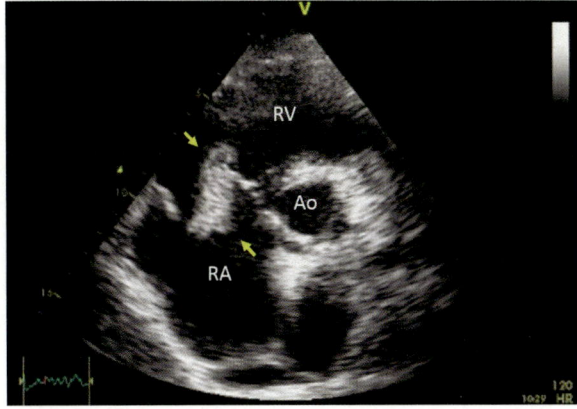

observed by TOE on prosthetic valves, particularly in the early postoperative months [11].

In a large series of prosthetic endocarditis, TOE showed 86–94 % sensitivity and 88–100 % specificity for vegetation diagnosis, while TTE sensitivity was only 36–69 % [12]. Bioprosthetic valve leaflets may become infected with secondary destruction of leaflet tissue. The distinction between wear-and-tear degeneration of tissue valves and endocarditis is often difficult. TOE also led to improved diagnostic accuracy in the diagnosis of endocarditis on bioprosthetic valves [5].

Right-Sided Endocarditis and Pacemaker Lead Infections

TTE permits easy and correct diagnosis of tricuspid vegetations, probably because the majority of patients with tricuspid endocarditis are young intravenous drug abusers with large vegetations (Fig. 5.4, Video 5.4). The vegetations are located on

Fig. 5.5 4-Chamber
apical view on TTE
revealing a large
vegetation (*arrow*) in the
pacemaker lead live (*small
arrow*). *LV* left ventricle,
RV right ventricle, *LA* left
atrial, *RA* right atrial

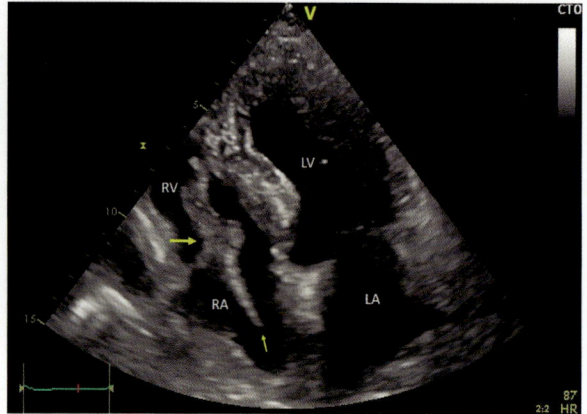

the atrial side of the tricuspid valve, in the trajectory of the regurgitant jet. San Roman et al. [13] showed that TOE did not improve on the accuracy of TTE in the detection of vegetations in tricuspid endocarditis. However, despite the low number of cases described, TOE appears to be more sensitive than TTE in the diagnosis of pulmonary valve endocarditis.

Infection or endocarditis on a pacemaker lead are difficult to diagnose by TTE since pacemaker leads produce reverberations and artefacts that may mask or render difficult the recognition of vegetations close to these structures. In addition, when vegetations were visualised, it was difficult to determine whether tricuspid valve endocarditis, lead infection or both were present. TOE was clearly superior to TTE in this clinical setting (sensitivity 23 % versus 94 %) (Fig. 5.5, Video 5.5).

Negative Blood Culture Endocarditis

In those cases, echo is crucial in the diagnosis of infectious endocarditis. The two main causes of negative blood culture endocarditis are: previous antibiotic treatment or infection by fastidious microorganisms, with limited capability for growth in conventional culture media (Fig 5.6, Video 5.6).

Abscess Formation and Paravalvular Extension of Infection

The second major echocardiographic criterion for endocarditis is the presence of perivalvular abscesses. Perivalvular abscesses are considered to be present when a definite region of reduced echo density, without colour flow detected inside, is found on the echocardiogram (Fig. 5.7, Video 5.7). They are more frequently observed in aortic valve IE and prosthetic valve IE. Sensitivity and specificity of

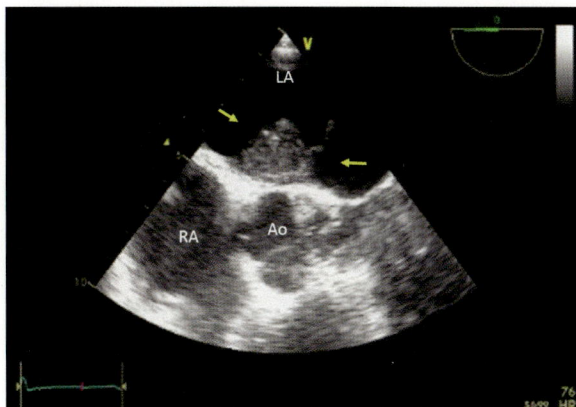

Fig. 5.6 Mural vegetation (*arrows*) located on the anterior wall of the left atrium visualised by TOE in an *Aspergillus* endocarditis. *LA* left atrial, *RA* right atrial, *Ao* aortic valve

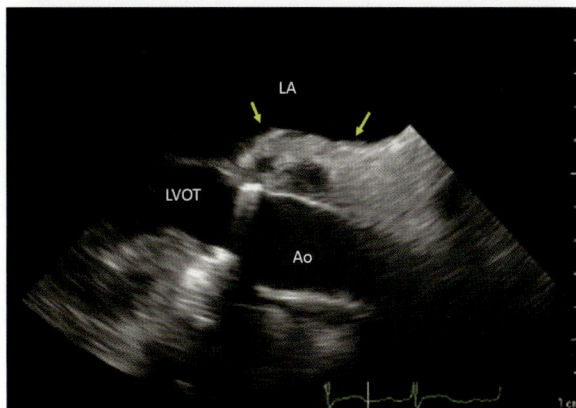

Fig. 5.7 Periannular aortic abscess (*arrows*) visualised by TOE extending throughout the graft in ascending aorta. *LA* left atrial, *Ao* ascending aorta, *LVOT* left ventricle outflow tract

TTE for abscess detection were 28 and 99 % respectively, compared to 87 and 95 % of TOE. TOE was particularly useful in prosthetic endocarditis. The diagnosis of aortic abscesses was easier than mitral abscesses, both with TTE (42 % vs 9 %) and TOE (86 % vs 57 %). The additional value of TOE is significantly higher for the diagnosis of abscesses than for the diagnosis of vegetations. For this reason, TOE must be systematically performed in aortic valve IE and as soon as an abscess is suspected.

Pseudoaneurysm is characterised anatomically by a perivalvular cavity communicating with the cardiovascular lesion. The echocardiographic hallmark of pseudoaneurysm is the presence of a pulsatile perivalvular echo-free space with colour Doppler within. The echocardiographic appearance of partial systolic collapse proves that the abscess communicates with the cardiovascular lumen (Fig. 5.8, Video 5.8). Perivalvular cavities are formed when annular infections break through and spread into contiguous tissue. In native aortic valve endocarditis, the generally occur through the weakest portion of the annulus, which is near the membranous septum.

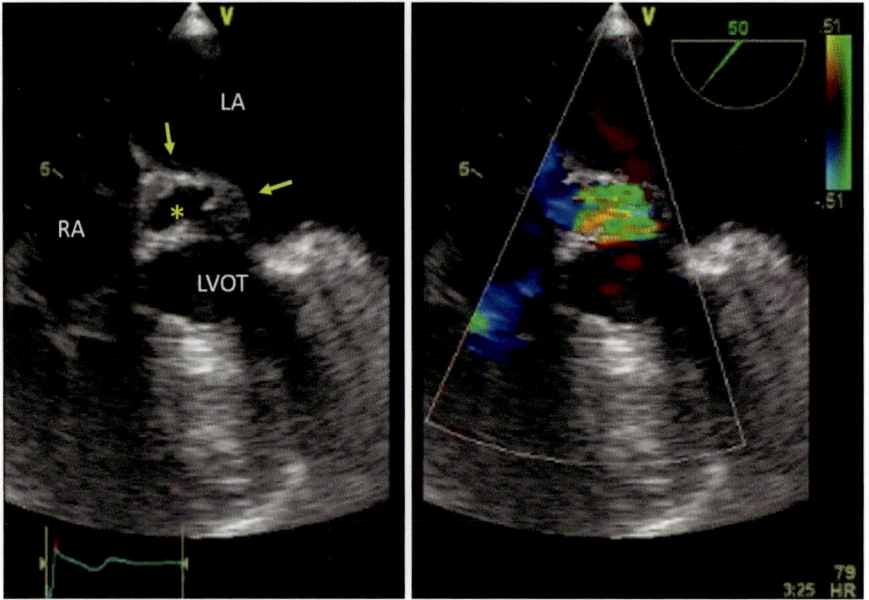

Fig. 5.8 Periannular aortic cavity with pulsatility and flow signal within (*asterisk*). Arrow shows the communication through which the pseudoaneurysm fills and empties. *LA* left atrial, *RA* right atrial, *LVOT* left ventricle outflow tract

Secondary involvement of the mitral-aortic intervalvular fibrosa and anterior mitral leaflet occurs as a result of direct extension of the infection from the aortic valve or as a result of an infected aortic regurgitant jet. The abscess can expand to form a pseudoaneurysm and can subsequently cause a perforation and communication between the left ventricle and left atrium. An intervalvular pseudoaneurysm was defined as an echo-free cavity located posteriorly in the intervalvular fibrosa region, just below the aortic annulus, and bound by the base of the anterior mitral leaflet, the medial wall of the left atrium and the posterior aortic root (Fig. 5.9, Video 5.9). Karalis et al. [3] described 24 (44 %) complications involving 55 consecutive cases of aortic endocarditis, including 8 abscesses and aneurysms in interfibrosa, 7 interfibrosa perforations into the adjacent left atrium and 9 anterior mitral aneurysms and perforation. TTE detected 43 % of these complications while TOE identified 90 % [14].

Both aortic root abscesses and pseudoaneurysms may rupture into adjacent chambers and therefore create intracardiac fistulous tracts (Fig. 5.10, Video 5.10). These fistulae may be single or multiple and generally extend from the aorta to the right ventricle or the right or left atrium [15]. Using colour Doppler, the site of the communication of the ruptured intervalvular pseudoaneurysms is usually well defined. By continuous-wave Doppler, systolic high-velocity flow suggests an abnormal communication between the aorta and either the left or right atria. Eccentric mitral regurgitation-type systolic jets by colour flow Doppler should suggest the possibility of interfibrosa perforation and should undergo further evaluation by TOE.

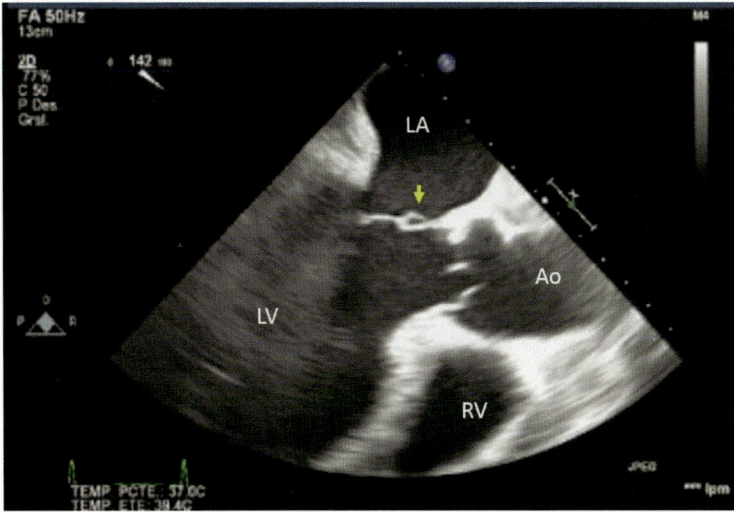

Fig. 5.9 Pseudoaneurysm located in the mitro-aortic interfibrosa (*arrow*) in a patient with a mitral and aortic endocarditis. Note the small vegetation on the ventricular side of the native aortic valve. *LA* left atrial, *Ao* ascending aorta, *LV* left ventricle, *RV* right ventricle

Fig. 5.10 Mitro-aortic endocarditis with a fistulised aortic periannular abscess (*arrows*) causing a communication between the aorta and the left atrium. *LA* left atrial, *Ao* ascending aorta, *LV* left ventricle, *RV* right ventricle

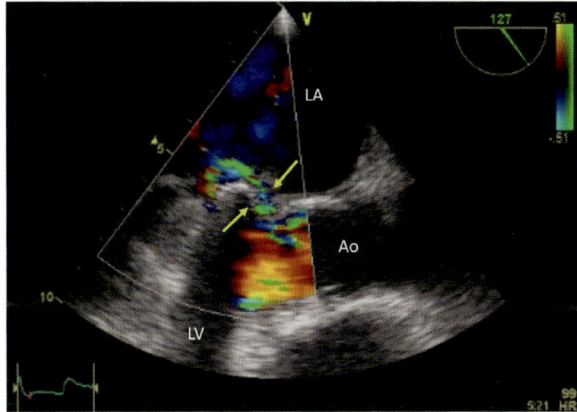

Prosthetic Valve Dehiscence

This represents the third main diagnostic criterion for IE. IE must be suspected in the presence of a new perivalvular regurgitation, even in the absence of vegetation or abscess. TOE has better sensitivity than TTE for the diagnosis, especially in mitral prosthetic valve infective endocarditis. Dehiscence of a prosthetic valve due to IE is a serious complication. Dehiscence is generally defined fluoroscopically as a rocking motion of the prosthetic valve more than 15° in any one plane. This complication may lead to a gross separation of the prosthetic annulus from the native tissue.

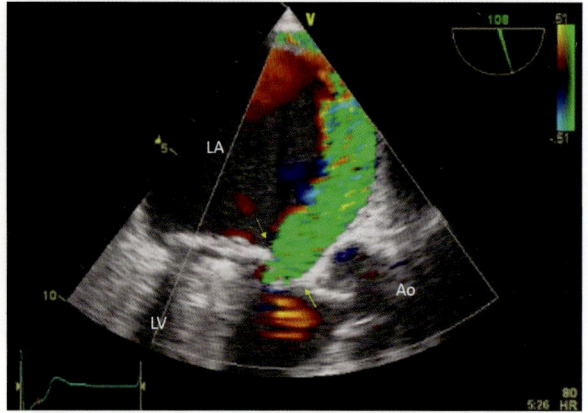

Fig. 5.11 Severe mitral periprosthetic leak (*arrows*) in a patient with suspected mitral prosthetic endocarditis. *LA* left atrial, *Ao* aortic valve, *LV* left ventricle

Prosthetic valve dehiscence is invariably associated with significant paravalvular regurgitation and is usually associated with haemodynamic compromise (Fig. 5.11, Video 5.11). Significant dehiscence in acute IE represents an urgent indication for surgical therapy.

Diagnosis of Other Complications

Valvular Complications

Regurgitation of the infected valve is almost constant and results from a variety of mechanisms. The vegetations themselves may prevent proper leaflet or cusp coaptation. Some degree of valvular destruction is commonly seen and may vary from a small perforation in a cusp to a complete flail leaflet. Valvular perforation is a frequent complication that may cause severe insufficiency with acute onset and precipitate heart failure (Fig. 5.12a, b, Video 5.12). In aortic endocarditis cusp perforation, flail or both may occur in up to 50 % of cases. Severe aortic insufficiency as estimated by Doppler has been associated with poor prognosis. In this setting, early diastolic closure of the mitral valve identifies patients with unstable haemodynamic status. Perforation of the mitral leaflets is less common, occurring only in 15 % of patients with mitral valve endocarditis (Fig. 5.13a, b, Video 5.13). Progressive destruction of the mitral valve results initially in ruptured chordae tendinae and ultimately flail leaflet.

TTE appears more useful in detecting mitral than aortic perforations. Colour flow Doppler imaging permits the location of abnormal flows in the areas of anatomic interruption and therefore aids the differentiation between mitral cusp perforation and true mitral regurgitation. TOE is recommended if a valve perforation is suspected and TTE is negative or equivocal.

TOE colour-flow mapping is of particular value in patients with a mechanical mitral prosthesis and paravalvular regurgitation. The presence of a new or increasing paravalvular regurgitation or valve dehiscence is a major criterion for the diagnosis

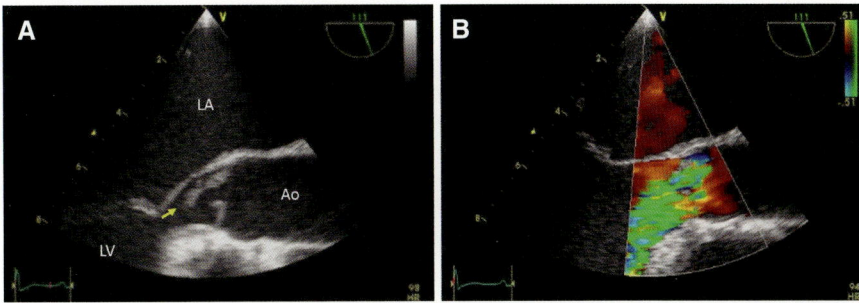

Fig. 5.12 (**a**) TOE showing the eversion of the non-coronary aortic sigmoid (*arrow*). (**b**) Colour Doppler detected severe aortic regurgitation. *LA* left atrial, *Ao* ascending aorta, *LV* left ventricle

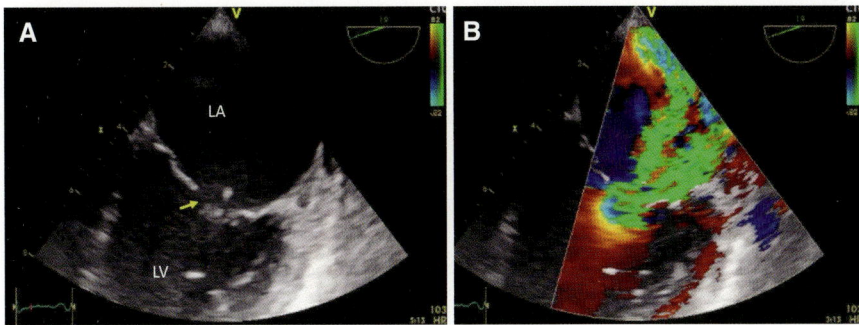

Fig. 5.13 (**a**) Anterior mitral valve perforation (*arrow*). (**b**) Colour Doppler shows 2 mitral regurgitant jets, one with flow through the perforation (*arrow*) in the anterior mitral valve. *LA* left atrial, *LV* left ventricle

of endocarditis. Khanderia et al. [16] reported that the transoesophageal approach had overall sensitivity of 96 % in the evaluation of mitral prostheses. The demonstration of aortic prosthetic paravalvular regurgitation is rather easy from the precordium as the colour-encoded regurgitant jets may be visualised from both the apical and parasternal views.

Echocardiography for Risk Stratification

Heart failure, perivalvular extension and embolic events represent the three most frequent and severe complications of IE. Echocardiography plays a key role in the management of these complications by aiding decision-making regarding valve surgery and its optimal timing. See Table 5.2.

Heart failure represents the main indication for valve surgery in IE [17] and the operation is usually indicated in an emergency (within 24 h) or urgent (within a few days) setting. TOE allows identification of the mechanisms responsible for these complications, such as acute valve regurgitation or intracardiac fistulae. TTE may

Table 5.2 Echocardiography recommendations in IE

Diagnosis
TTE: recommended as a first technique in the suspicion of IE
TOE: recommended in high suspicion of IE and negative TTE
Repeat TTE/TOE at 7–10 days when after an initial negative echocardiography a high suspicion of IE persists
TOE: in adult patients with positive TTE in order to improve the diagnosis of abscesses and the size of vegetations in prosthesis, aortic endocarditis and atrio-ventricular block
Follow-up in patients with medical treatment
Repeat TTE/TOE whenever there is a suspicion of complication (new murmur, persistent fever, AV block)
Intraoperative echocardiography
Intraoperative TOE is recommended in all patients who require surgical treatment
Follow-up at the end of treatment
TTE is recommended at the end of antibiotic treatment

provide criteria of poor haemodynamic tolerance, even in the absence of clinical congestive signs and the presence of these echocardiographic signs suggests the need for valve surgery since evolution to heart failure is inevitable.

Perivalvular extensions, discussed previously, are present in around 20 % of cases and indicate valve surgery owing to the risk of heart failure due to prosthetic valve dehiscence, fistulae or persistence of infection [18].

The second most common cardiac complication of IE is embolization. Embolic events are frequent and are symptomatic in around 20–25 % of cases and silent in almost 50 %. The risk of embolization appears much greater for mitral than for aortic valve endocarditis. The rate of embolic events declines rapidly after the initiation of effective antibiotics, dropping from an initial 13 events per 1000 patients-days in the first week to less than 1.2 events per 1000 patients-days after 2 weeks of therapy. Echocardiography, especially TOE, is useful for the evaluation of embolic risk at admission. The size and mobility of the vegetations are the best predictors of embolism, although several factors have been associated with an increased risk of embolism, including the location of the vegetation on the mitral valve. Careful measurement of the maximum vegetation size at the time of diagnosis and during follow-up is strongly recommended as part of the risk stratification, using both TTE and TOE. A recent study demonstrated that early surgery in patient with large vegetations reduced the risk of death and embolic events compared with conventional therapy. A vegetation size >10 mm following one or more embolic episode, or associated with another complicated course should indicate earlier surgery. In cases with a very large vegetation >15 mm, surgery may be indicated when valve repair seems possible, particularly in mitral valve IE. However, that result was obtained in a population with a very low operative risk. Nevertheless, the prediction of embolism remains challenging and should take into account other criteria such as the type of microorganism and conditions associated with a prothrombotic state.

Intraoperative TOE is very useful in patients operated on for IE, since it provides final anatomical evaluation of valvular and perivalvular damage, and for assessing the immediate result of conservative surgery. After hospital discharge, a clinical and echocardiographic periodic close follow-up at 1, 3, 6 and 12 months is mandatory during the first year post-discharge.

Conclusions

Echocardiography plays a key role not only in the diagnosis of IE but also in the prognostic assessment and follow-up under therapy and during surgery. Any patient suspected of having infective endocarditis by clinical criteria should be screened by TTE. When the images are of good quality and the study is negative an alternative diagnosis should be sought if the clinical suspicion is low. If the clinical suspicion is high, TOE should be performed. TOE should also be performed if the results of TTE are equivocal owing to underlying structural abnormalities or poor acoustic windows.

If TOE is negative, observation or re-evaluation of the clinical data is warranted. If the suspicion of endocarditis is high, TOE should be repeated after 7–10 days to allow potential vegetations to become more apparent. A repeated negative study should virtually rule out the diagnosis unless TOE images are of poor quality.

TOE should also be performed to provide a more detailed anatomical assessment when perivalvular complications are suspected particularly in the setting of aortic or prosthetic valve endocarditis or in infections caused by virulent microorganisms such as *S aureus*.

References

1. Durack DT, Lukes AS, Bright DK. New criteria for diagnosis of infective endocarditis: utilization of specific echocardiographic findins: Duke endocarditis service. Am J Med. 1994;96:200–9.
2. Li JS, Suton DJ, Mick N, et al. Proposed modifications to the Duke criteria for the diagnosis of infective endocarditis. Clin Infect Dis. 2000;30:633–8.
3. Karalis DG, Bansal RC, Hauck AJ, et al. Transesophageal echocardiographic recognition of subaortic complications in aortic valve endocarditis. Circulation. 1992;86:353–62.
4. Mügge A, Daniel WG, Frank G, Lichtlen PR. Echocardiography in infective endocarditis: reassessment of prognostic implications of vegetation size determined by the transthoracic and the tranesophageal approach. J Am Coll Cardiol. 1989;14:631–8.
5. Shively BK, Gurule FT, Roldan CA, Leggett JH, Schiller NB. Diagnostic value of tranesophageal compared with transthoracic echocardiography in infective endocarditis. J Am Coll Cardiol. 1991;18:391–7.
6. Habib G, Badano L, Tribouilloy C, Vilacosta I, Zamorano JL, Galderisi M, Voigt JU, Sicari R, Cosyns B, Fox K, Aakhus S, European Association of Echocardiography. Recommendations for the practice of echocardiography in infective endocarditis. Eur J Echocardiogr. 2010;11(2): 202–19.
7. Habib G, Lancellotti P, Antunes MJ, Bongiorni MG, Casalta JP, Del Zotti F, et al. 2015 ESC Guidelines for the management of infective endocarditis: The Task Force for the Management

of Infective Endocarditis of the European Society of Cardiology (ESC). Eur Heart J. 2015;36(44):3075–128.

8. Shapiro SM, Young E, De Guzman S, Ward J, Chiu C, Ginzton LE, Bayer AS. Transesophageal echocardiography in diagnosis of infective endocarditis. Chest. 1994;105:377–82.

9. Erbel R, Rohmann S, Drexler M, et al. Improved diagnostic value of echocardiography in patients with infective endocarditis by transoesophageal approach. A prospective study. Eur Heart J. 1988;9:43–53.

10. Sochowski RA, Chan K-L. Implication of negative results on a monoplane trnsesophageal echocardiographic study in patients with suspected infective endocarditis. J Am Coll Cardiol. 1993;21:216–21.

11. Lengyel M. The impact of transesophageal echocardiography on management of prosthetic valve endocarditis: experience of 31 cases and review of the literature. J Heart Valve Dis. 1997; 6:204–11.

12. Rozich JD, Edwards WD, Hanna RD, Laffey DM, et al. Mechanical prosthetic valve associated strands: pathologic correlates to tranesophageal echocardiography. J Am Soc Echocardiogr. 2003;16:97–100.

13. San Roman JA, Vilacosta I, Zamorano JL, Almeria C, Sanchez-Harguindey L. Transesophageal echocardiography in right-sided endocarditis. J Am Coll Cardiol. 1993;21:1226–30.

14. Chan KL. Early clinical course and long-term outcome of patients with infective endocarditis complicated by perivalvular abscess. CMAJ. 2002;167:19–24.

15. Năstase O, Rădulescu B, Serban M, Lăcău IS, Bubenek S, Popescu BA, et al. Pseudoaneurysm in the mitral-aortic intervalvular fibrosa-case report and literature review. Echocardiography. 2015;32:570–4.

16. Khanderia BK, Seward JB, Oh JK, Freeman WK, Nichols BA, Sinak LJ, Miller FA, Tajik AJ. Value and limitations of transesophageal echocardiography in assessment of mitral valve prostheses. Circulation. 1991;83:1956–68.

17. Tornos P, Almirante B, Olona M, Permanyer G, González T, Carballo J, Pahissa A, Soler-Soler J. Clinical outcome and long-term prognosis of late prosthetic valve endocarditis: a 20-year experience. Clin Infect Dis. 1997;24(3):381–6.

18. Chirillo F, Scotton P, Rocco F, Rigoli R, Pedrocco A, Martire P, et al. Manegement strategies and outcome for prosthetic valve endocarditis. Am J Cardiol. 2013;112:1177e–81.

Chapter 6
Other Imaging Modalities in Infective Endocarditis Diagnosis

Paola Anna Erba, Martina Sollini, Roberto Boni, and Elena Lazzeri

Introduction

The use of diagnostic imaging has increased significantly over the past decade in all fields of medical science. For more than a century, X-rays technology was the only available modality allowing doctors to observe the inner workings of the human body. Today, a new generation of imaging devices is probing even deeper and transforming medicine in the process. Indeed, recent advances in imaging technology – such as CT scans, MRIs, SPECT and PET scans, and other techniques – have had a major impact on the diagnosis and treatment of disease.

Infectious endocarditis (IE) represents an emblematic example where the use of nuclear molecular techniques is evolving as an important supplementary method for patients with suspected IE and diagnostic difficulties. The recent development of hybrid molecular imaging equipment for both conventional nuclear medicine (e.g., SPECT/CT) and PET (e.g., PET/CT) has raised evidence of the impact of SPECT and PET performed with suitable infection imaging agents and co-registered with

P.A. Erba, MD, PhD (✉)
Department of Translational Research and New Technology in Medicine,
University of Pisa, Pisa, Italy
e-mail: paola.erba@unipi.it

M. Sollini, MD
Department of Nuclear Medicine, IRCCS MultiMedica, Sesto San Giovanni, Italy
e-mail: martinasollini@msn.com

R. Boni, MD
Department of Nuclear Medicine, Department of Translational Research and New
Technology in Medicine, University of Pisa, Pisa, Italy
e-mail: robertoboni77@gmail.com

E. Lazzeri, MD, PhD
Department of Nuclear Medicine, Azienda Ospedaliero Universitaria Pisana, Pisa, Italy
e-mail: E_lazzeri@hotmail.com

© Springer International Publishing Switzerland 2016
G. Habib (ed.), *Infective Endocarditis*, DOI 10.1007/978-3-319-32432-6_6

CT in the diagnosis of IE. In fact, such technology allows the three-dimensional reconstruction of small regions of interest and precise localization of the site(s) of abnormal radiopharmaceutical accumulation, overcoming the long established paradigm of low diagnostic performance of nuclear medicine procedures that have been rather limited their application in the daily clinical routine.

Metabolic and functional imaging techniques have been evaluated in cases of IE with difficult clinical presentations [1]. Their unique whole-body exploring ability, i.e., to detect multiple sites of disease with a single examination, has been proven effective in guiding clinical management of patients in view of the selection of optimal treatment strategy [2]. This new approach to the IE patient where imaging techniques such as magnetic resonance imaging (MRI), multislice computed tomography (CT), and nuclear imaging are getting more and more important is based on the concept that IE is not a single disease but, rather, may present with very different aspects, depending on the first organ involved, the underlying cardiac disease (if any), the microorganism involved, the presence or absence of complications, and the patient's characteristics. Therefore, a very high level of expertise is needed, coming from practitioners from several specialties, including microbiologists, imagers, clinical expertees and surgeon. Including all these specialists into the patients' management is fundamental.

Despite IE and cardiovascular device (CIED) infection share a number of similar clinical and diagnostic aspects that makes often common their discussion in the same context, the different pathogenesis, clinical appearance and prognosis of CIED infections require specific diagnostic and therapeutic management [3]. Therefore, in this chapter we are not including CIED infections, limiting the discussion to IE.

Multislice Computed Tomography (MSCT) and Magnetic Resonance Imaging (MRI)

Recent advances in MSCT scanners allow high-resolution cardiac imaging. A CT scan of the heart can be performed with acquisition time of a single to a few heart beats, and with high spatial and temporal resolution. A complete examination of thorax takes a few minutes at the exposure of only 2–3 mSV of radiation.

MSCT is primarily deserved in IE patients to provide information about preoperative coronary assessment and silent embolic events. However it may also be used to evaluate abscess, valvular and perivalvular damage [4].

A key use of CT in patients with IE is the non-invasive assessment of the coronary arteries prior to surgery, particularly in patients at low risk of coronary artery disease and in patients with extensive aortic valve IE where coronary angiography is associated with risk of systemic embolism of vegetations and aortic wall perforation. In the same CT study, a cerebral or abdominal CT scan can be obtained in order to detect silent embolism. In fact, MSCT is well suited also for monitoring extra-cardiac manifestations/complications over time. All the patients with symptoms pointing towards a systemic dissemination should be carefully examined.

However, despite asymptomatic neurological lesions can be detected using systematic CT in 5–10 % of patients [5], routine CT-screening is not yet recommended [6].

MSCT angiography allowed the complete visualization of the intracranial vascular tree. The lower contrast burden and risk of permanent neurological damage as compared to conventional digital subtraction angiography, with a sensitivity of 90 % and specificity of 86 % makes MSCT the first choice procedure in this clinical setting [7]. However, in case of subarachnoid and/or intraparenchymal haemorrhage, other vascular imaging, such as angiography, is required to diagnose/exclude a mycotic aneurysm if not detected on MSCT. MRI has a clear advantage in term of sensitivity for the detection of cerebral lesions as compared to MSCT, also in the setting of IE [8]. However, for a critically ill patient, MSCT is more feasible and practical, and is an acceptable alternative when MRI is not available.

For the diagnosis of splenic and other abscesses, contrast-enhanced MSCT has high sensitivity and specificity [9]. However, the differentiation with infarction can be challenging, and the use of multiplanar 3D contrast-enhanced angiographic would allow vascular mapping with identification and characterization of peripheral vascular complications of IE and their follow up [10].

In addition to these well-established clinical indications for MSCT, it can be also used to assess the local extension of the disease. Indeed, the characteristic of valvular vegetations can be easily seen at MSCT as irregular masses protruding from the valve leaflets [11]. In native (NVE) and prosthetic valve infective endocarditis (PVE), MSCT provide comparable results in terms of detection of valvular abnormalities, abscesses and pseudoaneurysms to TEE [12]. MSCT seems to have an advantage compared to TEE in patients with more extensive calcification of the valves, in the assessment of the extent and consequences of any perivalvular extension, including the anatomy of pseudoaneurysms, abscesses and fistulae. In aortic IE, CT may additionally be useful to define the size, anatomy and calcification of the aortic valve, root and ascending aorta, which may be used to inform surgical planning. In pulmonary/right-sided endocarditis, CT may reveal concomitant pulmonary disease, including abscesses and infarct(s) [13]. In PVE where acoustic shadowing can decrease the sensitivity of TEE MSCT may be an equivalent/superior technique to echocardiography for the demonstration of prostheses-related vegetations, abscess, and dehiscence, and may be superior for the detection of pseudoaneurysm [14].

MSCT is limited by the use of iodine contrast, and the method is therefore not applicable in patients with renal failure, in patients with unstable haemodynamics, and with iodine allergy.

In some cases, the indications for a CT scan might be limited to the brain and its arteries. Specific recommendations are needed to clearly define the appropriate situations in which this modality should be used [14].

MRI, a non-ionizing imaging technique, is essentially deserved to diagnose complications of IE, particularly clinical and subclinical cerebral embolic events.

MRI allows an accurate diagnosis showing neurological involvement when it is present [15]. By systematic use of MRI, cerebral lesions have been demonstrated in as many as 82 % of IE patients [16], and subclinical cerebrovascular events have been found in 30–40 % of IE patients [17]. Cerebral MRI is in the majority of cases abnormal in IE patients with neurological symptoms. It has higher sensitivity than MSCT in the diagnosis of the culprit lesion, in particular with regard to stroke, transient ischaemic attack, and encephalopathy. MRI may also detect additional cerebral lesions that are not related to clinical symptoms. Cerebral MRI has no impact on the diagnosis of IE in patients with neurological symptoms since they already have one minor Duke criterion, but MRI impact therapeutic strategy, particularly timing of surgery [18].

Systematic cerebral MRI has an impact on the diagnosis of IE since it adds one minor Duke criterion [19] in patients who have cerebral lesions without neurological symptoms. In one study, findings of cerebral MRI upgraded the diagnosis of IE in 25 % of patients presenting initially with non-definite IE, thereby leading to earlier diagnosis [16]. Also cerebral microbleeds (small areas of haemosiderin deposits considered as an indicator of small vessel disease detected at gradient echo T2* sequences) have been found in 50–60 % of IE patients, but they should not be considered as a minor criterion in Duke classification [19]. Although detection of cerebral complications in IE may influence the clinical decisions, routine MRI screening is not recommended [14]. Vertebral osteomyelitis is another frequent complication in IE where the use of MRI is mandatory [20]. Systematic abdominal MRI detects lesions in 1 out 3 patients evaluated, most often affecting the spleen [21]. Ischaemic lesions are the most frequent, followed by abscesses and haemorrhagic lesions. However, abdominal MRI findings have no incremental impact on the diagnosis of IE when taking into account the findings of cerebral MRI.

The identification of silent cerebral complications appears to be MRI main utility although several reports demonstrate how MRI can identify valvular and perivalvular damage in IE [11]. Infection-related endothelial damage leads to cell death and surface deterioration [22]. Damage and infarction may occur if endocarditis progresses into myocarditis or if vegetation causes coronary artery embolization. This damage and infarction may be seen on cardiac MRI. Myocardial damage can be demonstrated noninvasively by detecting gadolinium contrast enhancement in the late phase [23]. These areas of late-phase contrast enhancement have been shown to be consistent with irreversible myocardial damage and fibrosis [24]. However, delayed contrast enhancement of the endothelial lining in IE has not extensively studied [25, 26]. While most of the known complications of IE are observed far from the source of infection due to distribution by blood flow, some complications have been shown to occur in close proximity to the source. For instance, regurgitant jet flows and intracardiac shunt may lead to development of lesions. Infections in the right ventricle that form due to jet flows in ventricular septal defects (VSDs) with left-to-right shunt can be attributed to the relative blood stasis in these areas. Endocarditis of the tricuspid valve and the right ventricular wall has been reported in such small high-flow VSDs [26]. However, direct endothelial damage can occur in any high-pressure flow area [24, 27]. In the presence of VSD, delayed contrast enhancement may be detected on the lateral wall of the right ventricle due to high-pressure jet causing direct endothelial damage and on the right surface of the proximal interventricular septum adjacent to the VSD secondary to the stasis. Endocardial jet lesions can also be found in patients with aortic regurgitation. Regurgitant jets may lead to infection, aneurysm, and perforation of the anterior mitral leaflet and chordae tendinea [26]. Cardiac MRI can depict the retrograde or antegrade dissemination of the infection regardless of the presence of vegetation or embolization. It was possible to detect the paravalvular extension of the infection by MRI, depicting delayed contrast enhancement on the paravalvular tissues. MRI may also miss the vegetations; however, the determination of delayed contrast enhancement of the endothelial lining can reveal the diagnosis of endocarditis [26]. Differential diagnosis of vegetation includes myxomas, thrombi, lipomas, and papillary fibroelastomas [28]. Myxomas usually demonstrate characteristic mobility on cine gradient-echo images. They show early moderate heterogeneous enhancement and delayed high heterogeneous enhancement after contrast administration. Contrast-enhanced cardiac MRI reveals thrombi as low-signal-intensity, because they are avascular. Lipomas demonstrate signal suppression on fat-saturated sequences. Papillary fibroelastomas appear as hypointense mobile masses on cine gradient-echo images which show high signal intensity after contrast administration [29, 30]. Metallic artifacts due to prosthetic valves may limit the diagnostic value of MRI examination. Cardiac MRI can be a valuable examination method to detect vegetations in patients with suspected IE. Furthermore, MRI can give valuable diagnostic and prognostic information about the disease by depicting features such as the antegrade and retrograde dissemination, paravalvular tissue extension, and subendocardial and vascular endothelial involvement on delayed contrast-enhanced images [26].

As a final note, it should be underline that MRI is limited by availability and is more time consuming compared with MSCT. Owing to magnetic field interference MRI cannot be used in patients with certain cardiac implantable electronic devices (CIEDs) [14].

Nuclear Molecular Imaging

Based on evidence in literature, radiolabeled leukocytes scintigraphy and [18F] FDG-PET/CT have been recently proposed as diagnostic tools in the diagnostic flow chart of IE (see Chap. 7) [5]. In particular, molecular imaging techniques have been proposed to confirm/exclude IE in case of "possible" or "rejected" IE (as for FUO), and to asess the embolic burden in case of "definite" IE [5]. The main added value of using these techniques are the reduction of the rate of misdiagnosed IE, classified in the 'Possible IE' category by using the Duke criteria alone and the detection of peripheral embolic and metastatic infectious events [31]. Evidence is higher in case of and prosthetic valve IE (PVE) [32, 33]; however, data show increased accuracy also in presence of native IE (NVE) and unconclusive clinical findings [34].

Radiolabeled leucocyte scintigraphy is more specific for the detection of infectious foci than [18F]FDG-PET/CT, and should be preferred in all situations that require enhanced specificity [32, 34]. Disadvantages of scintigraphy with radiolabelled WBC are the requirement of blood handling for radiopharmaceutical preparation, duration of the procedure that is more time consuming as compared to PET/CT, and a slightly lower spatial resolution and photon detection efficiency compared with PET/CT. On the other hand, patients who have recently undergone cardiac surgery might present post-operative inflammatory that results in non-specific [18F]FDG uptake in the immediate post-operative period. Furthermore, a number of pathological conditions can mimic the pattern of focally increased [18F]FDG uptake that is typically observed in IE, such as active thrombi, soft atherosclerotic plaques, vasculitis, primary cardiac tumours, cardiac metastasis from a non-cardiac tumour, post-surgical inflammation, and foreign body reactions [32]. Finally, due to the high physiological uptake of this tracer in the brain cortex, and to the fact that at this site, metastatic infections are generally <5 mm, the spatial resolution threshold of current PET/CT scanners localization of septic emboli in the brain might be challenging.

Such limitation and pittfalls of each techniques have to be carefully considered for the choice of the procedure and the final decision should be always be tailored on patients clinical condition, specific clinical questions and local available resources.

Scintigraphy

The identification of inflammatory cells early at the site of IE can prompt timely medical and/or surgical intervention before the development of morphologic damages from the infectious process. The use of gallium-67 or radiolabeled (using 111In- or 99mTc-) leukocytes (WBC) scintigraphy in infection is supported by the pathogenesis of infection itself. In fact, the infectious process determines the recruitment of inflammatory cells in the site of injury.

Gallium-67 scintigraphy has been used (Table 6.1) for the detection of NVE and PVE with a quite low specificity [5] while discordant results have been reported using radiolabeled WBC scintigraphy (Table 6.2). The main disadvantage of the use of gallium-67 or radiolabeled WBC scintigraphy in IE was the relatively low spatial resolution of 2D planar images, which translate in a low sensitivity and poor image quality. The introduction of the hybrid scanners (SPECT/CT) and the improvement of the equipment with high-performances CT component, overcame this drawback allowing a three-dimensional re- construction of small regions of interest and precise localization of the site(s) as demonstrated [35]. However, no data are available for 67Ga-SPECT/CT in IE, with the exception of a single case report [36]. On the contrary, adding the SPECT/CT acquisition(s) to planar images the sensitivity of 99mTc-WBC scintigraphy for IE increased up to 90 % (with 100 % specificity) [32, 34]. Nonetheless, 99mTc-WBC scintigraphy offers the possibility in the same examination to reveal the presence of septic embolism in up to 41 % of cases [34] (with the exception of CNS and spondilodyscitis), impacting on patients' management [33].

Table 6.1 Summary of literature for gallium-67 scintigraphy in IE

Reference	Patient(s)	Site of IE	Microbiology	Scintigraphic finding	Echocardiography
Wiseman et al. [68]	n = 11	Unknown	Unknown	63 % sensitivity	Unknown
Melvin et al. [69]	n = 33	Mixed	Unknown	2/33 pts positive	80 % sensitivity
Martin et al. [70]	80 year, M	Mitral, NVE	Staphylococcus aureus	Pericardium, mitral valve and knee	Negative
Miller et al. [71]	66 year, M	Aortic	Escherichia coli	Right side of the heart	Negative
Hardoff et al. [72]	3 months, M	Mitral, NVE	Staphylococcus aureus	Knee, hip, hearth	Mitral valve vegetation
O'Brien et al. [73]	52 year, M	Aortic, PVE	Staphylococcus aureus	Site of aortic valve	No vegetation; mitral and aortic insufficiency
Desai et al. [74]	62 year, F	Aortic, NVE	Enterococcus spp	Abscess aortic valve, pericarditis	Aortic valve vegetation
Vandenbos et al. [75]	61 year, F	Ventricular patch	Propinibacterium acnes	Left ventricle, patch	Negative (TTE, TEE)
Pena et al. [76]	28 year, M	Aortic, PVE	Staphylococcus spp	Site of aortic valve	Vegetation (TEE)
Salem et al. [77]	44 year, M	Aortic, PVE	Unknown	Periaortic valve abscess	Negative (TTE, TEE)
Thomson et al. [78]	70 year, M	Aortic, PVE	Enterococcus spp	Aortic root, spine	Perivalvular aortic root abscess (TEE)
Yavari et al. [79]	70 year, M	Aortic, PVE	Coagulase negative Staphylococcus	Aortic prosthesis disappearing at FU scan	Negative (TEE)
McWilliams et al. [36]	67 year, F	Aortic, PVE	Unknown	Aortic, prosthesis	No vegetation, suspicious of abscess (TEE)

TTE transthoracic echography, *TEE* transesophageal echography, *NVE* native vave endocarditis, *PVE* prosthetic valve endocarditis

Table 6.2 Radiolabeled WBC Scintigraphy in IE

Reference	Patient(s)	Site of IE	Microbiology	Radiopharmaceutical and acquisition	Scintigraphic finding	Echocardiography
O'Doherty et al. [80]	52 year, F	NVE	Staphylococcus aureus	^{111}In-oxine WBCs + ^{99m}Tc-colloids planar	Spleen abscesses	Unknown
Oates et al. [81]	n = 1	Mitral native	Unknown	^{111}In-oxine WBCs	Valve	Positive
Cerqueira et al. [82]	n = 3	Aortic PVE (2) Mitral NVE (1)	Unknown	^{111}In-oxine WBCs, planar	Valve (2) Valve + spleen embolism (1)	Nondiagnostic
Borst et al. [83]	n = 30	Unknown	Unknown	^{111}In-oxine/^{99m}Tc-HMPAO WBCs	Sensitivity = 67 %, specificity = 95 %	Unknown
Ramackers et al. [84]	72 year, M	EC	Staphylococcus aureus	^{99m}Tc-HMPAO WBCs	Right atrium, PM pocket	Vegetation in right atrium at EC
Adams [85]	56 year, M	Unknown	Staphylococcus aureus	^{99m}Tc-HMPAO WBCs	Myocardial abscess, spleen infarcts	Unknown
Campeau et al. [86]	49 year, M	Aortic, NVE	Staphylococcus aureus	^{111}In-oxine WBCs	Peristernal, hearth region	TTE: aortic sclerosis. TEE: perivalvular abscess
Ellemann et al. [87]	n = 6	Unknown	Unknown	^{99m}Tc-HMPAO WBCs, planar + SPECT	All negative scans	6/6 positive TTE or TEE
McDermott et al. [88]	n = 7	Aortic NVE + PVE, mitral NVE	Staphylococcus spp, Serratia, Streptococcus pneumoniae	^{111}In-oxine WBCs, planar	All negative scans	Vegetations (5–15 mm)

Erba et al. [34]	n = 131	Aortic and mitral PVE	Mixed	99mTc-HMPAO WBCs, planar + SPECT/CT	90% sensitivity, 100% specificity, 100% PPV, 94% NNP, 41% septic embolism	40/51 Positive
Hyafil et al. [33]	n = 42	Aortic and mitral PVE	Mixed	99mTc-HMPAO WBCs planar + SPECT/CT	Valve-perivalvular (14), impact on pts' management in 29%	TEE sensitivity 67% for abscess detection
Rouzet et al. [32]	n = 39	PVE	Mixed	99mTc-HMPAO WBCs (vs. [18F]FDG-PET) planar + SPECT/CT	65% sensitivity, 100% specificity, 100% PPV 81% NPV, 86% accuracy	Vegetation (12) Abscess (2) Partial valve deishence (2) New valve regurgitation (7) Perivalvular thickening (12) Pseudoaneurysm (4)

TTE transthoracic echography, *TEE* transesophageal echography, *NVE* native vave endocarditis, *PVE* prosthetic valve endocardits *EC* electrocatheter

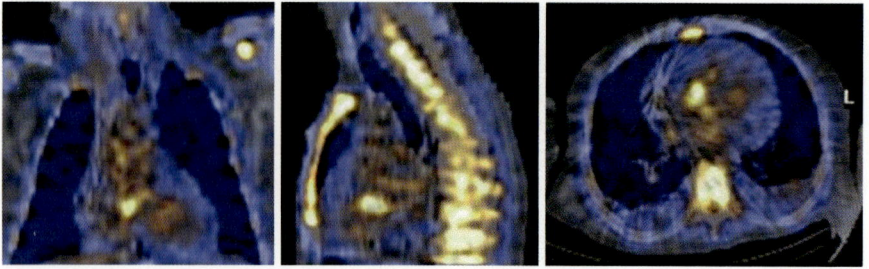

Fig. 6.1 Example of radiolabelled leukocyte scintigraphy in a patient with native valve endocarditis: from *left* to *right*, superimposed coronal, sagittal and transaxial SPECT/CT

^{99m}Tc-WBC scintigraphy consists of sequential acquisition that include whole body scan and spot planar imahes of the thorax and any additional region of interest (ROI) at 30 min (early), 4–6 (late images) and 20–24 h (delayed images, if needed) after the reinfusion of 370–555 MBq of ^{99m}Tc-HMPAO-WBC. SPECT/CT of the chest-upper abdomen is generally obtained at 4–6 h and repeated at 24 h in case of negative or doubtful imaging at 6 h. If necessary, additional SPECT/CT might be acquired at the same time point [34].

The scintigraphic studies arew classified as negative when no sites of abnormal uptake are observed, or positive for infection when at least one focus of abnormal uptake characterized by time-dependent increase in radioactivity from early planar to delayed images was observed [34]. This time-dependent pattern of uptake is especially relevant for the cardiac region, considering that physiologic accumulation of radiolabeled leukocytes in the bone marrow (as in the sternum, overlying the heart) early after reinfusion can interfere with interpretation of the planar images. To this issue, acquisition of images in time-mode, compensating for isotope decay at each time point and their analysis using the same scale frame to identify any focal area of activity that increases over time or shows a change in shape from early to late images are recommended [34].

When present, focal uptake indicating infection is further classified as pertaining to the heart (Fig. 6.1) and/or to extracardiac sites (Fig. 6.2) by SPECT/CT. To this respect using ^{99m}Tc-WBC scintigraphy sites of embolism might appear as areas of increased uptake as in the case of lung (hot spot) wherease for spleen and vertebral embolisms the typical finding at WBC scan is represented by a fotopenic area (cold spot). However, the detection of cold spots is not itself indicative of septic embolism since it might be present in a number of other clinical conditions (i.e., metastasis, angiomas, vertebral crushes); therefore, this needs further confirmation using CT or MR. Analysis of the SPECT/CT images includes visual inspection to exclude misregistration between the SPECT and the CT components and side by side inspection of both attenuation-corrected and noncorrected CT images, to minimize metal-related artifacts. SPECT/CT is mandatory to correctly interpret and localize the site and extent of radiolabeled leukocyte uptake indicating infection

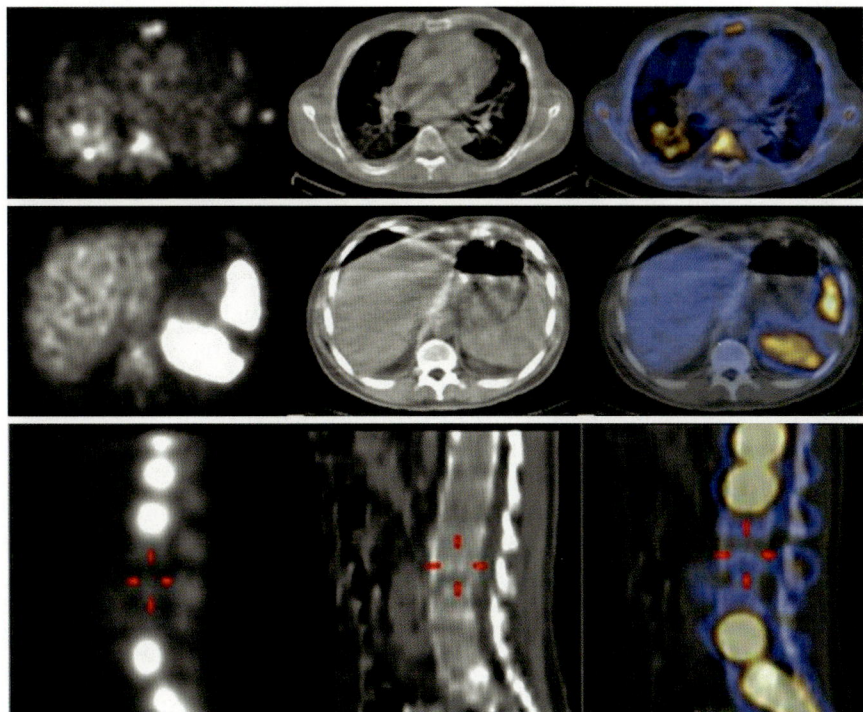

Fig. 6.2 Examples of the use of radiolabelled WBC scan to detect septic embolisms and metastatic sites of infection in patients with endocarditis: Lung (*upper panel*), spleen (*middle panel*), vertebral (*lower panel*) embolisms as were detected as final results based on radiolabelled leukocyte scan findings. Images demonstrate the focal area of increase uptake at basal right lung (left column SPECT images, middle column CT images and right column SPECT/CT images) while for spleen and vertebral embolisms the typical finding at WBC scan is represented by a fotopenic area

and to discriminate involvement of the heart valve or prosthesis from uptake around the prosthesis [34].

The effective dose equivalent for ^{99m}Tc-WBC scintigraphy is 0.011 mSv/MBq [37] that for a standard examination correspond to about 4–6 mSv; the corresponding effective dose equivalent for the CT is about 1.5–2 mSv.

Factors that may limit the sensitivity of radiolabeled WBC scan include the viability of the WBC after in vitro labeling process and the migration rate of the cells to the infection site. The latter becomes a particular concern in presence of microorganisms (i.e., Candida spp, Enterococcus spp, S.epidermis) able to escape the host defence mechanisms [38, 39] or in patients who are on antibiotic treatment, in whom cell chemotaxis may decrease. In addition, technical drawbacks or scintigraphy with WBC are due to the labeling process of cells that is time consuming, labor intensive, and costly and that examination goes on up to 24 h after injection of the radiolabeled WBC or longer [40].

[^{18}F]FDG-PET/CT

PET technology delivers high-resolution images by the use of biologically active compounds labeled with positron emitters. PET associated with computed tomography (CT), named PET/CT leads to many advantages in terms of optimal spatial resolution and accurate anatomical localization of abnormalities. Recent PET/CT scanner together with high spatial resolution can provide whole-body analysis in a single exam session of about 15 min. Images acquisition starts about 45–60 min after the radiopharmaceutical injection that is in case of IE, 2-deoxy-2-(^{18}F) fluoro-D-glucose ([^{18}F]FDG), a radiolabeled glycogen analogue. [^{18}F]FDG accumulated into cell that present with increased intracellular glucose metabolism, such as malignant cells [41]. Membrane transport via glucose transport proteins (GLUTs) and the intracellular phosphorylation by hexokinase have been identified as key steps for subsequent tissue accumulation in cells. Inflammatory cells involved in host response to infectious agents present enhanced glucose metabolism, too [42]. Therefore together with the well established role in the management of patients with malignancies evidence is also increasing regarding the value of PET/CT for assessing inflammatory and infectious conditions [1]. However, kidneys, bladder, brain, and meninges have a high metabolism in normal condition and [^{18}F]FDG-PET/CT results can therefore be difficult to interpret for those tissues or organs.

The use of [^{18}F]FDG-PET/CT in patients with suspected IE has rapidly grown in the last recent years (Table 6.3). In NVE, the use of [^{18}F]FDG-PET/CT is not yet established. On the contrary, in PVE the introduction of the finding of increased [^{18}F]FDG uptake around the prosthetic valve (Figs. 6.3a–d and 6.4a–c) as new major criterion, increased the sensitivity of the modified Duke criteria from 70 to 97 % by reducing the number of patients classified as "possible" [31]. In addition the use of [^{18}F]FDG-PET/CT in patients with fever or pyrexia of unknown origin may reveal embolic infectious foci (Table 6.4), as reported in 24–57 % of cases [2, 43, 44] with high diagnostic performances (87 % sensitivity, 97 % specificity and 52 % PPV) [45], supporting the diagnosis of IE. In case of [^{18}F]FDG-PET/CT the pattern of uptake at site of embolism is characterized by increased uptake of the radiopharmaceutical irrespective of the location (hot spot *versus* cold spot at ^{99m}Tc-WBC scintigraphy) (Figs. 6.3a–d through 6.5a–c).

The low-dose CT routinely used for attenuation correction during [^{18}F]FDG PET/CT is neither electrocardiogram gated nor contrast enhanced, therefore often unable to detect vegetations [46]. For this reason, the addition of electrocardiogram-gated computed tomography angiography (CTA) as been evaluated as tool to detect vegetations, anatomic aortic root abnormalities and coronary artery obstructions [46]. We can also argue that performing at the same time [^{18}F]FDG-PET/CT and contrast-enhanced-CT (ceCT) might result in a one-stop-shop imaging modality allowing the comprehensive evaluation of the whole body (including the CNS and the kidney) at the same time.

Table 6.3 [18F]FDG-PET or [18F]FDG-PET/CT = imaging in IE

Reference	Patient(s)	Site of IE	Microbiology	[18F]FDG PET or PET/CT findings	Echocardiography
NVE					
Yen et al. [89]	**n = 4**	Aortic (1)	Staphylococcus epidermidis	Valve	Perivalvular mass
		Tricuspid (1)	Staphylococcus aureus		Vegetation
		Mitral (2)	Escherichia coli (1) Negative culture (1)		Thrombus
Ho et al. [90]	**40 year, F**	Mitral	Haemophilus parainfluenzae	Base of left ventricle, cardiac fibrous ring near aortic root, Spleen embolism	Negative
Vind et al. [91]	**47 year, F**	Aortic	Haemophilus infuenzae + Staphylococcus spp.	Valve	No vegetation (stenosis); repeat TEE Post PET/CT: pseudoaneurysm
Sankatsing et al. [92]	**64 year, M**	Aortic (bicuspid valve)	Negative culture (final diagnosis: Bartonella henselae)	Sigmoid diverticulosis (FN)	Negative, repeat TTE (1 m) after positive serology: vegetation
Yeh et al. [93]	**87 year, F**	Mitral	Pseudomonas aeruginosa	Valve, Spleen embolism	Negative (calcification) Repeat post PET/CT: vegetation
Masuda et al. [94]	**Unknown**	Mitral	Streptococcus viridans	Valve, bone marrow, spleen	Vegetation + severe mitral regurgitation
Teoh et al. [95]	**61 year, M**	Aortic + CIED	Staphylococcus epidermidis	Valve, Mesenteric artery aneurysms, Spleen embolism	Vegetations

(continued)

Table 6.3 (continued)

Reference	Patient(s)	Site of IE	Microbiology	[18F]FDG PET or PET/CT findings	Echocardiography
Ricciardi et al. [96]	n = 7	Aortic (5), Aortic + mitralic (1), Mitralic (1)	Enterococcus faecalis (1), Staphylococcus haemolyticus(1), Streptococcus oralis (1), Streptococcus parasanguinis (1), Enterocuccus spp (1), Negative culture (3)	Negative	Vegetation (6), Flail posterior leaflet (1)
Wang et al. [97]	55 year, M	Aortic	Coxiella burnetii	Valve, lymph nodes	Vegetation + paravalvular abscess
PVE					
Belohlavek et al. [98]	Unknown	Aortic biological	Staphylococcus aureus	Valve, Left knee	Unknown
Love et al. [99]	Unknown	Mitral (unknown)	Positive culture (organism unknown)	Intracardiac uptake	Valvular vegetations and mitral annular abscess
Klingensmith et al. [100]	77 year, M	Unknown	Enterococcus spp.	Valve, Lung embolism	Unknown
Moghadam-Kia et al. [101]	82 year, M	Aortic mechanical	Streptococcus viridans	Right lateral atrial wall and left atrial appendage/pulmonary outflow tract, Lumbar embolism	No vegetation, mild aortic regurgitation, aortic leaflet thickening
Huyge et al. [102]	71 year, M	Aortic biological	Oxacillin resistant Staphylococcus epidermidis	Valve, Mediastinal lns	Negative
Kenzaka et al. [103]	35 year, M	Pulmonary mechanical	Streptococcus viridans	Artificial blood vessel site of right ventricular outflow tract	Negative
Plank et al. [104]	63 year, M	Mitral biological	Negative culture	Valve	Inconclusive

Yedidya et al. [105]	24 year, M	Pulmonary biological	Haemophilus parainfluenzae	Pulmonic stent	Negative
Wallner et al. [106]	75 year, M	Aortic biological	Candida parapsilosis	Valve	Negative
Feuchtner et al. [107]	74 year, M	Aortic mechanical	Negative culture	Valve	Paravalvular leak
Klaipetch et al. [108]	64 year, M	Aortic mechanical	Unknown	Valve, decreased after antibiotic therapy	Negative
Pons et al. [109]	30 year, F	Aortic mechanical	Streptococcus sanguinis	Valve	No vegetations, thickened area at noncoronary sinus of Valsalva
Gouriet et al. [110]	84 year, F	Mitral biological+PM	Morganella morganii+Enterococcus fecalis	Valve+lead	Mitral regurgitation+prolapsing cusp
Caldarella et al. [111]	70 year, M	Aortic mechanical	Streptococcus	Positive (late imaging)	Perivalvular thickening and abscess (TEE)
Saby et al. [31]	n=72	Bioprosthetic (44) Mechanical (28)	Staphylococcus aureus (16) Enterococcus faecalis (7) Streptococcus bovis (4) Other bacteria (5)	73% sensitivity 80% specificity 85% PPV 67% NPP 76% overall accuracy	Vegetation (27) Periannular complications (8) New partial dehiscence (13) LVEF<45% (7)
Tanis et al. [46]	n=4	Bileaflet aortic mechanical PVE (4) Biological aortic PVE (1)	Staphylococcus aureus (3) Streptococcus pneumoniae (1) Negative (1)	Aortic valve (2) Perivalvular abscess (1) Perivalvular abscess+toe osteomyelitis (1) Perivalvular abscess+spleen abscess (1)	Unremarkable (TTE/TEE) (1) Aortic root abnormalities (TTE) (1) Vegetation (TEE) (1) Vegetation+perivalvular abscess (TEE) (1) Perivalvular abscess (TEE) (1)

(continued)

Table 6.3 (continued)

Reference	Patient(s)	Site of IE	Microbiology	[¹⁸F]FDG PET or PET/CT findings	Echocardiography
Ricciardi et al. [96]	n = 13	Aortic (10) Aortic + mitralic (1) Mitralic (2)	Candida parapsilosis (2) Enterococcus faecalis (4) Streptococcus mutans (1) Streptococcus mitis (1) Staphylococcus epidermidis (1) Staphylococcus hominis (1) hVISA (1) MSSA (1) Negative colture (1)	Valve (18) Perivalvular abscess (1) Negative (4)	Vegetation (3) Fistula (1) Abscess (1) Negative (8)
Bartoletti et al. [112]	n = 3	Mechanic aortic (1) Biological aortic (2)	MRSE (1) Candida albicans (1) Staphylococcus lugdnensis (1)	Valve (3)	Negative (in 2 case positivity 2–3 we after PET/CT)
Chirillo et al. [113]	76 year, M	Aortic	Streptococcus anginosus	Valve + spleen + tonsil	Inconclusive
Gouriet et al. [114]	56 year, M	Biological aortic	Bartonella henselae	Valve	Tickened and partial aortic stenosis
Rouzet et al. [32]	n = 39	PVE	Mixed	93 % sentitivity 71 % specificity 68 % PPV 94 % NPV 80 % accuracy	Vegetation (12) Abscess (2) Partial valve deishence (2) New valve regurgitation (7) Perivalvular thickening (12) Pseudoaneurysm (4)

Prosthesis of aortic valve, aortic root and ascending aorta (Bentall's procedure)

Yen et al. [89]	n = 2	Aortic	Staphylococcus spp. Salmonella spp.	Aortic valve + aortic root	Inconclusive
Vind et al. [91]	47 year, F	Aortic	Staphylococcus aureus	Valve + base of ascending aorta/aortic wall/graft + aorta (atherosclerotic changes, FP)	Negative
El Hajjaji et al. [115]	56 year, M	Aortic	Cardiobacterium hominis	Aortic graft	No vegetations, non-specific thickening of aortic root
Tanis et al. [46]	n = 2	Aortic	Staphylococcus aureus (1) Actinobacillus (1)	Valve (1) Valve, Bentall (1)	Inconclusive (2)
Ricciardi et al. [96]	n = 7	Aortic	Enterococcus faecalis (1) Pseudomonas aeruginosa (2) Staphylococcus haemolyticus (1) Streptococcus bovis (1) MSSA (1) Negative colture (1)	Valve (5) Valve, Bentall (2)	Vegetation (2) Leak prosthetic valve + aortic aneurysm (1) Pseudo-aneurysm (1) Negative (3)
Bartoletti et al. [112]	n = 3	Aortic	Pseudomonas aeruginosa (2) Streptococcus bovis (1)	Valve + ascending aorta (1) Prosthetic wall + peri-valvular tissue (1) Valve + spleen (1)	Negative (in 1 case positivity after PET/CT)

TTE transthoracic echography, *TEE* transesophageal echography, *NVE* native vave endocarditis, *PVE* prosthetic valve endocarditis, *NPV* negative predictive value, *PPV* positive predictive value, *LVEF* left ventricle ejection fraction, *FP* false positive, *hVISA* Heteroresistan vancomycin intermediate Staphylococcus aureus, *MSSA* Methicillin-sensitive Staphylococcus aureus, *PM* pacemaker

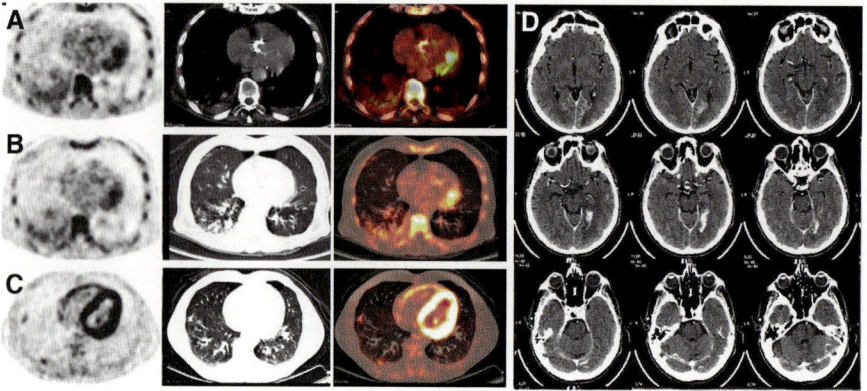

Fig. 6.3 (**a–d**) Examples of pattern of [^{18}F]FDG uptake at PET/CT in patients with IE and concomitant lung and brain embolism. (**a**) Mechanical aortic prosthesis with linear focal uptake in the anteromedial portion. (**b**, **c**) examples of septic embolisms detection at right lung using [^{18}F]FDG-PET/CT appearing as area of focal increase of the radiofarmaceutical corresponding to micronodular lesions at the CT component. (For **a–c** *left column* emission images, *middle column* CT images and *right column* fused PET/CT images.) (**d**) ceCT of the brain showing recent ischemic lesion at the left parahippocampal girus, occipito-basal and occipito-mesial cortex

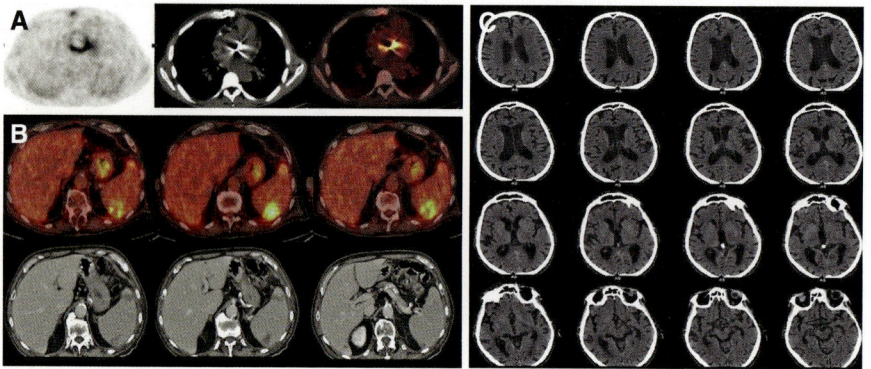

Fig. 6.4 (**a–c**) Examples of pattern of [^{18}F]FDG uptake at PET/ceCT in patients with IE and concomitant spleen embolism. (**a**) Mechanical aortic prosthesis with linear focal uptake in the posterior and lateral portion (*left column* emission images, *middle column* CT images and *right column* fused PET/CT images). (**b**) Example of septic embolisms detection at the spleen [^{18}F]FDG PET/ceCT appearing as area of focal increase of the radiofarmaceutical corresponding to hypodens lesions at the CT component (*upper column* fused transaxial PET/CT images, lower column transaxial ceCT). (**c**) ceCT of the brain showing a normal pattern

An additional promising role of [^{18}F]FDG-PET/CT may be seen in patients with established IE, in whom it could be used to monitor response to antimicrobial treatment [47].

Also in the case of [^{18}F]FDG for the diagnosis of IE pitfalls should be considered when interpreting the scan to avoid potential sources of false-positive findings in

PET studies. First, variable focal of diffuse physiological [^{18}F]FDG uptake is often observed in the normal myocardium of fasting non-diabetic patients (6–12 h to overnight) with normal glucose levels [48]. Accumulation of [^{18}F]FDG is most notable in the left ventricular myocardium, which has a greater muscle mass than other cardiac chambers. Uptake in the wall of the right ventricle is typically equal to or less intense than that in the left ventricular myocardium; uptake in the wall of the right and left atria is usually not detected. Factors possibly influencing myocardial uptake of [^{18}F]FDG include patients' age, fasting time, blood glucose levels, and a low-carbohydrate diet. In particular, age and fasting time do not affect physiological [^{18}F]FDG uptake in the myocardium, whereas blood glucose levels may have a non-linear effect on myocardial uptake [49]. Within physiologic Free Fatty Acid (FFA) and insulin levels, FFA concentrations exert a major influence on myocardial glucose uptake through an effect on the hexokinase reaction [50]. When serum insulin concentrations exceed 100 pmol/L and FFA concentrations are suppressed, a further increase of myocardial glucose uptake is achieved by a direct effect of insulin at membrane level. At supraphysiologic insulin concentrations, phosphorylation is increasingly rate limiting because insulin has little direct effect on hexokinase activity or compartmentalized fractions of hexokinase [51].

Low-carbohydrate diet [52] and very high-fat, low-carbohydrate, protein-permitted meal followed by fasting for 3–6 h [53] before [^{18}F]FDG injection might be adopted to decrease myocardial uptake. However, no specific protocol has yet been standardized or recommended or both to reduce the nonspecific myocardial uptake when assessing cardiac infection with [^{18}F]FDG-PET/CT. Alternatively, unfractionated heparin (50 IU/kg iv) could be administered before [^{18}F]FDG injection [54]. Heparin acts activating lipoprotein lipase and hepatic lipase, enhances plasma lipolytic activity and elevates plasma levels of FFA [55].

Another potential confounding factor for [^{18}F]FDG-PET/CT is represented by increased metabolic activity along the posterior aspect of the heart, where lipomatous hypertrophy of the interatrial septum may appear as a fat-containing mass with increased [^{18}F]FDG uptake [56]. A number of pathologic conditions can mimic the pattern of focally increased [^{18}F]FDG uptake that is typically observed in IE: active thrombi [48], soft atherosclerotic plaques [57], vasculitis [58], primary cardiac tumors [59], cardiac metastasis from a noncardiac tumor [60], postsurgical inflammation [61], and foreign body reactions (such as BioGlue, a surgical adhesive used to repair the aortic root) [62]. All these clinical conditions should be considered in the differential diagnosis and excluded before diagnosis IE. Results from studied in literature are not jet able to indicate a time-line after surgery when the risk of false positive results at [^{18}F]FDG PET/CT is minimized; therefore, at least 3 months from surgical procedure are suggested [32]. Indeed, high specificity for IE using [^{18}F] FDG can be achieved only by adopting accurate patients selection and inclusion criteria. On the contrary, the use of [^{18}F]FDG-PET/CT in patients with lower pretest probability would rely on the high negative predictive value of this imaging procedure.

The effective dose equivalent for [^{18}F]FDG-PET is 0.02 mSv/MBq that correspond to about 3–4 mSv for an administered activity of 185 MBq [63]. In this case

Table 6.4 [^{18}F]FDG-PET/CT imaging in the detection of septic embolism in IE

Reference	Patient(s)	Site of IE	Microbiology	[^{18}F]FDG-PET/CT findings	Echocardiography (TTE/TEE)
Van Riet et al. [116]	**n = 25**	NVE unknown (15) PVE unknown (10)	Staphylococcus aureus (4) Streptococcus spp. (10) Enterococcus faecalis (9) Escherichia coli (1) Negative culture (1)	12 % IE 44 % septic embolism of metastatic infection	25 positive, unspecified
Gheysens et al. [117]	**59 year, F**	NVE	MRSA	Left ventricle + lung embolism + septic arthritis + muscle abscess	Vegetation, perforation of the posterior leaflet and severe mitral regurgitation
Özcan et al. [45]	**n = 72**	NVE (52), PVE (12) CIED (2) Other (6)	Staphylococcus aureus (24) Coagulase-negative staphylococcus (5) Viridans group streptococci (9) Enterococcus species (12) Other streptococci (13) HACEK (1) Other bacteria (4)	IE: 18 % sensitivity and 100 % PPV Septic embolism: 87 % sensitivity, 97 % specificity and 52 % PPV	Unknown
Bonfiglioli et al. [43]	**n = 71**	NVE (38) PVE (33)	Mixed	24 % unexpected semptic embolism	Unknown
Kouijzer et al. [118]	**n = 18**	NVE (18) PVE (2)	Staphylococcus aureus (10) Streptococcus spp. (8)	39 % sensitivity, 93 % specificity 64 % PPV, 82 % NPV	Positive for IE at TTE or TEE (6) Positive for IE at TTE + TEE (12)
Asmar et al. [119]	**n = 72**	Mixed	Mixed	1/7 pts important findings	TTE + TEE 67 % sensitivity

Study	n	Population	Microorganisms	Outcomes	Imaging findings
Kestler et al. [2]	n=47	NVE (23) PVE/CIED (24) Control (94)	Enterococcus faecalis (11) Staphylococcus spp. (9) Streptococcus spp. (12) Abiotrophia defective (1) Pseudomonas aeruginosa (2) Haemophilus aphrophillus (1) Coagulase-negative Staphylococcus (1) Aggregatibacter actinomycetemcomitans (1) Bacteroides thetaiotaomicron (1) Clostidium perfringens (1) Lactobacillus paracasei (1) Propionibacterium acnes (1) Fungi (2) Polymicrobial (1) Blood-culture negative (2)	57% septic embolism Two-fold reduction number of relapses Significantly more infectious complications diagnosed	Unspecified
Orvin et al. [44]	n=40	NVE (32), PVE (8); concomitant endovascular devices (14)	Streptococcus viridans (4) Staphylococcus aureus (8) Streptococcus spp. (6) Enterococcus faecalis (5) HACEK (2) Coxiella burnetii (2) Listeria spp. (1) Bartonella spp. (1) Coagulase-negative Staphylococcus (4) Propionibacterium acnes (1) Diphtheroids spp. (1) Blood-culture negative (6)	42.5% septic embolism, treatment planning modified in 35%	Vegetation on native (15) and prosthetic (8) valve, on EC (3); perivalvular abscess (2), new valvular insufficiency (8) No findings (4) Vegetation size (mm) 9.8±6.7

TTE transthoracic echography, *TEE* transesophageal echography, *NVE* native valve endocarditis, *PVE* prosthetic valve endocarditis, *PPV* positive predictive value, *LVEF* left ventricle ejection fraction, *CIED* cardiac-implatable electronic device, *HACEK* Haemophilus species (Haemophilus parainfluenzae, Haemophilus aphrophilus, Haemophilus paraphrophilus), Actinobacillus actinomycetemcomitans, Cardiobacterium hominis, Eikenella corrodens, and Kingella species, *EC* electrocatheter, *MRSA* Methicillin-resistant Staphylococcus aureus, *NPV* negative predictive value

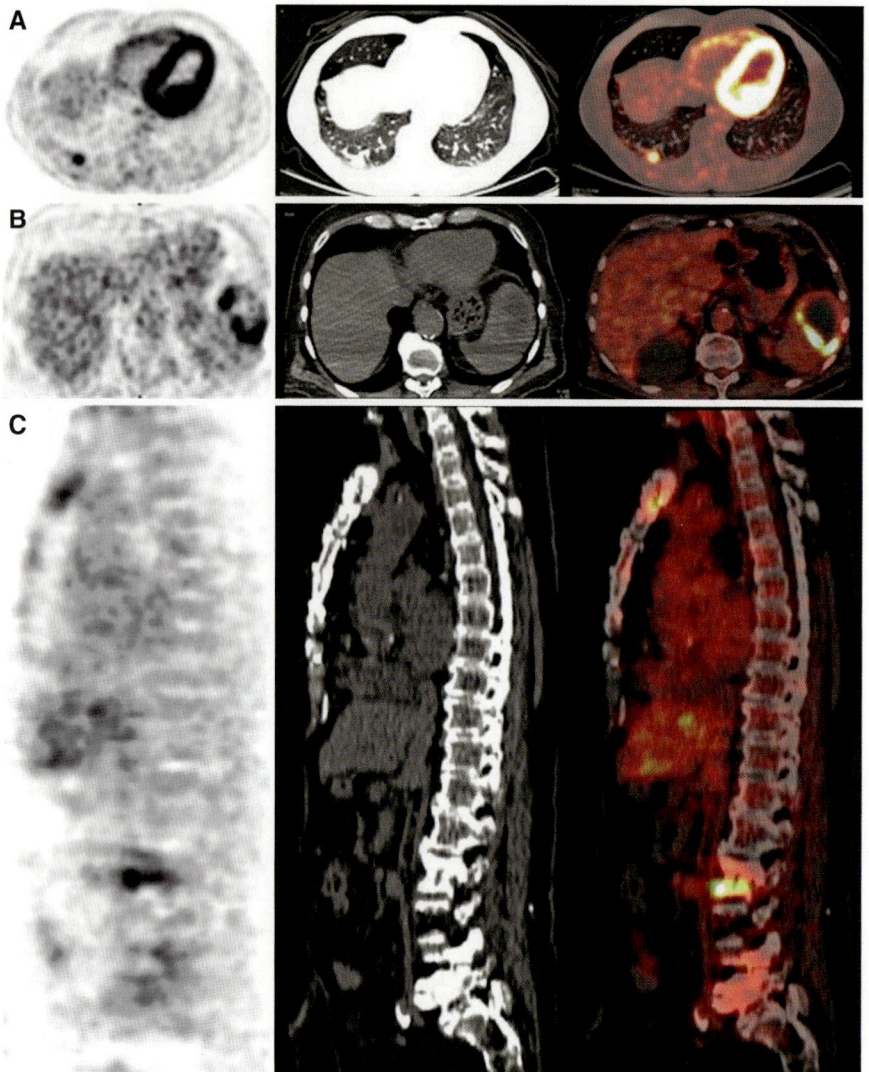

Fig. 6.5 (**a–c**) Examples of septic embolisms detection using [¹⁸F]FDG PET/CT. [¹⁸F]FDG PET/CT uptake in a micro-nodular lesion at the right lung (**a**), in a splenic abscess appearing as rim of increase radiopharmaceutical accumulation around a cold area (**b**), and at spine where uptake involve the inferior portion of the vertebral body of L3 and the superior portion of the vertebral body of L4 identifying spondylodiscitis (**c**). *Left column* emission transaxial images, *middle column* CT transaxial images, *right column* transaxial superimposed PET/CT images

is more difficult to estimate the corresponding effective dose equivalent for the CT component since it could range from 1 to 20 mSv and may be even higher for a high resolution diagnostic CT scan. Given the variety of CT systems and protocols the radiation exposure for a PET/CT examination should be estimated specific to the system and protocol being used.

Future Directions

Multimodality imaging may be further improved by the combination of PET or SPECT imaging with MRI. Such combination might take advantages of the superb ability of MRI to differentiate soft-tissue bound-aries [64] and of the addition of a molecular MRI agent to trace two biological targets simultaneously [65]. Particularly, the combination of PET radiopharmaceuticals (not only [^{18}F]FDG) to MRI imaging could significantly improve the sensitivity and specificity of the diagnosis and follow-up treatment of infectious and inflammatory diseases. Preliminary results in cardiac PET/MRI imaging, despite limited to few centers and only to specific clinical applications (i.e. perfusion, viability, atherosclerosis, myocarditis, sarcoidosis and amyloidosis), support the advantages of PET/MRI as compared to other hybrid techniques [66] not only in terms of more accurate assessment and better anatomical localization of lesions in soft tissues. In fact, MRI offers the opportunity to gather functional MRI (fMRI), which includes diffusion-weighted imaging (DWI), magnetic resonance spectroscopy (MRS) and perfusion imaging. Recent improvements in MRI contrast agents, in particular new trends in designing dual probe "RARE, RAdioREsonance molecular probes," which can be used simultaneously for PET/MRI imaging may lead to even more insights into the dynamics and characteristics of the inflammatory process. A third interesting feature of PET/MRI is motion correction based on MRI, which would allow more accurate quantification of PET data, leading to better treatment monitoring and the possibility of earlier response evaluation.

In the field of IE combining the strengths of PET and MRI modalities combined in a simultaneous PET/MRI study could be of significant relevance in the evaluation of local extension of infection at heart site as well as for the detection of IE complications such as CNS septic embolism and spondylodiscitis [67].

References

1. Revest M, Patrat-Delon S, Devillers A, Tattevin P, Michelet C. Contribution of 18fluoro-deoxyglucose PET/CT for the diagnosis of infectious diseases. Med Mal Infect. 2014; 44:251–60.
2. Kestler M, Muñoz P, Rodríguez-Créixems M, Rotger A, Jimenez-Requena F, Mari A, et al. Role of 18 F-FDG PET in patients with infectious endocarditis. J Nucl Med. 2014;55:1093–8.
3. Millar BC, Prendergast BD, Alavi A, Moore JE. 18FDG-positron emission tomography (PET) has a role to play in the diagnosis and therapy of infective endocarditis and cardiac device infection. Int J Cardiol. 2013;167:1724–36.
4. Feuchtner GM, Stolzmann P, Dichtl W, Schertler T, Bonatti J, Scheffel H, et al. Multislice computed tomography in infective endocarditis. J Am Coll Cardiol. 2009;53:436–44.
5. Iung B, Erba PA, Petrosillo N, Lazzeri E. Common diagnostic flowcharts in infective endocarditis. Q J Nucl Med Mol Imaging. 2014;58:55–65.
6. Colen TW, Gunn M, Cook E, Dubinsky T. Radiologic manifestations of extra-cardiac complications of infective endocarditis. Eur Radiol. 2008;18:2433–45.
7. Goddard AJ, Tan G, Becker J. Computed tomography angiography for the detection and characterization of intra-cranial aneurysms: current status. Clin Radiol. 2005;60:1221–36.

8. Cruz-Flores S. Neurologic complications of valvular heart disease. Handb Clin Neurol. 2014;119:61–73.
9. Grob A, Thuny F, Villacampa C, Flavian A, Gaubert JY, Raoult D, et al. Cardiac multidetector computed tomography in infective endocarditis: a pictorial essay. Insights Imaging. 2014;5:559–70.
10. Huang JS, Ho AS, Ahmed A, Bhalla S, Menias CO. Borne identity: CT imaging of vascular infections. Emerg Radiol. 2011;18:335–43.
11. Rajiah P, Nazarian J, Vogelius E, Gilkeson RC. CT and MRI of pulmonary valvular abnormalities. Clin Radiol. 2014;69:630–8.
12. Fagman E, Perrotta S, Bech-Hanssen O, Flinck A, Lamm C, Olaison L, et al. ECG-gated computed tomography: a new role for patients with suspected aortic prosthetic valve endocarditis. Eur Radiol. 2012;22:2407–14.
13. Ortiz J. Isolated pulmonic valve infective endocarditis: a persistent challenge. Infection. 2004;32:170–5.
14. Bruun NE, Habib G, Thuny F, Sogaard P. Cardiac imaging in infectious endocarditis. Eur Heart J. 2014;35:624–32.
15. Belzunegui J. Infectious spondylodiskitis. Reumatol Clin. 2008;4:13–7.
16. Duval X, Iung B, Klein I, Brochet E, Thabut G, Arnoult F, et al. Effect of early cerebral magnetic resonance imaging on clinical deci- sions in infective endocarditis: a prospective study. Ann Intern Med. 2010;152:497–504.
17. Snygg-Martin U, Gustafsson L, Rosengren L, Alsiö A, Ackerholm P, Andersson R, et al. Cerebrovascular complications in patients with left-sided infective endo- carditis are common: a prospective study using magnetic resonance imaging and neurochemical brain damage markers. Clin Infect Dis. 2008;47:23–30.
18. Goulenok T, Klein I, Mazighi M, Messika-Zeitoun D, Alexandra JF, Mourvillier B, et al. Infective endocarditis with symptomatic cerebral complications: contribution of cerebral magnetic resonance imaging. Cerebrovasc Dis. 2013;35:327–36.
19. Li JS, Sexton DJ, Mick N, Nettles R, Fowler Jr VG, Ryan T, et al. Proposed modifications to the Duke criteria for the diagnosis of infective endocarditis. Clin Infect Dis. 2000;30:633–8.
20. Jutte P, Lazzeri E, Sconfienza LM, Cassar-Pullicino V, Trampuz A, Petrosillo N, et al. Diagnostic flowcharts in osteomyelitis, spondylodiscitis and prosthetic joint infection. Q J Nucl Med Mol Imaging. 2014;58:2–19.
21. Iung B, Klein I, Mourvillier B, Olivot JM, Detaint D, Longuet P, et al. Respective effects of early cerebral and abdominal magnetic resonance imaging on clinical decisions in infective endocarditis. Eur Heart J Cardiovasc Imaging. 2012;13:703–10.
22. Bashore TM, Cabell C, Fowler Jr V. Update on infective endocarditis. Curr Probl Cardiol. 2006;31:274–352.
23. Rehwald WG, Fieno DS, Chen EL, Kim RJ, Judd RM. Myocardial magnetic resonance imaging contrast agent concentrations after reversible and irreversible ischemic injury. Circulation. 2002;105:224–9.
24. Kim RJ, Wu E, Rafael A, Chen EL, Parker MA, Simonetti O, et al. The use of contrast-enhanced magnetic resonance imaging to identify reversible myocardial dysfunction. N Engl J Med. 2000;343:1445–53.
25. Dursun M, Yilmaz S, Ali Sayin O, Olgar S, Dursun F, Yekeler E, et al. A rare cause of delayed contrast enhance- ment on cardiac magnetic resonance imag- ing: infective endocarditis. J Comput Assist Tomogr. 2005;29:709–11.
26. Dursun M, Yılmaz S, Yılmaz E, Yılmaz R, Onur İ, Oflaz H, et al. The utility of cardiac MRI in diagnosis of infective endocarditis: preliminary results. Diagn Interv Radiol. 2015;21: 28–33.
27. Gregory SA, Yepes CB, Byrne JG, D'Ambra MN, Chen MH. Atrial endocarditis – the importance of the regurgitant jet lesions. Echocardiography. 2005;22:426–30.
28. Eslami-Varzaneh F, Brun EA, Sears-Rogan P. An unusual case of multiple papillary fibroelastoma, review of literature. Cardiovasc Pathol. 2003;12:170–3.

29. O'Donnell DH, Abbara S, Chaithiraphan V, Yared K, Killeen RP, Cury RC, et al. Cardiac tumors: optimal cardiac MR sequences and spectrum of imaging appearances. AJR Am J Roentgenol. 2009;193:377–87.
30. Sparrow PJ, Kurian JB, Jones TR. Siva- nanthan MU. MR imaging of cardiac tumors. Radiographics. 2005;25:1255–76.
31. Saby L, Laas O, Habib G, Cammilleri S, Mancini J, Tessonnier L, et al. Positron emission tomography/computed tomography for diagnosis of prosthetic valve endocarditis: increased valvular 18 F-fluorodeoxyglucose uptake as a novel major criterion. J Am Coll Cardiol. 2013;61:2374–82.
32. Rouzet F, Chequer R, Benali K, Lepage L, Ghodbane W, Duval X, et al. Respective performance of 18 F-FDG PET and radiolabeled leukocyte scintigraphy for the diagnosis of prosthetic valve endocarditis. J Nucl Med. 2014;55:1980–5.
33. Hyafil F, Rouzet F, Lepage L, Benali K, Raffoul R, Duval X, et al. Role of radiolabelled leucocyte scintigraphy in patients with a suspicion of prosthetic valve endocarditis and inconclusive echocardiography. Eur Heart J Cardiovasc Imaging. 2013;14:586–94.
34. Erba PA, Conti U, Lazzeri E, Sollini M, Doria R, De Tommasi SM, et al. Added value of 99mTc-HMPAO-labeled leukocyte SPECT/CT in the characterization and management of patients with infectious endocarditis. J Nucl Med. 2012;53:1235–43.
35. Bar-Shalom R, Yefremov N, Guralnik L, Keidar Z, Engel A, Nitecki S, et al. SPECT/CT using 67Ga and 111In-labeled leukocyte scintigraphy for diagnosis of infection. J Nucl Med. 2006;47:587–94.
36. McWilliams ET, Yavari A, Raman V. Aortic root abscess: multimodality imaging with computed tomography and gallium-67 citrate single-photon emission computed tomography/computed tomography hybrid imaging. J Cardiovasc Comput Tomogr. 2011;5:122–4.
37. International Commission on Radiological Protection; J Valentin, editor. Annals of the ICRP, publication 80, Radiation dose to patients from radiopharmaceuticals. Oxford: Elsevier Science; 1999. p. 67.
38. Cheung GY, Rigby K, Wang R, Queck SY, Braughton KR, Whitney AR, et al. Staphylococcus epidermidis strategies to avoid killing by human neutrophils. PLoS Pathog. 2010;6:e1001133.
39. Thurlow LR, Thomas VC, Narayanan S, Olson S, Fleming SD, Hancock LE. Gelatinase contributes to the pathogenesis of endocarditis caused by Enterococcus faecalis. Infect Immun. 2010;11:4936–43.
40. Chen W, Kim J, Molchanova-Cook OP, Dilsizian V. The potential of FDG PET/CT for early diagnosis of cardiac device and prosthetic valve infection before morphologic damages ensue. Curr Cardiol Rep. 2014;16:459.
41. Avril N, Menzel M, Dose J, Schelling M, Weber W, Janicke F, et al. Glucose metabolism of breast cancer assessed by 18 F-FDG PET: histologic and immunohistochemical tissue analysis. J Nucl Med. 2001;42:9–16.
42. Kumar R, Basu S, Torigian D, Anand V, Zhuang H, Alavi A. Role of modern imaging techniques for diagnosis of infection in the era of 18 F- fluorodeoxyglucose positron emission tomography. Clin Microbiol Rev. 2008;21:209–24.
43. Bonfiglioli R, Nanni C, Morigi JJ, Graziosi M, Trapani F, Bartoletti M, et al. ^{18}F-FDG PET/CT diagnosis of unexpected extracardiac septic embolisms in patients with suspected cardiac endocarditis. Eur J Nucl Med Mol Imaging. 2013;40:1190–6.
44. Orvin K, Goldberg E, Bernstine H, Groshar D, Sagie A, Kornowski R, et al. The role of FDG-PET/CT imaging in early detection of extra-cardiac complications of infective endocarditis. Clin Microbiol Infect. 2015;21:69–76.
45. Özcan C, Asmar A, Gill S, Thomassen A, Diederichsen AC. The value of FDG-PET/CT in the diagnostic work-up of extra cardiac infectious manifestations in infectious endocarditis. Int J Cardiovasc Imaging. 2013;29:1629–37.
46. Tanis W, Scholtens A, Habets J, van den Brink RB, van Herwerden LA, Chamuleau SA, et al. CT angiography and ^{18}F-FDG-PET fusion imaging for prosthetic heart valve endocarditis. JACC Cardiovasc Imaging. 2013;6:1008–13.

47. Vaidyanathan S, Patel CN, Scarsbrook AF, Chowdhury FU. FDG PET/CT in infection and inflammation-current and emerging clinical applications. Clin Radiol. 2015;70:787–800. pii: S0009-9260(15)00106-3.
48. Shreve PD, Anzai Y, Wahl RL. Pitfalls in oncologic diagnosis with FDG PET imaging: physiologic and benign variants. Radiographics. 1999;19:61–77.
49. de Groot M, Meeuwis AP, Kok PJ, Corstens FH, Oyen WJ. Influence of blood glucose level, age and fasting period on non-pathological FDG uptake in heart and gut. Eur J Nucl Med Mol Imaging. 2005;32:98–101.
50. Knuuti MJ, Mäki M, Yki-Järvinen H, Voipio-Pulkki LM, Härkönen R, Haaparanta M, et al. The effect of insulin and FFA on myocardial glucose uptake. J Mol Cell Cardiol. 1995; 27:1359–67.
51. Russell RR, Mrns JM, Mommessin JI, Taegtmeyer H. Compartmentation of hexokinase in rat heart: a critical factor for tracer kinetic analysis of myocardial glucose metabolism. J Clin Invest. 1992;90:1972–7.
52. Lum D, Wandell S, Ko J, Coel M. Positron emission tomography of thoracic malignancies: reduction of myocardial fluorodeoxyglucose uptake artifacts with a carbohydrate restricted diet. Clin Positron Imaging. 2000;3:155.
53. Williams G, Kolodny GM. Suppression of myocardial 18 F-FDG uptake by preparing patients with a high-fat, low-carbohydrate diet. AJR Am J Roentgenol. 2008;190:W151–6.
54. Minamimoto R, Morooka M, Kubota K, Ito K, Masuda-Miyata Y, Mitsumoto T, et al. Value of FDG-PET/CT using unfractionated heparin for managing primary cardiac lymphoma and several key findings. J Nucl Cardiol. 2011;18:516–20.
55. Persson E. Lipoprotein lipase, hepatic lipase and plasma lipolytic activity effects of heparin and low molecular weight heparin fragment (Fragmin). Acta Med Scand Suppl. 1988; 724:1–56.
56. Fan CM, Fischman AJ, Kwek BH, Abbara S, Aquino SL. Lipomatous hypertrophy of the interatrial septum: Increased uptake on FDG PET. AJR Am J Roentgenol. 2005;184: 339–42.
57. Williams G, Kolodny GM. Retrospective study of coronary uptake of 18 F-fluorodeoxyglucose in association with calcification and coro- nary artery disease: a preliminary study. Nucl Med Commun. 2009;30:287–91.
58. Kobayashi Y, Ishii K, Oda K, Nariai T, Tanaka Y, Ishiwata K, et al. Aortic wall inflammation due to Takayasu arteritis imaged with 18 F-FDG PET coregistered with enhanced CT. J Nucl Med. 2005;46:917–22.
59. Kaderli AA, Baran I, Aydin O, Bicer M, Akpinar T, Ozkalemkas F, et al. Diffuse involvement of the heart and great vessels in primary cardiac lymphoma. Eur J Echocardiogr. 2010; 11:74–6.
60. García JR, Simo M, Huguet M, Ysamat M, Lomeña F. Usefulnessof 18-fluorodeoxyglucose positron emission tomography in the evaluation of tumor cardiac thrombus from renal cell carcinoma. Clin Transl Oncol. 2006;8:124–8.
61. Abidov A, D'agnolo A, Hayes SW, Berman DS, Waxman AD. Uptake of FDG in the area of a recently implanted bioprosthetic mitral valve. Clin Nucl Med. 2004;29:848.
62. Schouten LR, Verberne HJ, Bouma BJ, van Eck-Smit BL, Mulder BJ. Surgical glue for repair of the aortic root as a possible explanation for increased F-18 FDG uptake. J Nucl Cardiol. 2008;15:146–7.
63. ICRP. Radiation dose to patients from radiopharmaceuticals. Addendum 3 to ICRP publication 53. ICRP publication 106. Approved by the commission in october 2007. Ann ICRP. 2008;38:1–197.
64. Judenhofer MS, Wehrl HF, Newport DF, Catana C, Siegel SB, Becker M, et al. Simultaneous PET-MRI: a new approach for functional and morphological imaging. Nat Med. 2008;14:459–65.
65. Majmudar MD, Nahrendorf M. Cardiovascular molecular imaging: the road ahead. J Nucl Med. 2012;53:673–6.

66. Rischpler C, Nekolla SG, Kunze KP, Schwiger M. PET/MRI of the heart. Semin Nucl Med. 2015;45:234–47.
67. Glaudemans AW, Quintero AM, Signore A. PET/MRI in infectious and inflammatory diseases: will it be a useful improvement? Eur J Nucl Med Mol Imaging. 2012;39:745–9.
68. Wiseman J, Rouleau J, Rigo P, Strauss HW, Pitt B. Gallium-67 myocardial imaging for the detection of bacterial endocarditis. Radiology. 1976;120:135–8.
69. Melvin ET, Berger M, Lutzker LG, Goldberg E, Mildvan D. Noninvasive methods for detection of valve vegetations in infective endocarditis. Am J Cardiol. 1981;47:271–8.
70. Martin P, Devriendt J, Goffin Y, Verhas M. Gallium 67 scintigraphy in fibrinous pericarditis associated with bacterial endocarditis. Eur J Nucl Med. 1982;7:192–3.
71. Miller SW, Palmer EL, Dinsmore RE, Brady TJ. Gallium-67 and magnetic resonance imaging in aortic root abscess. J Nucl Med. 1987;28:1616–9.
72. Hardoff R, Luder AS, Lorber A, Dembo L. Early detection of infantile endocarditis by gallium-67 scintigraphy. Eur J Nucl Med. 1989;15:219–21.
73. O'Brien K, Barnes D, Martin RH, Rae JR. Gallium-SPECT in the detection of prosthetic valve endocarditis and aortic ring abscess. J Nucl Med. 1991;32:1791–3.
74. Desai SP, Yuille DL. The unsuspected complications of bacterial endocarditis imaged by gallium-67 scanning. J Nucl Med. 1993;34:955–7.
75. Vandenbos F, Roger PM, Mondain-Miton V, Dunais B, Fouché R, Kreitmann P, et al. Ventricular patch endocarditis caused by Propionibacterium acnes: advantages of gallium scanning. J Infect. 2001;43:249–51.
76. Pena FJ, Banzo I, Quirce R, Vallina NK, Hernández A, Guede C, et al. Ga-67 SPECT to detect endocarditis after replacement of an aortic valve. Clin Nucl Med. 2002;27:401–4.
77. Salem R, Boucher L, Laflamme L. Dual Tc-99 m sestamibi and Gallium-67 SPECT localize a myocardial abscess around a bioprosthetic aortic valve. Clin Nucl Med. 2004;29:799–800.
78. Thomson LE, Goodman MP, Naqvi TZ, Feldman R, Buchbinder NA, Waxman A, D'Agnolo A. Aortic root infection in a prosthetic valve demonstrated by gallium-67 citrate SPECT. Clin Nucl Med. 2005;30:265–8.
79. Yavari A, Ayoub T, Livieratos L, Raman V, McWilliams ET. Diagnosis of prosthetic aortic valve endocarditis with gallium-67 citrate single-photon emission computed tomography/ computed tomography hybrid imaging using software registration. Circ Cardiovasc Imaging. 2009;2:e41–3.
80. O'Doherty MJ, Page C, Croft D. 111In-leukocyte imaging: intrasplenic abscesses. Eur J Nucl Med. 1985;11:141–2.
81. Oates E, Sarno RC. Detection of bacterial endocarditis with indium-111 labeled leukocytes. Clin Nucl Med. 1988;13:691–3.
82. Cerqueira MD, Jacobson AF. Indium-111 leukocyte scintigraphic detection of myocardial abscess formation in patients with endocarditis. J Nucl Med. 1989;30:703–6.
83. Borst U, Becker W, Maisch B, Börner W, Kochsiek K. Indium-111 or Tc-99 m-HMPAO marked granulocytes as specific markers of florid stage endocarditis – results comparing clinical, histological and scintigraphic findings in 30 patients with suspected endocarditis. Z Kardiol. 1992;81:432–7.
84. Ramackers JM, Kotzki PO, Couret I, Messner-Pellenc P, Davy JM, Rossi M. The use of technetium-99 m hexamethylpropylene amine oxime labelled granulocytes with single-photon emission tomography imaging in the detection and follow-up of recurrence of infective endocarditis complicating transvenous endocardial pacemaker. Eur J Nucl Med. 1995;22:1351–4.
85. Adams BK. Tc-99 m leukocyte scintigraphy in infective endocarditis. Clin Nucl Med. 1995;20:395–7.
86. Campeau RJ, Ingram C. Perivalvular abscess complicating infective endocarditis: complementary role of echocardiography and indium-111-labeled leukocytes. Clin Nucl Med. 1998;23:582–4.
87. Ellemann A, Rubow S, Erlank P, Reuter H. Is there a role for 99mTc-HMPAO leucocyte scintigraphy in infective endocarditis? Cardiovasc J S Afr. 2003;14:199–203.

88. McDermott BP, Mohan S, Thermidor M, Parchuri S, Poulose J, Cunha BA. The lack of diagnostic value of the indium scan in acute bacterial endocarditis. Am J Med. 2004;117:621–3.
89. Yen RF, Chen YC, Wu YW, Pan MH, Chang SC. Using 18-fluoro-2-deoxyglucose positron emission tomography in detecting infectious endocarditis/endoarteritis: a preliminary report. Acad Radiol. 2004;11:316–21.
90. Ho HH, Cheung CW, Yeung CK. Septic peripheral embolization from Haemophilus parainfluenzae endocarditis. Eur Heart J. 2006;27:1009.
91. Vind SH, Hess S. Possible role of PET/CT in infective endocarditis. J Nucl Cardiol. 2010;17:516–9.
92. Sankatsing SU, Kolader ME, Bouma BJ, Bennink RJ, Verberne HJ, Ansink TM, et al. 18 F-fluoro-2-deoxyglucose positron emission tomography-negative endocarditis lenta caused by Bartonella henselae. J Heart Valve Dis. 2011;20:100–2.
93. Yeh CL, Liou JY, Chen SW, Chen YK. Infective endocarditis detected by ^{18}F-fluoro-2-deoxy-D-glucose positron emission tomography/computed tomography in a patient with occult infection. Kaohsiung J Med Sci. 2011;27:528–31.
94. Masuda A, Manabe O, Naya M, Oyama-Manabe N, Yamada S, Matsushima S, et al. Whole body assessment by ^{18}F-FDG PET in a patient with infective endocarditis. J Nucl Cardiol. 2013;20:641–3.
95. Teoh EJ, Backhouse L, Chandrasekaran B, Sabharwal NK, Beale AM, Gleeson FV, et al. Mycotic aneurysm of the superior mesenteric artery and other sequelae of prosthetic valve endocarditis on ^{18}F-FDG PET/CT. Eur J Nucl Med Mol Imaging. 2014;41:1993–4.
96. Ricciardi A, Sordillo P, Ceccarelli L, Maffongelli G, Calisti G, Di Pietro B, et al. 18-Fluoro-2-deoxyglucose positron emission tomography-computed tomography: an additional tool in the diagnosis of prosthetic valve endocarditis. Int J Infect Dis. 2014;28:219–24.
97. Wang SX, Zhang XC, Wang SY, Shun TT, He YL. 18 F-FDG PET/CT localized valvular infection in chronic Q fever endocarditis. J Nucl Cardiol. 2015;22(6):1320–2.
98. Belohlavek O, Votrubova J, Skopalova M, Fencl P. The detection of aortic valve infection by FDG-PET/CT in a patient with infection following total knee replacement. Eur J Nucl Med Mol Imaging. 2005;32:518.
99. Love C, Tomas MB, Tronco GG, Palestro CJ. FDG PET of infection and inflammation. Radiographics. 2005;25:1357–68.
100. Klingensmith 3rd WC, Perlman D, Baum K. Intrapatient comparison of 2-deoxy-2-[F18] fluoro-D-glucose with positron emissiontomography/computed tomography to Tc-99 m fanolesomab (NeutroSpec) for localization of infection. Mol Imaging Biol. 2007;9:295–9.
101. Moghadam-Kia S, Nawaz A, Millar BC, Moore JE, Wiegers SE, Torigian DA, et al. Imaging with (18)F-FDG-PET in infective endocarditis: promising role in difficult diagnosis and treatment monitoring. Hell J Nucl Med. 2009;12:165–7.
102. Huyge V, Unger P, Goldman S. Images in radiology. A bright spot. Am J Med. 2010; 123:37–9.
103. Kenzaka T, Shimoshikiryo M, Kitao A, Kario K, Hashimoto M. Positron emission tomography scan can be a reassuring tool to treat difficult cases of infective endocarditis. J Nucl Cardiol. 2011;18:741–3.
104. Plank F, Mueller S, Uprimny C, Hangler H, Feuchtner G. Detection of bioprosthetic valve infection by image fusion of (18)fluorodeoxyglucose-positron emission tomography and computed tomography. Interact Cardiovasc Thorac Surg. 2012;14:364–6.
105. Yedidya I, Stein GY, Vaturi M, Blieden L, Bernstine H, Pitlik SD, et al. Positron emission tomography/computed tomography for the diagnosis of endocarditis in patients with pulmonic stented valve/pulmonic stent. Ann Thorac Surg. 2011;91:287–9.
106. Wallner M, Steyer G, Krause R, Gstettner C, von Lewinski D. Fungal endocarditis of a bioprosthetic aortic valve. Pharmacological treatment of a Candida parapsilosis endocarditis. Herz. 2013;38:431–4.
107. Feuchtner G, Plank F, Uprimny C, Chevtchik O, Mueller S. Paravalvular prosthetic valve abscess detected with 18FDG-PET/128-slice CT image fusion. Eur Heart J Cardiovasc Imaging. 2012;13:276–7.

108. Klaipetch A, Manabe O, Oyama-Manabe N, Chiba S, Naya M, Yamada S, et al. Cardiac (18) F-FDG PET/CT with heparin detects infective vegetation in a patient with mechanical valve replacement. Clin Nucl Med. 2012;37:1184–5.
109. Pons J, Morin F, Bernier M, Perron J, Sénéchal M. Diagnostic challenge of annular abscess in a patient with prosthetic aortic valve: can F-fluorodeoxyglucose positron emission tomography be helpful? Rev Esp Cardiol (Engl Ed). 2012;65:296–8.
110. Gouriet F, Bayle S, Le Dolley Y, Seng P, Cammilleri S, Stein A, et al. Infectious endocarditis detected by PET/CT in a patient with a prosthetic knee infection: case report and review of the literature. Scand J Infect Dis. 2013;45:570–4.
111. Caldarella C, Leccisotti L, Treglia G, Giordano A. Which is the optimal acquisition time for FDG PET/CT imaging in patients with infective endocarditis? J Nucl Cardiol. 2013;20: 307–9.
112. Bartoletti M, Tumietto F, Fasulo G, Giannella M, Cristini F, Bonfiglioli R, Raumer L, Nanni C, Sanfilippo S, Di Eusanio M, Scotton PG, Graziosi M, Rapezzi C, Fanti S, Viale P. Combined computed tomography and fluorodeoxyglucose positron emission tomography in the diagnosis of prosthetic valve endocarditis: a case series. BMC Res Notes. 2014;7:32.
113. Chirillo F, Boccaletto F, Scotton P, Possamai M, Olivari Z. Complete and partly unexpected diagnostic findings at 18 F-FDG-PET/CT scanning in patients with suspected prosthetic valve endocarditis. Eur Heart J Cardiovasc Imaging. 2014;15:1057.
114. Gouriet F, Fournier PE, Zaratzian C, Sumian M, Cammilleri S, Riberi A, Casalta JP, Habib G, Raoult D. Diagnosis of Bartonella henselae prosthetic valve endocarditis in man. France Emerg Infect Dis. 2014;20:1396–7.
115. El Hajjaji I, Mansencal N, Dubourg O. Diagnosis of Cardiobacterium hominis endocarditis: usefulness of positron emission tomography. Int J Cardiol. 2012;160:e3–4.
116. Van Riet J, Hill EE, Gheysens O, Dymarkowski S, Herregods MC, Herijgers P, et al. (18) F-FDG PET/CT for early detection of embolism and metastatic infection in patients with infective endocarditis. Eur J Nucl Med Mol Imaging. 2010;37:1189–97.
117. Gheysens O, Lips N, Adriaenssens T, Pans S, Maertens J, Herregods MC, et al. Septic pulmonary embolisms and metastatic infections from methicillin-resistant Staphylococcus aureus endocarditis on FDG PET/CT. Eur J Nucl Med Mol Imaging. 2012;39:183.
118. Kouijzer IJ, Vos FJ, Janssen MJ, van Dijk AP, Oyen WJ, Bleeker-Rovers CP. The value of 18 F-FDG PET/CT in diagnosing infectious endocarditis. Eur J Nucl Med Mol Imaging. 2013;40:1102–7.
119. Asmar A, Ozcan C, Diederichsen AC, Thomassen A, Gill S. Clinical impact of 18 F-FDG-PET/CT in the extra cardiac work-up of patients with infective endocarditis. Eur Heart J Cardiovasc Imaging. 2014;15:1013–9.

Chapter 7
Diagnostic Criteria for Infective Endocarditis

Franck Thuny

In cases where the suspicion of IE is high, the appropriate antibiotics must be used as soon as possible because a delay in antibiotic therapy has negative effects on clinical outcomes in acute bacterial infectious diseases. Thus, efforts should be made to rapidly identify patients with a definite or highly probable diagnosis of IE and the causative pathogen to ensure that the appropriate antibiotic therapy begins promptly. See Tables 7.1 and 7.2, respectively, for the definition of infective endocarditis according to the modified Duke criteria and the definition of the terms used in the ESC 2015 modified criteria for the diagnosis of IE, which can help with this diagnostic process.

A diagnosis of IE usually relies on the association of an infectious syndrome and a recent endocardial involvement. This association is the cornerstone of the successive classifications and scores proposed to facilitate the difficult diagnosis of the disease. During the past decades, these classifications have been modified with the progress of the microbiological testing and the cardiac imaging techniques (Fig. 7.1). Thus, the first clinical diagnostic criteria of Von Reyn and colleagues only used the results of blood cultures to define the bacterial infection and the presence of a new regurgitant murmur or a predisposing heart disease to define the endocardial involvement [1]. With the emergence of echocardiography, the subsequent published criteria of the Duke University included the echo detection of the typical endocardial lesions (vegetations, abscess, new prosthetic dehiscence) as a major criterion of the diagnosis [2]. In 2002, these criteria were modified, especially to include the results of the *Coxiella burnetii* serology as a new major criterion [3]. This latter classification has a sensitivity of approximately 80 % overall when the criteria are evaluated at the end of patient follow-up in epidemiological studies [4]. However, in clinical practice, the modified Duke criteria show a lower diagnostic accuracy for early diagnosis, especially in the case of prosthetic valve endocarditis

F. Thuny, MD, PhD
Unit of Heart Failure and Valve Heart Disease, Nord Hospital, Marseille, France
e-mail: Franck.thuny@gmail.com

© Springer International Publishing Switzerland 2016
G. Habib (ed.), *Infective Endocarditis*, DOI 10.1007/978-3-319-32432-6_7

Table 7.1 Definition of infective endocarditis according to the modified Duke criteria

Definite IE
Pathological criteria
Microorganisms demonstrated by culture or histological examination of a vegetation, a vegetation that has embolized, or an intracardiac abscess specimen; or
Pathological lesions; vegetation or intracardiac abscess confirmed by histological examination showing active endocarditis
Clinical criteria
2 major criteria; or
1 major criterion and 3 minor criteria; or
5 minor criteria
Possible IE
1 major criterion and 1 minor criterion; or
3 minor criteria
Rejected IE
Firm alternate diagnosis; or
Resolution of IE syndrome with antibiotic therapy for ≤4 days; or
No pathological evidence of IE at surgery or autopsy, with antibiotic therapy for ≤4 days; or
Does not meet criteria for possible IE, as above

IE infective endocarditis
From Li et al. [3]. With permission of Oxford University Press

(PVE) and pacemaker/defibrillator leads IE, for which echocardiography is normal or inconclusive in up to 30 % of cases [5, 6]. Recent advances in imaging techniques have resulted in an improvement in identification of endocardial involvements and extracardiac complications of IE [7–9]. Thus, recent works have demonstrated that cardiac/whole body CT scan, cerebral MRI, ^{18}F-FDG PET/CT, and radiolabelled leukocytes SPECT/CT improve the detection of silent vascular phenomena (embolic events or infectious aneurysms) as well as endocardial lesions, especially in cases of prosthetic valves or pacemaker/defibrillator [10–22]. Given the recent published data, the 2015 ESC Guidelines propose the implementation of three additional points in the diagnostic criteria:

1. The identification of paravalvular lesions by cardiac CT is now considered as a major criterion;
2. In the setting of suspicion of endocarditis on a prosthetic valve, an abnormal activity around the site of implantation detected by ^{18}F-FDG PET/CT (only if the prosthesis was implanted for more than 3 months) or radiolabelled leukocytes SPECT/CT is now considered as a major criterion;
3. The identification of recent embolic events or infectious aneurysms (IAs) only by imaging (silent events) is now considered as a minor criterion.

See Fig. 7.2 for the ESC diagnostic algorithm including the ESC 2015 modified diagnostic criteria.

Table 7.2 Definition of the terms used in the ESC 2015 modified criteria for diagnosis of IE

Major criteria
1. Blood cultures positive for IE
(a) Typical microorganisms consistent with IE from 2 separate blood cultures:
Viridans streptococci, *Streptococcus gallolyticus (S bovis),* HACEK group, *S. aureus*; or
Community-acquired enterococci, in the absence of a primary focus; or
(b) Microorganisms consistent with IE from persistently positive blood cultures:
≥2 positive blood cultures of blood samples drawn >12 h apart; or
All of 3 or a majority of ≥4 separate cultures of blood (with first and last samples drawn ≥1 h apart); or
(c) Single positive blood culture for *Coxiella burnetii* or phase I IgG antibody titre >1:800
2. Imaging positive for IE
(a) Echocardiogram positive for IE:
Vegetation;
Abscess, pseudoaneurysm, intracardiac fistula;
Valvular perforation or aneurysm;
New partial dehiscence of prosthetic valve
(b) **Abnormal activity around the site of prosthetic valve implantation detected by ^{18}F-FDG PET/CT (only if the prosthesis was implanted for >3 months) or radiolabelled leukocytes SPECT/CT**
(c) **Definite paravalvular lesions by cardiac CT**
Minor criteria
1. Predisposition such as predisposing heart condition, or injection drug use
2. Fever defined as temperature >38 °C
3. Vascular phenomena **(including those detected only by imaging)**: major arterial emboli, septic pulmonary infarcts, infectious (mycotic) aneurysm, intracranial haemorrhage, conjunctival haemorrhages, and Janeway's lesions
4. Immunological phenomena: glomerulonephritis, Osler's nodes, Roth's spots, and rheumatoid factor
5. Microbiological evidence: positive blood culture but does not meet a major criterion as noted above or serological evidence of active infection with organism consistent with IE

The three-implemented criteria over the modified Duke criteria (Li) are shown in boldface
From Li et al. [3]. With permission of Oxford University Press
CT computed tomography, *ESC* European Society of Cardiology, *FDG* fluorodeoxyglucose; *HACEK Haemophilus parainfluenzae*, *H. aphrophilus*, *H. paraphrophilus*, *H. influenzae*, *Actinobacillus actinomycetemcomitans*, *Cardiobacterium hominis*, *Eikenella corrodens*, *Kingella kingae*, and *K. denitrificans*, *Ig* immunoglobulin, *PET* positron emission tomography, *SPECT* single photon emission computerized tomography

Evidence of endocardial lesions

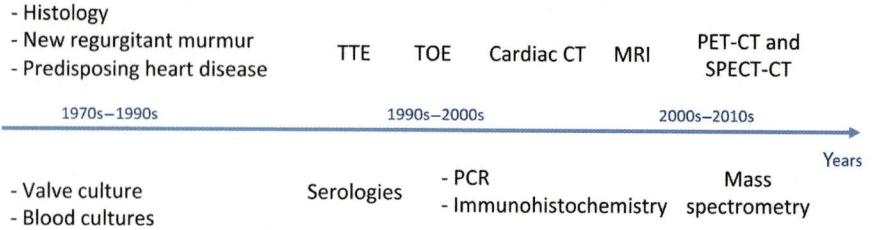

Fig. 7.1 Evolution of the diagnostic methods used to diagnose infective endocarditis during the last decades. *TTE* transthoracic echocardiography, *TOE* trans-oesophageal echocardiography, *CT* computed tomography, *PET* positron emission tomography

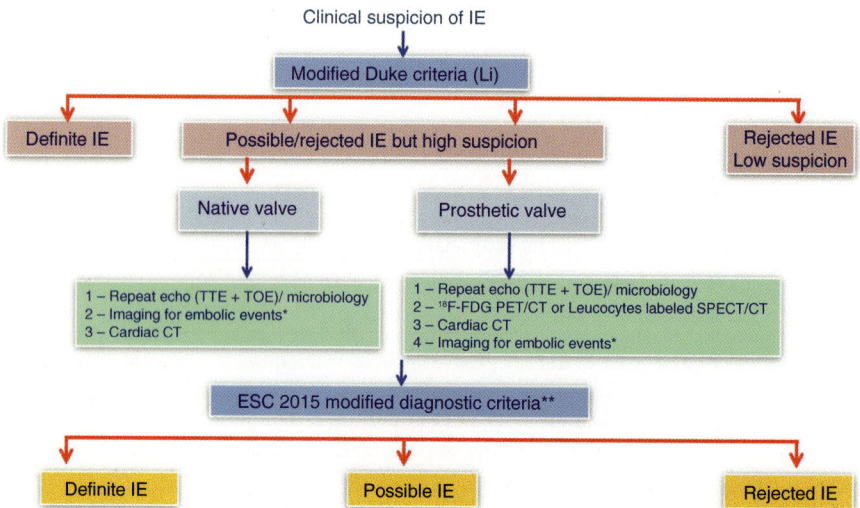

Fig. 7.2 ESC diagnostic algorithm including the ESC 2015 modified diagnostic criteria. The diagnosis of IE is still based upon classical Duke criteria, with a major role of echocardiography and blood cultures. When the diagnosis remains possible or even rejected but with a persisting high level of clinical suspicion, echocardiography and blood culture should be repeated, and other imaging techniques should be used, either for diagnosis of cardiac involvement (cardiac CT, 18F-FDG PET/CT or leukocytes-labelled SPECT/CT) or for imaging embolic events (cerebral MRI, whole body CT, and/or PET/CT). *May include Cerebral MRI, Whole Body CT, and/or PET/CT. ** see Table 7.2. *CT* computed tomography, *ESC* European Society of Cardiology, *FDG* fluorodeoxyglucose, *IE* infective endocarditis, *PET* positron emission tomography, *SPECT* single photon emission computerized tomography, *TOE* transoesophageal echocardiography, *TTE* transthoracic echocardiography (From Habib et al. [23]. Used with permission of Oxford University Press)

References

1. von Reyn FC, Arbeit RD, Friedland GH, et al. Criteria for the diagnosis of infective endocarditis. Clin Infect Dis. 1994;19:368–70.
2. Durack DT, Lukes AS, Bright DK. New criteria for diagnosis of infective endocarditis: utilization of specific echocardiographic findings. Duke endocarditis service. Am J Med. 1994; 96:200–9.
3. Li JS, Sexton DJ, Mick N, et al. Proposed modifications to the duke criteria for the diagnosis of infective endocarditis. Clin Infect Dis. 2000;30:633–8.
4. Habib G, Derumeaux G, Avierinos JF, et al. Value and limitations of the duke criteria for the diagnosis of infective endocarditis. J Am Coll Cardiol. 1999;33:2023–9.
5. Hill EE, Herijgers P, Claus P, et al. Abscess in infective endocarditis: the value of transesophageal echocardiography and outcome: a 5-year study. Am Heart J. 2007;154:923–8.
6. Vieira ML, Grinberg M, Pomerantzeff PM, et al. Repeated echocardiographic examinations of patients with suspected infective endocarditis. Heart. 2004;90:1020–4.
7. Thuny F, Grisoli D, Collart F, et al. Management of infective endocarditis: challenges and perspectives. Lancet. 2012;379:965–75.
8. Thuny F, Gaubert JY, Jacquier A, et al. Imaging investigations in infective endocarditis: current approach and perspectives. Arch Cardiovasc Dis. 2013;106:52–62.
9. Bruun NE, Habib G, Thuny F, et al. Cardiac imaging in infectious endocarditis. Eur Heart J. 2014;35:624–32.
10. Feuchtner GM, Stolzmann P, Dichtl W, et al. Multislice computed tomography in infective endocarditis: comparison with transesophageal echocardiography and intraoperative findings. J Am Coll Cardiol. 2009;53:436–44.
11. Fagman E, Perrotta S, Bech-Hanssen O, et al. Ecg-gated computed tomography: a new role for patients with suspected aortic prosthetic valve endocarditis. Eur Radiol. 2012;22:2407–14.
12. Snygg-Martin U, Gustafsson L, Rosengren L, et al. Cerebrovascular complications in patients with left-sided infective endocarditis are common: a prospective study using magnetic resonance imaging and neurochemical brain damage markers. Clin Infect Dis. 2008;47:23–30.
13. Cooper HA, Thompson EC, Laureno R, et al. Subclinical brain embolization in left-sided infective endocarditis: results from the evaluation by mri of the brains of patients with left-sided intracardiac solid masses (embolism) pilot study. Circulation. 2009;120:585–91.
14. Duval X, Iung B, Klein I, et al. Effect of early cerebral magnetic resonance imaging on clinical decisions in infective endocarditis: a prospective study. Ann Intern Med. 2010;152:497–504.
15. Iung B, Klein I, Mourvillier B, et al. Respective effects of early cerebral and abdominal magnetic resonance imaging on clinical decisions in infective endocarditis. Eur Heart J Cardiovasc Imaging. 2012;13:703–10.
16. Saby L, Le Dolley Y, Laas O, et al. Early diagnosis of abscess in aortic bioprosthetic valve by 18f-fluorodeoxyglucose positron emission tomography-computed tomography. Circulation. 2012;126:e217–20.
17. Saby L, Laas O, Habib G, et al. Positron emission tomography/computed tomography for diagnosis of prosthetic valve endocarditis: increased valvular (18)f-fluorodeoxyglucose uptake as a novel major criterion. J Am Coll Cardiol. 2013;61:2374–82.
18. Erba PA, Conti U, Lazzeri E, et al. Added value of 99mtc-hmpao-labeled leukocyte spect/ct in the characterization and management of patients with infectious endocarditis. J Nucl Med. 2012;53:1235–43.
19. Gahide G, Bommart S, Demaria R, et al. Preoperative evaluation in aortic endocarditis: findings on cardiac CT. AJR Am J Roentgenol. 2010;194:574–8.
20. Thuny F, Avierinos JF, Tribouilloy C, et al. Impact of cerebrovascular complications on mortality and neurologic outcome during infective endocarditis: a prospective multicentre study. Eur Heart J. 2007;28:1155–61.

21. Bensimhon L, Lavergne T, Hugonnet F, et al. Whole body [(18) f]fluorodeoxyglucose positron emission tomography imaging for the diagnosis of pacemaker or implantable cardioverter defibrillator infection: a preliminary prospective study. Clin Microbiol Infect. 2010;17:836–44.
22. Sarrazin JF, Philippon F, Tessier M, et al. Usefulness of fluorine-18 positron emission tomography/computed tomography for identification of cardiovascular implantable electronic device infections. J Am Coll Cardiol. 2012;59:1616–25.
23. Habib G, et al. 2015 ESC guidelines for the management of infective endocarditis. The task force for the management of infective endocarditis of the European Society of Cardiology (ESC). Eur Heart J. 2015;36(44):3075–128.

Part IV
Prognostic Assessment

Chapter 8
Prognosis in Infective Endocarditis

Isidre Vilacosta, Carmen Olmos Blanco, Cristina Sarriá Cepeda, Javier López Díaz, Carlos Ferrera Durán, David Vivas Balcones, Luis Maroto Castellanos, and José Alberto San Román Calvar

Introduction

Infective endocarditis (IE) still is a very serious and challenging disease. Despite diagnostic and therapeutic improvements, IE remains associated with high mortality and severe complications. The in-hospital mortality rate of patients with IE varies from 15 to 30 % [1]. Being such a complex disease, it is difficult to establish a clear-cut prognosis for a given patient. However, at present we have enough data to approximately predict the outcome of most patients with this disease.

When assessing the prognosis of patients with IE, three different clinical periods should be distinguished (Fig. 8.1): prognostic assessment at admission, early risk reassessment during the first week of antibiotics, and short and long-term prognosis after discharge [1]. In addition, for those patients facing surgery in the active phase of the disease, an accurate surgical risk score would be desirable.

In this chapter, we will focus on the prognosis of patients with left-sided IE; right-sided IE is being addressed in Chap. 15.

I. Vilacosta, MD, PhD (✉) • C. Olmos Blanco, MD, PhD • C. Ferrera Durán, MD
D. Vivas Balcones, MD, PhD • L. Maroto Castellanos, MD, PhD
Department of Cardiology, Hospital Clínico San Carlos, Madrid, Spain
e-mail: i.vilacosta@gmail.com; Carmen.olmosblanco@gmail.com; Carlosferreraduran@gmail.com; dvivas@secardiologia.es; Luis.maroto@salud.madrid.org

C. Sarriá Cepeda, MD, PhD
Department of Internal Medicine and Infectious Diseases,
Hospital Universitario de la Princesa, Madrid, Spain
e-mail: csarriac@gmail.com

J. López Díaz, MD, PhD • J.A. San Román Calvar, MD, PhD
Instituto de Ciencias Del Corazón (ICICOR), Hospital Clínico Universitario de Valladolid,
Valladolid, Spain
e-mail: javihouston@yahoo.es; asanroman@secardiologia.es

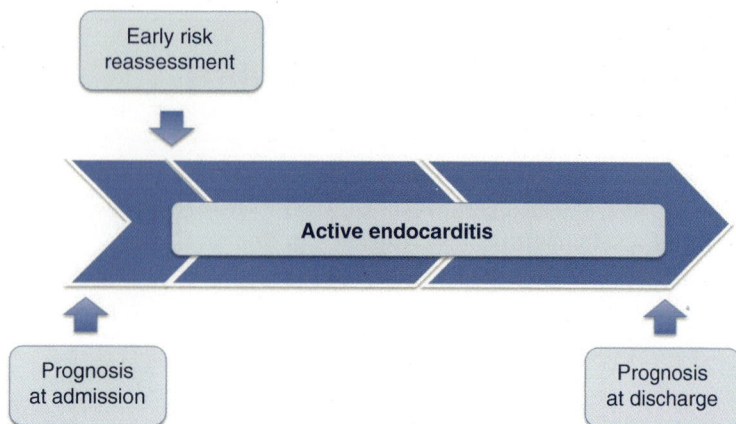

Fig. 8.1 Diagram representing the three clinical periods on which prognosis assessment during hospitalization for active endocarditis should be performed

Prognostic Assessment at Admission

In-hospital prognosis in IE is influenced by four main factors: patients' characteristics, the presence or absence of cardiac and non-cardiac complications, the infecting microorganism, and the echocardiographic findings (Table 8.1) [1].

The risk of patients with left-sided IE has been assessed according to these factors [2–4]. In each case, in-hospital outcome may be advanced by the association of several prognostic markers present at the time of diagnosis. Quick identification of patients at highest risk of death or severe complications (septic shock, embolism) may offer the opportunity to change the course of the disease (emergent or urgent surgery) and thereby, improve prognosis [2].

Several groups have attempted to find out predictors of poor in-hospital prognosis and identified three available within 72 h after admission: heart failure, periannular complications (Fig. 8.2), and *S. aureus* infection [4–7]. In one study, combining these factors to stratify the patients' risk, the authors found that, when all three are present, the risk of death or need for surgery reaches 79 % [4]. It is noteworthy that these three cornerstones in the diagnosis of IE are also pivotal regarding prognosis (Fig. 8.3).

Several attempts have been done in order to identify laboratory parameters useful for risk stratification. Among others, thrombocytopenia is a well known risk factor for death in sepsis [8] that has been included in several sepsis severity scores, such as the sequential organ failure assessment (SOFA) and the multiple organ dysfunction score [9, 10]. Thrombocytopenia is common in IE although rarely very severe [11]. Thrombocytopenic patients have higher mortality rate compared with patients without thrombocytopenia [11, 12]. Patients with thrombocytopenia presented more frequently with a severe clinical picture: acute onset of symptoms, acute renal failure, septic shock, confusional syndrome, and coma. In addition, higher mortality was associated with the degree of thrombocytopenia [11]. Apparently, thrombocytopenia could be a manifestation of the severity of the underlying septic condition. Serial measurements of the platelet count are better predictors of outcome than a

Table 8.1 Predictors of poor outcome present at the time of diagnosis

Patient characteristics
Older age
Prosthetic valve endocarditis
Diabetes mellitus
Comorbidities (e.g., frailty, immunosuppression, renal or pulmonary disease)
Clinical complications of infective endocarditis
Heart failure
Renal failure
Large area of ischemic stroke
Brain haemorrhage
Septic shock
Thrombocytopenia
Microorganisms
Staphylococcus aureus
Fungi
Non-HACEK gram-negative bacilli
Echocardiographic findings
Periannular complications
Severe left-sided valve regurgitation
Low left ventricular ejection fraction
Pulmonary hypertension
Very large vegetations
Severe prosthetic dysfunction
Premature mitral valve closure

From Habib et al. [1]. Used with permission of Oxford University Press

single measurement [12]. Why other laboratory parameters such as C-reactive protein and neutrophilia have not been found to predict poor outcome is not clear [11].

Thus, thrombocytopenia could be added to the triad of clinical, microbiological, and echocardiographic parameters that rapidly, at admission, permits a prediction of patients' outcome in IE: the more variables present, the higher the risk. Naturally, these patients should be closely followed and referred to tertiary care centers with surgical facilities.

A number of studies have shown that older age, diabetes, septic shock, large ischaemic stroke, brain haemorrhage, the need for haemodialysis, or a high degree of co-morbidity are also predictors of poor in-hospital outcome [2, 3, 13–19]. Some of these prognostic factors are discussed in more detail below.

Older Age

The influence of age in a large cohort of patients with left-sided IE has been assessed [20]. As expected, older patients have a higher percentage of prosthetic and degenerative valves, higher rates of nosocomial endocarditis and predisposing diseases

Fig. 8.2 Transesophageal image on an enormous abscess

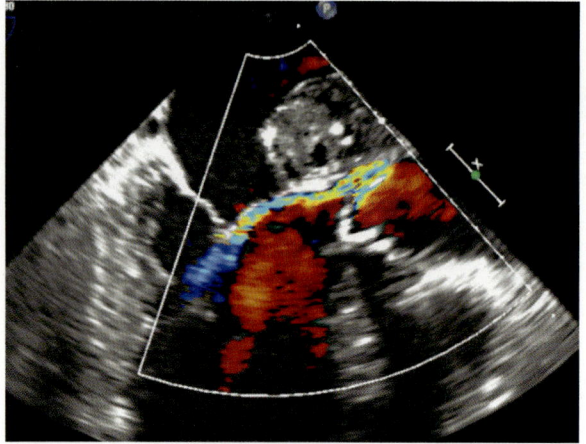

Fig. 8.3 Schematic diagram showing the cornerstones in diagnosis and prognosis of patients with endocarditis

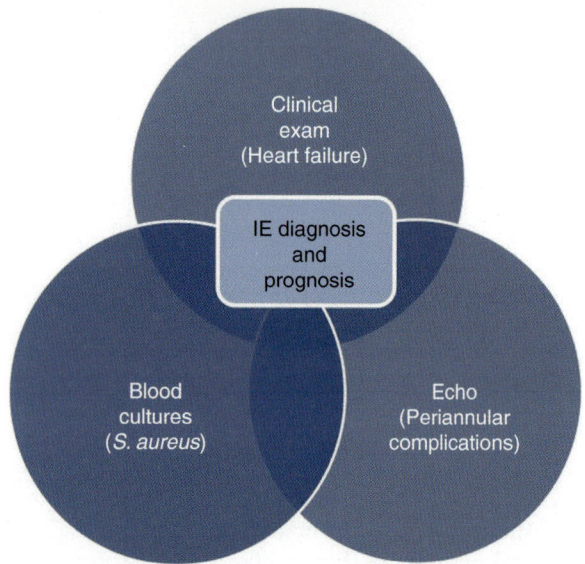

such as diabetes and cancer, and an increase in *S. bovis* and enterococci infections. An increase in mortality is observed with increasing age [20]. This is probably related to an increased mortality among older patients who undergo urgent and elective surgery. Importantly, the percentage of patients with surgical indications who are rejected for surgery increases significantly with age [20].

Diabetes

It is well known that individuals with diabetes have a greater frequency and severity of infections and that infection is one of the leading causes of death in hospitalized patients with diabetes [21, 22]. Among the reasons for this susceptibility to severe infections are abnormalities in cell-mediated immunity and phagocyte function, diminished vascularization, and increased rate of colonization of *S. aureus* [21, 22]. It has been well documented that patients with type 2 diabetes mellitus have a significantly higher prevalence of IE [23, 24]. In addition, diabetes has been identified as an independent risk factor of mortality in different bacterial infections including IE [17, 25–27]. It has been found that the cause of death among diabetics with IE was mostly related to infection [25, 28]. Therefore, the prognostic relevance of diabetes in patients with IE may be due to the relationship of diabetes with septic shock [28].

Septic Shock

One of the factors more tightly related to mortality in IE is the development of septic shock [16, 18, 28, 29]. Diabetes, acute renal insufficiency, *S. aureus* infection, large vegetation size, and especially signs of persistent infection have been associated with the development of septic shock [14]. These patients undergo surgery much less frequently and have a higher mortality than those without [14]. In addition, patients with septic shock who undergo surgery have a mortality rate lower than that of those who receive medical therapy alone [14]. It is not fully established if surgery improves prognosis in these patients, since surgery under this circumstances is associated with high mortality rate.

Neurological Complications

In a recent and large series [15], 25 % of patients with left-sided IE suffered neurological complications. Independent risk factors found to be associated with all neurological complications include very large vegetation size ($\geq$3 cm), *S. aureus* infection, mitral valve involvement, and anticoagulant therapy. As expected, this latter variable is particularly related to hemorrhagic events. Overall mortality was 30 %, and neurological complications had a negative impact on outcome [15]. The outcome of these patients appears to depend on the type of neurological event [30], and, when graded, only moderate to severe ischemic strokes and brain hemorrhages are significantly associated with a worse prognosis [15].

Dialysis

Infection is, after cardiovascular disease, the leading cause of death in patients with end-stage renal disease [31]. The incidence of IE in dialysis patients is higher than in the general population [28, 32, 33]. Frequent episodes of bacteraemia related to dialysis access, and a higher rate of valvular heart disease predisposing the valves to bacterial seeding may explain the higher incidence of IE in dialysis patients [34,

35]. In addition, it has been well documented that those patients in dialysis who develop IE have a poorer prognosis. In fact, survival rates have barely changed in the last decades [31, 36]. Recently, Chou et al. analyzed 502 patients with IE from a total incident dialysis population of 68,426 adult subjects over 9 years. The incidence rate of IE was 201.4/100.000 person-years, and increased over the study period [31]. Being older, diabetic, and having baseline cardiovascular diseases, including heart failure, coronary artery disease, cerebrovascular accident, and valvular heart disease were independent risk factors for IE [31]. In this study, the authors found that patients on haemodialysis had a 42 % higher risk for IE than did those on peritoneal dialysis [31]. Other groups had similar experiences [37, 38]. Fernández-Cean et al. evaluated the relationship between dialysis modality and the outcome of IE. In-hospital mortality in patients switched to peritoneal dialysis was lower [8.3 %] than in those who stayed on haemodialysis [55.5 %]. The authors suggested that the high mortality of IE in chronic haemodialysis may be associated with the vascular access necessary for procedure [38].

In another very large series, 11,156 dialysis patients hospitalized for IE from 2004 to 2007 were analyzed [39]. During the study period, 11.4 % underwent valve replacement surgery (tissue valve, 44.3 %; non-tissue valve, 55.7 %). Other predictors of mortality in patients undergoing valve replacement included older age, diabetes mellitus, two valve replacement, S. aureus, and surgery during index hospitalization. Survival did not differ between tissue or non-tissue prosthesis [39, 40].

S. aureus (including methicillin-resistant strains) is the most common microorganism in dialysis patients with IE; Enterococcus faecalis and culture-negative IE are also frequently present [31, 36, 37].

Comorbidities

Charlson comorbidity scale score of 2 or greater, and abnormal mental status increase the probability of death [5]. However, few studies have investigated this relationship.

Systemic and Local Infection Response During the First Week of Treatment

Reassessment of Patient Risk

After a few days of medical treatment, basically antibiotics and diuretics when needed, it is very important to evaluate the systemic and local response of the infection, and the presence of hemodynamic deterioration. This should be done clinically, echocardiographically, and by the taking blood cultures. The appearance of signs of heart failure or lack of infection control worsen patient prognosis and exposes patients to a high risk of death from heart failure, embolism, severe sepsis, or complete atrioventricular block [14, 41].

Uncontrolled infection is one of the most feared complications of IE and is the second most frequent cause for surgery. It is suspected to be present when there are persisting signs of infection or when ongoing and progressive valvular or perivalvular echocardiographic signs of infection are present. Perivalvular extension of IE is the most common cause of uncontrolled infection and is associated with poor prognosis and a high likelihood of the need for surgery [4].

Persisting fever is a frequent problem observed during treatment of IE. Management of persisting fever includes replacement of intravenous lines, repeat laboratory measurements, blood cultures, echocardiography (intracardiac focus of infection), and searching for extracardiac foci of infection [1]. Increasing vegetation size is also a sign of locally uncontrolled infection that has been associated with an increased risk for embolism [42].

When treating patients with IE, an early negativization of blood cultures should be expected implying that the infection is under control. On the contrary, if they remain positive, a lack of control of the infection should be suspected. Persistently positive blood cultures 48–72 h after initiation of adequate antibiotic treatment is an independent risk factor for in-hospital mortality [43]. Besides, it has also been shown that surgical mortality in IE strongly depends on its indication [44]. Patients urgently operated on with IE and persistent infection have a four times higher risk of death after surgery than those who do not have persistent infection. These results suggest that surgery must be considered when blood cultures remain positive after 3 days of antibiotic therapy and other causes for persistently positive blood cultures (inadequate antibiotic regimen, metastatic foci, etc.) have been excluded. Thus, from a practical point of view, persisting positive blood cultures 2–3 days from the initiation of antibiotics should be taken into account when stratifying the risk of patients with IE.

Role of Risk Scoring Systems in Predicting Operative Mortality in Active Endocarditis

During the active phase of IE, when patients are on intravenous antibiotics, clinicians rely on a set of surgical indications that include heart failure or haemodynamic instability, lack of infection control, and a high risk of embolism [1]. Basically, surgery is being performed in patients in whom medical therapy has failed. However, it is difficult to establish the real impact of surgical treatment on the patient's prognosis, since surgery itself carries significant risks. In fact, surgical mortality in this situation is the highest of all surgeries performed in patients with valvular heart disease [45, 46].

Prognostic scoring systems, if accurate, could be of help in this scenario. Nonetheless, in most cases the scoring system will confirm what an experienced clinician suspects, that is, that the patient is at high risk. So the key clinical question is how to know, in a given patient with a surgical indication, that surgery is not a good choice. In other words, risk score systems should be able to recognize which patients should not be sent to surgery.

The ideal risk score model in this scenario should have at least three main characteristics: (1) it should be constructed from cardiac operations of patients with active IE exclusively; (2) many of the already existing parameters of cardiac surgery risk scores (impaired renal function, diabetes, etc.) are important risk factors and should be retained; and (3) variables unique to IE, such as type of microorganism, sepsis, perivalvular destruction, etc., should be well represented.

The performance of additive and logistic EuroSCORE I have been previously assessed in patients with IE with contradictory results [47–49]. EuroSCORE I, based on cardiac surgery undertaken in 1995, is nowadays outdated. Since the representation of cases with active IE in EuroSCORE II is minimal, it should be used with caution in these patients. In addition, for detecting operative mortality, EuroSCORE II was no better than EuroSCORE I [49].

Given that the Society of Thoracic Surgeons (STS) score [50] cannot be used either, Gaca et al. developed a risk score specific to IE using 19,543 patients from the STS database [51]. In this series, the overall mortality was 8.2 %, much lower than expected. The authors described a model with 14 variables to help in clinical decision-making. Unfortunately, there are a number of issues that prevent their daily applicability to our patients: only half of the patients had active IE, in fact 43 % of operations were elective, microbiologic information was not provided, and anatomic factors such as extensive periannular complications with abscesses and pseudoaneurysms were not considered. All these issues could be relevant when considering surgical outcome.

De Feo et al. also developed a risk score in their single center pilot study of 440 native valve IE patients undergoing surgery [52]. Six mortality predictors were identified, including age, renal failure, NYHA class IV, critical preoperative state, lack of preoperative attainment of blood culture negativity, and perivalvular involvement. Four risk classes were drawn ranging from very low risk (≤5 points, mean predicted mortality 1 %) to very high risk (≥20 points, 43 % mortality) [52]. This score has the advantage of being relatively simple with only six parameters, and it seems to be not inferior to the STS score [49]. However, it was derived exclusively from native infected valves, so it is not applicable to prosthetic valve IE; 17 % of cases were not on antibiotics, and right-sided infections were included.

PALSUSE is a recent risk score for in-hospital mortality developed from a multicenter cohort of 1000 consecutive patients with IE [53]. The score was developed using seven prognostic variables with a similar predictive value (OR between 1.7 and 2.3): prosthetic valve, age ≥70, large intracardiac destruction, *Staphylococcus* infection, urgent surgery, sex (female), and EuroSCORE ≥10. In-hospital mortality ranged from 0 % in patients with a PALSUSE score of 0–45.4 % in those with a score >3 [53]. Of note, although surgery was initially indicated in 630 patients

(63%), it was finally performed in 437 (43.7%), so 193 patients were considered inoperable or died before surgery. Surprisingly, although surgery was performed in the acute phase of IE, the mean period of time from diagnosis to surgery was very long (17.4±20.5 days). In a recent multicenter study, the median time from admission to surgery was 7 days [54]. In addition, this series included patients with possible IE (n=148), and patients with right-sided IE (pacemakers, etc.), which have a much better prognosis and should be studied separately [1, 55].

The SHARPEN clinical risk score is based on clinical and laboratory parameters from a small cohort of 233 patients with IE [56]. This 11-year study found that in-hospital mortality in IE remains high [23%]. Patients who underwent valvular surgery had a low mortality rate (7.8%). The main limitation of this study is that only 27% of patients with surgical indications underwent surgery [56]. Nowadays, 40–57% of patients with IE undergo cardiac surgery during hospitalization [13–16, 18, 28, 53, 54]. Obviously, this and other series have an insurmountable handicap, ie, higher risk cases have already been dismissed from surgery.

To summarize: all these studies have many limitations and pitfalls, and, in addition, all of them are limited by "survivor bias," where patients who are well enough to undergo surgery are more likely to survive than those who are too fragile or are complicated cases. Predictably, patients with an indication for surgery who cannot proceed due to prohibitive surgical risk have the worst prognosis [54, 57]. Therefore, the above-mentioned scores are far from being ideal, and they are probably not very useful for clinical decision making.

Short-Term Follow-Up After Discharge

Following in-hospital treatment, the main complications of patients with IE are recurrence of infection, heart failure, need for valve surgery, and death [1].

Patients should be aware of the risk of having a new episode of IE, and they need to be educated in recognizing the signs and symptoms of IE. The appearance of fever of unknown origin, chills, or other signs of infection requires immediate clinical evaluation and drawing blood cultures before using empirical antibiotics. The Task Force also recommends taking blood samples (white cell count, ESR, C-reactive protein, etc.) and blood cultures systematically at the initial follow-up visit for an early detection of recurrences [1]. The actual risk of recurrence amongst survivors of IE is low and varies from 2 to 11.7% [1, 58, 59]. Two main types of recurrence should be distinguished: relapse and reinfection. Although not systematically differentiated in the literature, the term relapse refers to a repeat episode of IE caused by the same microorganism, whilst reinfection corresponds to an infection caused by a different agent [1]. Relapses are most often due to inadequate antibiotic treatment, resistance to conventional antibiotic regimens, periannular extension of the infection, and a persistent focus of infection. Factors associated with an increased rate of relapse are listed in Table 8.2.

Table 8.2 Conditions associated with increased risk of relapse

Inadequate antibiotic treatment (agent, dose, duration)
Microorganisms difficult to treat with antibiotics alone, (i.e. *Coxiella burnetii*, fungi, *Bartonella* spp, *Brucella*)
Polymicrobial infection in intravenous drug users
Prosthetic valve endocarditis
Persistent metastatic foci of infection (abscesses)
Resistance to conventional antibiotic regimens
Positive valve cultures
Chronic dialysis

From Habib et al. [1]. Used with permission of Oxford University Press

As patients with previous IE are at risk of reinfection [58, 60], prophylactic measures should be followed as advised by the ESC guidelines [1]. Reinfection is more frequent in intravenous drug users [58, 60, 61], prosthetic valve IE [58, 62], in patients undergoing chronic dialysis [60, 63], and in those cases with large periannular extension of the infection [64]. Patients with reinfection are at higher risk of death and need for valve replacement [60]. Likewise, perivalvular destruction is associated with a higher rate of recurrence and a higher surgical mortality [64]. Importantly, the type of valve implanted has no clear effect on the risk of recurrent IE [65].

Once the patient has been discharged and during the firsts months of follow-up, residual severe valve regurgitation or progressive valve deterioration may decompensate left ventricular function leading to heart failure. To monitor ventricular function, clinical and echocardiographic evaluations should be serially repeated during the first year of follow-up for an early recognition of signs of heart failure or poor haemodynamic tolerance [1].

At this stage, after completion of antibiotic treatment, recommendations for valve surgery in these patients follow conventional guidelines [66, 67]. The need for late valve replacement is low, ranging from 3 to 8 % in recent series [63, 68, 69].

Long-Term Prognosis

In recent series, the crude long-term survival rates after discharge were estimated to be 80–90 % at 1 year, 70–80 % at 2 years, and 60–70 % at 5 years [60, 62, 64, 68–73]. The main predictors of long-term mortality are age, comorbidities, recurrences, and heart failure, especially when cardiac surgery cannot be performed [60, 68, 71]. So, at this point in time, mortality will be more patient-related (ie, related to the underlying patients condition) than disease-related (direct consequence of IE). In any case, compared with an age and sex-matched general population, patients surviving a first episode of IE, even those who underwent valve replacement, have a significantly worse survival [58, 70]. This excess mortality is especially high within the first few years after hospital discharge, and can be explained by late complications such as heart failure, sudden death, ventricular arrhythmias, and a new stroke [70, 72, 74].

Conclusion

In summary, a patient's prognosis should be assessed at three different time periods during hospitalization: at admission, during the first week after a few days of antibiotic treatment, and before discharge. Considering patients' prognosis will force clinicians to ponder the possible complications that a patient may face and this, ultimately, implies that we are thinking ahead and prepared.

References

1. Habib G, Hoen B, Tornos P, Thuny F, Prendergast B, Vilacosta I, et al. Guidelines on the prevention, diagnosis, and treatment of infective endocarditis (new version 2009): the task force on the prevention, diagnosis, and treatment of infective endocarditis of the European Society of Cardiology (ESC). Endorsed by the European Society of Clinical Microbiology and Infectious Diseases (ESCMID) and by the International Society of Chemotherapy (ISC) for Infection and Cancer. Eur Heart J. 2009;30(19):2369–413.
2. Thuny F, Beurtheret S, Mancini J, Gariboldi V, Casalta JP, Riberi A, et al. The timing of surgery influences mortality and morbidity in adults with severe complicated infective endocarditis: a propensity analysis. Eur Heart J. 2011;32(16):2027–33.
3. Chu VH, Cabell CH, Benjamin Jr DK, Kuniholm EF, Fowler Jr VG, Engemann J, et al. Early predictors of in-hospital death in infective endocarditis. Circulation. 2004;109(14):1745–9.
4. San Román JA, López J, Vilacosta I, Luaces M, Sarriá C, Revilla A, et al. Prognostic stratification of patients with left-sided endocarditis determined at admission. Am J Med. 2007; 120(4):369.e1–7.
5. Hasbun R, Vikram HR, Barakat LA, Buenconsejo J, Quagliarello VJ. Complicated left-sided native valve endocarditis. Risk classification for mortality. JAMA. 2003;289(15):1933–40.
6. Granowitz E, Longworth DL. Risk stratification and bedside prognostication in infective endocarditis. JAMA. 2003;289(15):1991–3.
7. Mansur AJ, Grinberg M, Cardoso HA, da Luz PL, Bellotti G, Pileggi F. Determinants of prognosis in 300 episodes of infective endocarditis. Thorac Cardiovasc Surg. 1996;44(1):2–10.
8. Levy MM, Fink MP, Marshall JC, Abraham E, Angus D, CooK D, et al. 2001 SCCM/ESICM/ACCP/ATS/SIS international sepsis definitions conference. Crit Care Med. 2003;31(4):1250–6.
9. Ferreira FL, Bota DP, Bross A, Mélot C, Vincent JL. Serial evaluation of the SOFA score to predict outcome in critically ill patients. JAMA. 2001;286(14):1754–8.
10. Marshall JC, Cook DJ, Christou NV, Bernard GR, Sprung CL, Sibbald WJ. Multiple organ dysfunction score: a reliable descriptor of a complex clinical outcome. Crit Care Med. 1995;23(10):1638–52.
11. Ferrera C, Vilacosta I, Fernández C, López J, Sarriá C, Olmos C, et al. Usefulness of thrombocytopenia at admission as a prognostic marker in native valve left-sided infective endocarditis. Am J Cardiol. 2015;115(7):950–5.
12. Sy RW, Chawantanpipat C, Richmond D, Kritharides L. Thrombocytopenia and mortality in infective endocarditis. J Am Coll Cardiol. 2008;51(18):1824–5.

13. Nadji G, Rusinaru D, Remadi JP, Jeu A, Sorel C, Tribouilloy C. Heart failure in left-sided native valve infective endocarditis: characteristics, prognosis, and results of surgical treatment. Eur J Heart Fail. 2009;11(7):668–75.
14. Olmos C, Vilacosta I, Fernández C, López J, Sarriá C, Ferrera C, et al. Contemporary epidemiology and prognosis of septic shock in infective endocarditis. Eur Heart J. 2013;34(26): 1999–2006.
15. García-Cabrera E, Fernández-Hidalgo N, Almirante B, Ivanova-Georgieva R, Noureddine M, Plata A, et al. Neurological complications of infective endocarditis. Risk factors, outcome, and impact of cardiac surgery: a multicenter observational study. Circulation. 2013;127(23): 2272–84.
16. Delahaye F, Alla F, Beguinot I, Bruneval P, Doco-Lecompte T, Lacassin F, et al. In-hospital mortality of infective endocarditis: prognostic factors and evolution over an 8-year period. Scand J Infect Dis. 2007;39(10):849–57.
17. Duval X, Alla F, Doco-Lecompte T, Le Moing V, Delahaye F, Mainardi JL, et al. Diabetes mellitus and infective endocarditis: the insulin factor in patient morbidity and mortality. Eur Heart J. 2007;28(1):59–64.
18. Gelsomino S, Maessen JG, van der Veen F, Livi U, Renzulli A, Lucà F, et al. Emergency surgery for native mitral valve endocarditis: the impact of septic and cardiogenic shock. Ann Thorac Surg. 2012;93(5):1469–76.
19. Olmos C, Vilacosta I, Pozo E, Fernández C, Sarriá C, López J, et al. Prognostic implications of diabetes in patients with left-sided endocarditis: findings from a large cohort study. Medicine (Baltimore). 2014;93(2):114–9.
20. López J, Revilla A, Vilacosta I, Sevilla T, Villacorta E, Sarriá C, et al. Age-dependent profile of left-sided infective endocarditis. A 3-center experience. Circulation. 2010;121(7):892–7.
21. Calvet HM, Yoshikawa TT. Infections in diabetes. Infect Dis Clin North Am. 2001;15(2): 407–21.
22. Joshi N, Caputo GM, Weitekamp MR, Karchmer AW. Infections in patients with diabetes mellitus. N Engl J Med. 1999;341(25):1906–12.
23. Movahed MR, Hashemzadeh M, Jamal MM. Increased prevalence of infectious endocarditis in patients with type II diabetes mellitus. J Diabetes Complications. 2007;21(6):403–6.
24. Strom BL, Abrutyn E, Berlin JA, Kinman JL, Feldman RS, Stolley PD, et al. Risk factors for infective endocarditis: oral hygiene and nondental exposures. Circulation. 2000;102(23): 2842–8.
25. Chirillo F, Bacchion F, Pedrocco A, Scotton P, De Leo A, Rocco F, et al. Infective endocarditis in patients with diabetes mellitus. J Heart Valve Dis. 2010;19(3):312–20.
26. Kourany WM, Miro JM, Moreno A, Corey GR, Pappas PA, Abrutyn E, et al. Influence of diabetes mellitus on the clinical manifestations and prognosis of infective endocarditis: a report from the International Collaboration on Endocarditis-Merged Database. Scand J Infect Dis. 2006;38(8):613–9.
27. Bertoni AG, Saydah S, Brancati FL. Diabetes and the risk of infection-related mortality in the U.S. Diabetes Care. 2001;24(6):1044–9.
28. Murdoch DR, Corey GR, Hoen B, Miró JM, Fowler Jr VG, Bayer AS, et al. Clinical presentation, etiology, and outcome of infective endocarditis in the 21st century. Arch Intern Med. 2009;169(5):463–73.
29. Mourviller B, Trouillet JL, Timsit JF, Baudot J, Chastre J, Regnier B, et al. Infective endocarditis in the intensive care unit: clinical spectrum and prognostic factors in 228 consecutive patients. Intensive Care Med. 2004;30(11):2046–52.
30. Parrino PE, Kron IL, Ross SD, Shockey KS, Kron AM, Towler MA, et al. Does a focal neurologic deficit contraindicate operation in a patient with endocarditis? Ann Thorac Surg. 1999;67(1):59–64.
31. Chou M-T, Wang J-J, Wu W-S, Weng S-F, Ho C-H, Lin Z-Z, et al. Epidemiologic features and long-term outcome of dialysis patients with infective endocarditis in Taiwan. Int J Cardiol. 2015;179:465–9.

32. Maraj S, Jacobs LE, Maraj R, Kotler MN. Bacteremia and infective endocarditis in patients on hemodialysis. Am J Med Sci. 2004;327(5):242–9.
33. Hoen B. Infective endocarditis: a frequent disease in dialysis patients. Nephrol Dial Transplant. 2004;19(6):1360–2.
34. Powe NR, Jaar B, Furth SL, Hermann J, Briggs W. Septicemia in dialysis patients: incidence, risk factors, and prognosis. Kidney Int. 1999;55(3):1081–90.
35. Umana E, Ahmed W, Alpert MA. Valvular and perivalvular abnormalities in end-stage renal disease. Am J Med Sci. 2003;325(4):237–42.
36. Shroff GR, Herzog CA, Ma JZ, Collins AJ. Long-term survival of dialysis patients with bacterial endocarditis in the United States. Am J Kidney Dis. 2004;44(6):1077–82.
37. Jones DA, McGill LA, Rathod KS, Matthews K, Gallagher S, Uppal R, et al. Characteristics and outcomes of dialysis patients with infective endocarditis. Nephron Clin Pract. 2013; 123(3–4):151–6.
38. Fernández-Cean J, Álvarez A, Burguez S, Baldovinos G, Larre-Borges P, Cha M. Infective endocarditis in chronic hemodialysis: two treatment strategies. Nephrol Dial Transplant. 2002;17(12):2226–30.
39. Leither MD, Shroff GR, Ding S, Gilbertson DT, Herzog CA. Long-term survival of dialysis patients with bacterial endocarditis undergoing valvular replacement surgery in the United States. Circulation. 2013;128(4):344–51.
40. Herzog CA, Ma JZ, Collins AJ. Long-term survival of dialysis patients in the United States with prosthetic heart valves: should ACC/AHA practice guidelines on valve selection be modified? Circulation. 2002;105(11):1336–41.
41. Thuny F, Habib G. When should we operate on patients with acute infective endocarditis? Heart. 2010;96(11):892–7.
42. Vilacosta I, Graupner C, San Román JA, Sarriá C, Ronderos R, Fernández C, et al. Risk of embolization after institution of antibiotic therapy for infective endocarditis. J Am Coll Cardiol. 2002;39(9):1489–95.
43. López J, Sevilla T, Vilacosta I, Sarriá C, Revilla A, Ortiz C, et al. Prognostic role of persistent positive blood cultures after initiation of antibiotic therapy in left-sided infective endocarditis. Eur Heart J. 2013;34(23):1749–54.
44. Revilla A, López J, Vilacosta I, Villacorta E, Rollán MJ, Echevarría JR, et al. Clinical and prognostic profile of patients with infective endocarditis who need urgent surgery. Eur Heart J. 2007;28(1):65–71.
45. Vikram HR, Buenconsejo J, Hasbun R, Quagliarello VJ. Impact of valve surgery on 6-month mortality in adults with complicated, left-sided native valve endocarditis: a propensity analysis. JAMA. 2003;290(24):3207–14.
46. Aksoy O, Sexton DJ, Wang A, Pappas PA, Kourany W, Chu V, et al. Early surgery in patients with infective endocarditis: a propensity score analysis. Clin Infect Dis. 2007;44(3):364–72.
47. Mestres CA, Castro MA, Bernabeu E, Josa M, Cartaná R, Pomar JL, et al. Preoperative risk stratification in infective endocarditis. Does the EuroSCORE model work? Preliminary results. Eur J Cardiothorac Surg. 2007;32(2):281–5.
48. Rasmussen RV, Bruun LE, Lund J, Larsen CT, Hassager C, Bruun NE. The impact of cardiac surgery in native valve infective endocarditis: can EuroSCORE guide patient selection? Int J Cardiol. 2011;149(3):304–9.
49. Wang TKM, Oh T, Voss J, Gamble G, Kang N, Pemberton J. Comparison of contemporary risk scores for predicting outcomes after surgery for infective endocarditis. Heart Vessels. 2014;30(2):227–34.
50. Shahian DM, O'Brien SM, Filardo G, Ferraris VA, Haan CK, Rich JB, et al. The Society of thoracic surgeons 2008 cardiac surgery risk models: part 1-coronary artery bypass grafting surgery. Ann Thorac Surg. 2009;88(1 Suppl):S2–22.
51. Gaca JG, Sheng S, Daneshmand MA, O'Brien S, Scott Rankin J, Matthew Brennan J, et al. Outcomes for endocarditis surgery in North America: A simplified risk scoring system. J Thorac Cardiovasc Surg. 2011;141(1):98–106.

52. De Feo M, Cotrufo M, Carozza A, De Santo LS, Amendolara F, Giordano S, et al. The need for a specific risk prediction system in native valve infective endocarditis surgery. Sci World J. 2012;2012:307571.
53. Martínez-Sellés M, Muñoz P, Arnáiz A, Moreno M, Gálvez J, Rodríguez-Roda J, et al. Valve surgery in active infective endocarditis: a simple score to predict in-hospital prognosis. Int J Cardiol. 2014;175(1):133–7.
54. Chu VH, Park LP, Athan E, Delahaye F, Freiberger T, Lamas C, et al. Association between surgical indications, operative risk, and clinical outcome in infective endocarditis. A prospective study from the International Collaboration on Endocarditis. Circulation. 2015;131(2): 131–40.
55. Olmos C, Vilacosta I, Sarriá C, Fernández C, López J, Ferrera C, et al. Characterization and clinical outcome of patients with possible infective endocarditis. Int J Cardiol. 2015;178: 31–3.
56. Chee Q-Z, Tan Y-QB, Ngiam JN, Win MTM, Shen X, Choo J-NJ, et al. The SHARPEN clinical risk score predicts mortality in patients with infective endocarditis: An 11-year study. Int J Cardiol. 2015;191:273–6.
57. Mirabel M, Sonneville R, Hajage D, Novy E, Tubach F, Vignon P, et al. Long-term outcomes and cardiac surgery in critically ill patients with infective endocarditis. Eur Heart J. 2014; 35(18):1195–204.
58. Shih C-J, Chu H, Chao P-W, Lee Y-J, Kuo S-C, Li S-Y, et al. Long-term clinical outcome of major adverse cardiac events in survivors of infective endocarditis: a nationwide population-based study. Circulation. 2014;130(19):1684–91.
59. Gálvez-Acebal J, Almendro-Delia M, Ruiz J, de Alarcón A, Martínez-Marcos FJ, Reguera JM, et al. Influence of early surgical treatment on the prognosis of left-sided infective endocarditis: a multicenter cohort study. Mayo Clin Proc. 2014;89(10):1397–405.
60. Alagna L, Park LP, Nicholson BP, Keiger AJ, Strahilevitz J, Morris A, et al. Repeat endocarditis: analysis of risk factors based on the International Collaboration on Endocarditis-Prospective Cohort Study. Clin Microbiol Infect. 2014;20(6):566–75.
61. Kaiser SP, Melby SJ, Zierer A, Schuessler RB, Moon MR, Moazami N, et al. Long-term outcomes in valve replacement surgery for infective endocarditis. Ann Thorac Surg. 2007;83(1): 30–5.
62. Heiro M, Helenius H, Makila S, Hohenthal U, Savunen T, Engblom E, et al. Infective endocarditis in a finnish teaching hospital: a study on 326 episodes treated during 1980-2004. Heart. 2006;92(10):1457–62.
63. Heiro M, Helenius H, Hurme S, Savunen T, Metsärinne K, Engblom E, et al. Long-term outcome of infective endocarditis: a study on patients surviving over one year after the initial episode treated in a Finnish teaching hospital during 25 years. BMC Infect Dis. 2008;8:49.
64. Fedoruk LM, Jamieson WR, Ling H, MacNab JS, Germann E, Karim SS, et al. Predictors of recurrence and reoperation for prosthetic valve endocarditis after valve replacement surgery for native valve endocarditis. J Thorac Cardiovasc Surg. 2009;137(2):326–33.
65. David TE, Gavra G, Feindel CM, Regesta T, Armstrong S, Maganti MD. Surgical treatment of active infective endocarditis: a continued challenge. J Thorac Cardiovasc Surg. 2007;133(1): 144–9.
66. Nishimura RA, Otto CM, Bonow RO, Carabello BA, Erwin 3rd JP, Guyton RA, et al. 2014 AHA/ACC guideline for the management of patients with valvular heart disease: a report of the American College of Cardiology/American Heart Association Task Force on Practice Guidelines. J Thorac Cardiovasc Surg. 2014;148(1):e1–132.
67. Vahanian A, Alfieri O, Andreotti F, Antunes MJ, Barón-Esquivias G, Baumgartner H, et al. Guidelines on the management of valvular heart disease (version 2012). Eur Heart J. 2012; 33(19):2451–96.
68. Martínez-Sellés M, Muñoz P, Estevez A, del Castillo R, García-Fernández MA, Rodríguez-Creixems M, et al. Long-term outcome of infective endocarditis in non-intravenous drug users. Mayo Clin Proc. 2008;83(11):1213–7.

69. Fernández-Hidalgo N, Almirante B, Tornos P, González-Alujas MT, Planes AM, Galiñanes M, et al. Immediate and long-term outcome of left-sided infective endocarditis. A 12-year prospective study from a contemporary cohort in a referral hospital. Clin Microbiol Infect. 2012;18(12):E522–30.
70. Thuny F, Giorgi R, Habachi R, Ansaldi S, Le Dolley Y, Casalta JP, et al. Excess mortality and morbidity in patients surviving infective endocarditis. Am Heart J. 2012;164(1):94–101.
71. Mokhles MM, Ciampichetti I, Head SJ, Takkenberg JJ, Bogers AJ. Survival of surgically treated infective endocarditis: a comparison with the general Dutch population. Ann Thorac Surg. 2011;91(5):1407–12.
72. Ternhag A, Cederstrom A, Torner A, Westling K. A nationwide cohort study of mortality risk and long-term prognosis in infective endocarditis in Sweden. PLoS One. 2013;8(7):e67519.
73. Bannay A, Hoen B, Duval X, Obadia JF, Selton-Suty C, Le Moing V, et al. The impact of valve surgery on short- and long-term mortality in left-sided infective endocarditis: do differences in methodological approaches explain previous conflicting results? Eur Heart J. 2011;32(16): 2003–15.
74. Fedeli U, Schievano E, Buonfrate D, Pellizzer G, Spolaore P. Increasing incidence and mortality of infective endocarditis: a population-based study through a record-linkage system. BMC Infect Dis. 2011;11:48.

Part V
Complications

Chapter 9
Hemodynamic Complications in Infective Endocarditis

Bernard Iung

Abbreviations

AR   Aortic regurgitation
BNP   B-type natriuretic peptide
ICE   International collaboration on infective endocarditis
IE   Infective endocarditis
NYHA   New York Heart Association
MR   Mitral regurgitation

Introduction

Hemodynamic complications are frequent and particularly severe consequences of infective endocarditis (IE). Heart failure occurring during the acute phase of IE most often presents as acute heart failure due to valve destruction. Pathophysiologic features account for particularities in clinical or echocardiographic presentation which are important to consider in order to avoid any delay in diagnosis. Hemodynamic complications of IE may provide an indication for valvular surgery during acute IE, often according to an emergency or urgent timing.

Electronic supplementary material The online version of this chapter (doi:10.1007/978-3-319-32432-6_9) contains supplementary material, which is available to authorized users.

B. Iung, MD
Department of Cardiology, Hôpital Bichat, DHU Fire and Paris Diderot University,
Paris, France
e-mail: bernard.iung@bch.aphp.fr

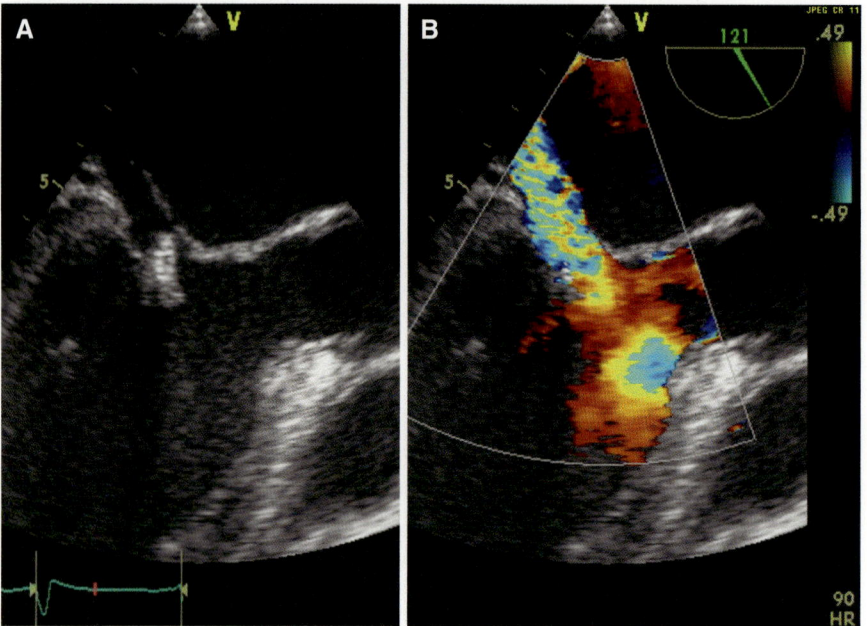

Fig. 9.1 (**a**, **b**). Endocarditis on a native mitral valve. Transesophageal echocardiography. (**a**) Perforation of the anterior leaflet with two adjacent vegetations. (**b**) Severe mitral regurgitation. See also Video 9.1

Pathophysiology

Valvular Lesions

The main mechanism involved in heart failure occurring during IE is acute regurgitation secondary to the direct consequences of infection of valvular tissue. The main structural lesions directly due to the infective process which cause regurgitation are leaflet perforation, leaflet tear, and chordal rupture on the mitral valve (Fig. 9.1a, b, Video 9.1). Similar leaflet lesions occur on the cusps of a bioprosthesis. Perivalvular lesions may also contribute to hemodynamic impairment when abscesses are fistulised in both upstream and downstream cardiac chambers, causing perivalvular regurgitations (Fig. 9.2a–c, Videos 9.2 and 9.3). Perivalvular lesions seldom result in severe regurgitations on native valves but are the main cause of severe regurgitations in prosthetic valve IE, in particular in the aortic position, and the only mechanism of regurgitation in IE on a mechanical prosthesis. Less frequently, fistulae may contribute to hemodynamic impairment through left-to-right shunts, for example between the aorta and right atrium.

Direct infection of valvular and/or perivalvular tissue explains the rapid development of regurgitation which is a specificity of IE and is a major difference with most other aetiologies of valvular regurgitations, which result in a slow process of chronic regurgitation.

Fig. 9.2 (**a–c**) Mycotic endocarditis (candida) on an aortic bioprosthesis. (**a**) Transthoracic echocardiography, parasternal short-axis view. Large and circumferential periprosthetic abscess. (**b**) Transthoracic echocardiography, parasternal short-axis view. Severe periprosthetic aortic regurgitation. (**c**) Transesophageal echocardiography: severe periprosthetic aortic regurgitation along the anterior leaflet of the mitral valve. See also Videos 9.2 and 9.3

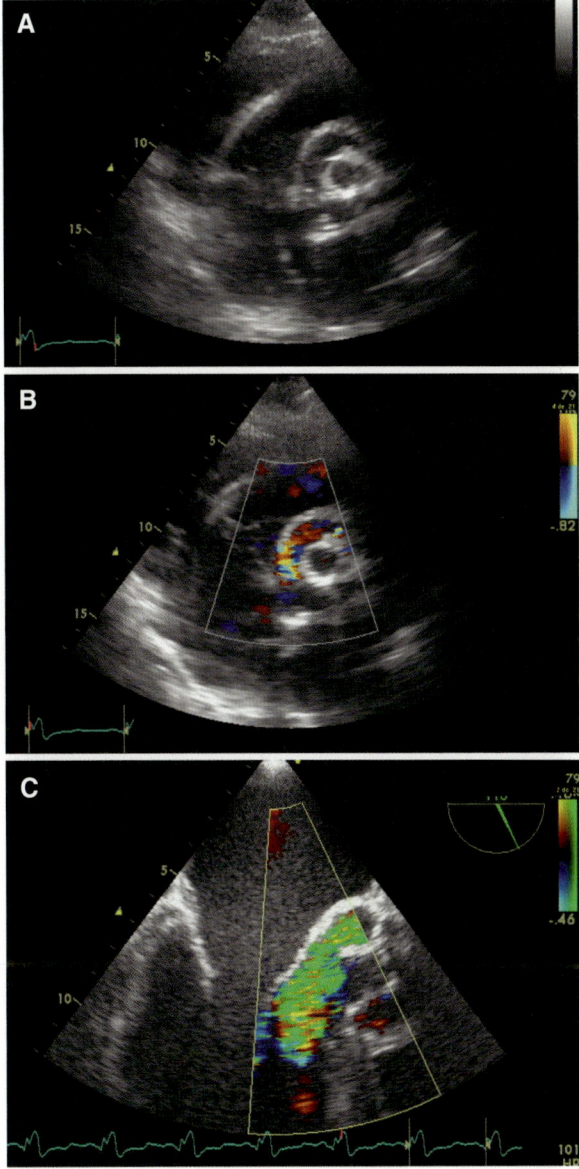

Hemodynamic Consequences

Despite differences between aortic regurgitation (AR) and mitral regurgitation (MR), the main hemodynamic features are common for acute AR and MR. They both result in left ventricular volume overload. However, acute regurgitations markedly differ from chronic regurgitations by the response of the left ventricle to volume overload.

In chronic regurgitation, progressive enlargement of the left ventricle allows for an increase in stroke volume which compensates for regurgitant volume, thereby enabling peripheral cardiac output to be preserved. In addition, despite left ventricular volume overload, the increase in end-diastolic left ventricular pressure is limited by compliance changes inherent to the enlargement of the left ventricular cavity. Limited impairment of cardiac output and filling pressures accounts for the good functional tolerance of chronic regurgitation, even when regurgitation is severe, provided left ventricular function is preserved.

In acute regurgitation, conversely, there is not enough time for the left ventricle to progressively enlarge in response to sudden volume overload [1]. Therefore, the absence of increase in forward stroke volume does not compensate for the regurgitant volume and peripheral cardiac output is decreased. Moreover, the non-dilated left ventricle cannot accommodate volume overload, which leads to a shift towards the steep part of the pressure-volume curve [1]. The sharp increase in left ventricular end-diastolic pressure largely offsets the positive hemodynamic effect of increased preload on stroke volume. Therefore, the two main components of hemodynamics, *i.e.* cardiac output and filling pressures, are rapidly and markedly impaired in acute regurgitation. In the absence of structural changes of the left ventricle, compensatory mechanisms are limited to the increase in sympathetic tone and the activation of the renin-angiotensin system [1]. This results in particular in tachycardia, which has a limited effect, and an increase in systemic vascular resistance increasing left ventricular afterload.

The rapid pressure increase in the upstream cavity (left ventricle for AR and left atrium for MR) and the simultaneous rapid pressure decrease in the downstream cavity (aorta for AR and left ventricle for MR) limits the pressure gradient driving regurgitation. This has important implications in patient presentation, accounting for frequent low-intensity and brief murmurs even in severe regurgitation [2, 3]. Rapid equalization of pressures also decreases orifice velocity and jet area, which may be misleading in the echocardiographic quantitation of regurgitation [2].

Additional consequences are specific to the location of valve regurgitation. They play a less important role in general hemodynamic impairment but account for particular features in clinical presentation. In acute AR, pulse pressure is not increased due to reduced forward stroke volume. The sharp increase in left ventricular end-diastolic pressure may cause premature closure of the mitral valve contributing to impaired left ventricular filling. Aortic regurgitant flow also accounts for a decrease in diastolic coronary perfusion and may cause myocardial ischaemia, in conjunction with increased myocardial oxygen consumption secondary to increased left ventricular filling pressures and tachycardia. In acute MR, regurgitation occurs in a non-dilated, non-compliant, left atrium. The increase in left atrium and pulmonary wedge pressures is therefore particularly pronounced [1].

Hemodynamic changes due to acute regurgitations may be influenced by pre-existing heart disease. Prior chronic valvular regurgitation associated with enlargement of the left ventricle tends to attenuate the consequences of superimposed acute regurgitation. Conversely, impairment of left ventricular compliance, for example in patients with hypertension or aortic stenosis, further worsens the tolerance of acute regurgitation.

Diagnosis

The diagnosis of hemodynamic complications of IE relies on two concomitant issues which are the diagnosis of IE and the diagnosis of heart failure. The attribution of a primary presentation of heart failure to IE may be difficult because of the highly polymorphic presentation of IE, in particular when signs of infection are not obvious. On the other hand, the diagnosis of heart failure may be missed or, more frequently, delayed in a patient primarily managed for IE, due to specificities of the presentation of heart failure in patients with acute IE.

Clinical Presentation

Clinical features of heart failure during IE are not specific and include the usual signs of left and/or right congestive heart failure. Dyspnea may be difficult to interpret in patients with severe sepsis. It is therefore necessary to systematically search for clinical and radiologic signs of congestion; biomarkers may also be useful in this setting.

Classically, cardiac murmur draws attention on the diagnosis of IE in patients presenting with sepsis and/or heart failure. Because of the specific pathophysiological features of acute regurgitation, cardiac murmurs are often of low-intensity and may be brief, occurring in early diastole for AR and in early systole for MR, which should not be misinterpreted as a marker of mild regurgitation. In a patient managed for IE, even mild and brief murmurs should raise the possibility of severe valvular dysfunction [1]. This highlights the need for careful daily clinical examination, in particular cardiac auscultation. This is particularly required in patients in whom rapid worsening of valvular regurgitation is a risk, such as those with staphylococcal IE. The awareness of mild changes in clinical cardiac examination during acute IE should prompt rapid investigation to avoid a delayed diagnosis at the stage of severe heart failure.

In acute AR, the reduced forward stroke volume accounts for a narrow pulse pressure and the lack of increased peripheral arterial pulsatility [1].

Cardiogenic shock is a less frequent presentation with hypotension and cutaneous signs reflecting vasoconstriction, which are the consequences of decreased cardiac output in acute valvular regurgitation. Differential diagnosis with septic shock may be difficult but is paramount given the different implications on patient management and outcome, in particular with regards to indications for early surgery [4, 5].

Electrocardiogram and Chest X-Ray

Electrocardiogram does not add a relevant contribution to the diagnosis of hemodynamic complications of IE in most cases. Sinus tachycardia is frequent but non-specific. Signs of left ventricular overload are often missing due to the rapid onset of left ventricular volume overload. However, repeated electrocardiograms are needed during IE to diagnose other complications, in particular conduction disturbances in aortic IE.

As in other heart failure settings, the main value of chest X-ray is to contribute to an early diagnosis by showing interstitial edema, which is generally not associated with pulmonary auscultation abnormalities. More severe heart failure is associated with alveolar edema. Signs of pulmonary congestion may be present even in patients with few or no symptoms in whom the diagnosis of heart failure may be missed otherwise [6]. Heart size is often normal, except in the case of pre-existing heart disease.

Echocardiography

When IE is revealed by acute heart failure, echocardiography plays a key role in the diagnosis of IE by showing specific lesions such as vegetations or abscesses which are major criteria in the Duke classification [7]. This is of particular importance when blood cultures are negative.

In a patient with known IE, the evaluation of valvular regurgitation and its hemodynamic consequences should take into account the pathophysiology of acute regurgitation. Spatial extension of the regurgitant jet, as assessed by colour Doppler, often tends to overestimate the degree of chronic regurgitation. Conversely, small areas of regurgitant jet may be observed in severe acute MR and eccentric jets may be difficult to quantitate (Fig. 9.3a, b, Videos 9.4 and 9.5) [8]. Quantitative measurements of effective regurgitant area and regurgitant volume may be influenced by loading conditions and the thresholds of severity used in chronic regurgitation have not been validated in acute regurgitation. In addition, even a "moderate" regurgitant volume may reflect severe regurgitation when it occurs in a non-dilated, noncompliant upstream cardiac chamber [8]. Semi-quantitative indices seem to be reliable in the setting of acute regurgitation [1, 2, 8]:

- vena contracta width >6 mm, holodiastolic flow reversal and short pressure half-time for AR (Fig. 9.4a–d, Videos 9.6 and 9.7),
- vena contracta width >7 mm and systolic pulmonary vein flow reversal for MR.

Potential difficulties in quantitating the severity of acute regurgitations highlight the need for an integrative approach combining different criteria for quantitation and an accurate assessment of the mechanisms of regurgitation. Transesophageal echocardiography should be widely considered in the assessment of patients presenting with acute regurgitation and/or acute IE [7].

The consequences of regurgitation should not be assessed from the size of cardiac chambers or left ventricular ejection fraction, which are often normal. Decreased cardiac output and, more importantly, increased systolic pulmonary pressure are reliable indices of poor hemodynamic tolerance of acute regurgitation. Premature mitral valve closure, as assessed by M-mode, is due to a marked increase in left ventricular diastolic pressure and is a marker of poor tolerance of acute AR [7].

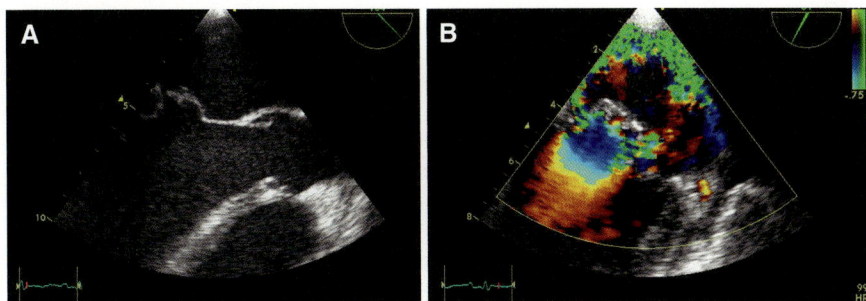

Fig. 9.3 (a, b) Endocarditis on a native mitral valve. Transesophageal echocardiography. (a) Paracommissural prolapse of the anterior leaflet (A3). (b) Eccentric regurgitant jet swirling in left atrium. See also Videos 9.4 and 9.5

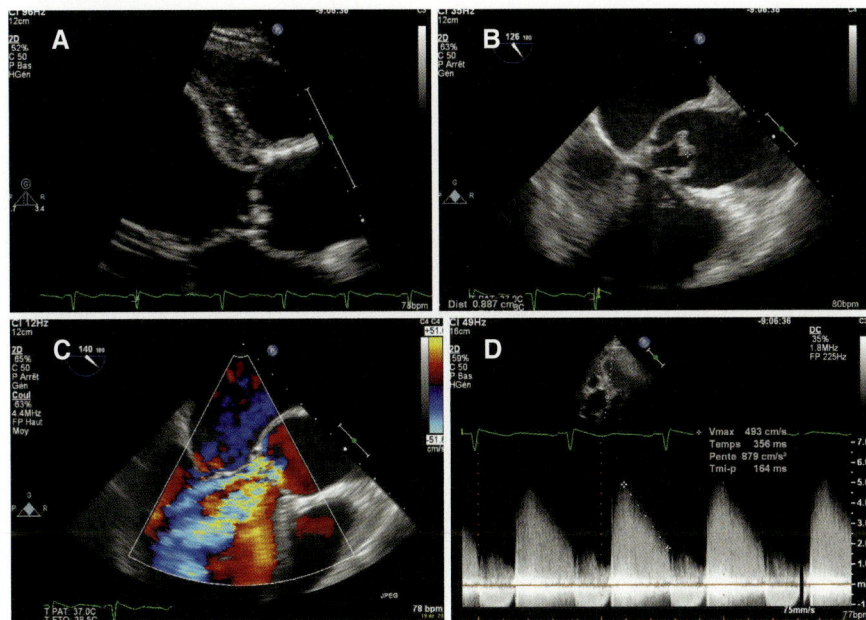

Fig. 9.4 (a–d) Endocarditis on a bicuspid aortic valve with severe regurgitation. (a) Transthoracic echocardiography, parasternal long-axis view. Vegetation on the posterior aortic cusp and prolapse of the anterior aortic cusp. (b) Transesophageal echocardiography: presence of two aortic vegetations on the anterior and posterior aortic cups. (c) Transesophageal echocardiography: severe regurgitation (vena contracta width 8 mm). (d) Doppler signal of the aortic jet with a short pressure half-time (164 ms). See also Videos 9.6 and 9.7

Biomarkers

Studies on B-type natriuretic peptide (BNP) in IE focused on their prognostic value [9]. BNP serum levels are particularly useful for the diagnosis of heart failure when symptoms may be difficult to interpret, for example in a context of severe sepsis or shock. Repeated assessments may contribute to an early diagnosis of hemodynamic decompensation.

Frequency of Heart Failure in Infective Endocarditis

The frequency of heart failure during IE is difficult to assess for different reasons. Firstly, the figures differ depending on whether the definition of heart failure is based on clinical signs of left or right congestive heart failure or New York Heart Association (NYHA) class. Secondly, referral bias is likely to occur in series from tertiary centres where patients are often referred because of complications. In a Spanish series, heart failure was diagnosed in 39 % of patients managed from the beginning of IE in a tertiary centre whereas its frequency was 68 % in patients who were transferred from another hospital [10].

Population-based series are theoretically the most suitable to estimate an unbiased frequency of heart failure but the few series available do not always report heart failure. Large multicentre registries are also informative. However, the lack of standardization of the definition of heart failure may account for discrepancies between series (Table 9.1) [6, 11–14]. Signs of congestive heart failure are reported in 15–36 % of patients, most often 30–35 %. NYHA class III-IV was reported in 22–52 % of patients. Discrepancies in rates of NYHA class may be due to difficulties in differentiating between NYHA class II and III dyspnea in patients hospitalized for IE, whose functional capacity is often limited by other factors than heart failure.

Prognostic Impact of Heart Failure

The overall relationship between heart failure and early, 1-year and long-term mortality has been shown in a number of series [13, 15–17]. Two specific analyses of

Table 9.1 Frequency of heart failure during acute infective endocarditis in population-based and multicentre series

	n=	Country	Years	Heart failure (%)	NYHA III–IV (%)
Population-based series					
Hoen et al. [11]	390	France	1999	34	–
Sy et al. [12]	1536	Australia	2000–2006	15	–
Selton-Suty et al. [13]	497	France	2008	34	22
Multicentre series/registries					
Kiefer et al. [6]	4075	International (ICE)	2000–2006	33	22
Tornos et al. [14]	159	Europe (Euro Heart Survey)	2001 (4 months)	36	52

NYHA New York Heart Association

ICE international collaboration on infective endocarditis

heart failure in IE have been issued from a tertiary centre on 259 patients and from the International Collaboration on Endocarditis (ICE) prospective cohort in 4075 patients [6, 18]. Of these 108 (42 %) and 1359 (34 %) patients were classified as having heart failure during index hospitalization, respectively. The strong relationship between heart failure and severe regurgitation, in contrast with the absence of significant difference in left ventricular ejection fraction, further highlights the key role of acute valvular regurgitation [18]. Both series reported consistent findings with in-hospital mortality rates of 24 % vs. 13 % and 30 % vs. 13 % in patients with and without heart failure, respectively. 1-year mortality was 37 % vs. 25 % [18].

The relationship between heart failure and outcome should take into account confounding factors since patients with heart failure also differ by other prognostic factors: older age, more frequent comorbidities, healthcare-associated IE and perivalvular complications, from those without heart failure [6, 18]. The prognosis of patients with heart failure is also dramatically influenced by the performance of early surgery. The relationship between heart failure and in-hospital and 1-year mortality remains, however, significant in multivariate analysis adjusting for patient characteristics, other complications of IE and the performance of early surgery [18].

The prognostic impact of heart failure is also attested in multivariate models aiming at predicting survival or adverse events in IE. Beyond the identification of predictive factors, their combination in multivariate models, which are then applied to other samples, validates the robustness of the predictive factors identified. Three multivariate scoring systems have been described in IE and validated on independent samples. Two models identified heart failure as an independent predictive factor of 6-month mortality [19, 20] with consistent adjusted hazard ratios between 2.1 and 2.6. Hazard ratio was higher (9.0) for patients presenting with heart failure at day 15, illustrating the particularly poor prognosis of persistent heart failure in IE [20]. In another externally validated model, heart failure at admission was a strong independent predictive factor of death or surgery during in-hospital stay, with an adjusted odds-ratio of 2.3 [21, 22].

A recent study suggested that serum BNP levels on admission have an incremental predictive value of in-hospital death over usual clinical, microbiological and echocardiographic variables, but these findings need to be confirmed in larger populations [9].

Impact of Early Surgery in Patients with Heart Failure

Early surgery was associated with a survival benefit in the two series analyzing patients with IE and heart failure [6, 18]. In the single-centre series of 259 patients, of whom 108 had heart failure, early surgery was associated with improved 1-year survival in multivariate analysis (adjusted hazard ratio 0.45, 95 % CI [0.22–0.93]) [18]. In the 1359 patients with heart failure in the ICE cohort, 1-year survival was 29 % in patients undergoing early surgery *vs.* 58 % in those who did not. In a propensity score-adjusted analysis, early surgery remained associated with a borderline reduction of in-hospital mortality (adjusted hazard-ratio 0.76, 95 % CI [0.58–0.99]) and a more pronounced reduction of 1-year mortality (adjusted hazard-ratio 0.44, 95 % CI [0.34–0.56]) [6].

Unlike for the prevention of embolism, no randomized trial has assessed the benefit of early surgery in patients with IE and heart failure. The assessment of the benefit of early surgery in IE from observational series is subject to a number of biases [23]. The long-term benefit of early surgery may be offset by operative mortality when analyzing only in-hospital outcome. At least 6-month follow-up is required to evaluate the benefit of early surgery [24]. The consistent benefit of early surgery on mid-term survival in patients with heart failure is a strong argument supporting wide indications for surgery in this context. A propensity-matched analysis accounting for differences in patient characteristics showed that the benefit of early surgery on 6-month survival was particularly pronounced in patients with moderate to severe heart failure [25].

Patients with cardiogenic shock have a particularly poor prognosis and derive benefit from early surgery, whereas surgery is associated with poor outcome in patients with septic shock [4]. This highlights the importance of an accurate early diagnosis of the respective contribution of complications of IE in critically ill patients.

Indications for Surgery in Patients with Heart Failure

Indications for early surgery in IE are detailed in Chap. 8. With regards to heart failure, European and American guidelines are fairly consistent in providing strong recommendations (class I) to operate on patients with symptoms of heart failure or cardiogenic shock caused by severe regurgitation or fistulae [3, 26]. In case of refractory pulmonary edema or cardiogenic shock, ESC guidelines advise emergency surgery, i.e., within 24 h [26]. Indications are debated in patients with severe AR or MR without heart failure. The poor hemodynamic tolerance of severe acute regurgitations is an incentive to consider early surgery before heart failure onset, in particular for severe AR and when the predicted operative risk is low.

Among patients operated during the acute phase of IE, heart failure represents the most frequent indication for surgery [13–15, 27]. This is in accordance with the high percentage of patients with heart failure, over 40 % in most series comparing the characteristics of operated and non-operated patients (Table 9.2) [14, 24, 25, 28–35]. This is also consistent with the high frequency of new-onset or severe valvular regurgitation in operated patients. However, heart failure is present in 10–30 % of non-operated patients, thereby raising concerns about the appropriateness of the management of patients with IE in practice.

A French Survey showed that certain patients with IE complicated by heart failure were inappropriately denied surgery [36]. In a recent study from the ICE cohort, 74 % of patients had a theoretical indication for surgery during the acute phase of IE [35]. The presence of new heart failure in NYHA class III or IV was associated with more frequent performance of surgery. Nevertheless, surgery was not performed in

24% of patients who had an indication. This may be due to comorbidities, which were more frequent in non-operated than in operated patients and to the fact that the most frequent reason for not performing surgery was a poor prognosis regardless of treatment, in 34% of patients. However, hemodynamic instability was given as the reason for not performing surgery in 20% of patients [35]. Hemodynamic instability increases operative risk but these patients also have a particularly poor spontaneous prognosis. Risk-benefit analysis favours indications for early surgery when hemodynamics is compromised by the consequences of valvular lesions [4]. Decision-making is difficult in acute IE due to the number of variables which may influence spontaneous prognosis and operative mortality. The use of a specific risk score contributes to improve the evaluation of operative mortality [37]. However, patients should not be denied surgery on the basis of a high operative risk alone. Patients with complicated IE often have both high operative risk and high mortality in the absence of surgery. In the ICE cohort, patients who did not undergo surgery despite a theoretical indication and who had a high predicted mortality were those who had the worst outcomes [35]. The poor prognosis of non-operated patients despite theoretical indications is also attested in critically ill patients [38].

Hemodynamic Complications During Follow-Up

Valvular lesions due to IE may be well-tolerated during the acute phase when regurgitation is not severe. Residual valvular lesions require close follow-up to allow for timely elective surgery. Indications are the same as for other chronic valvular diseases and are mainly based on the quantitation of regurgitation severity, symptoms and consequences on the left ventricle [3, 39].

A large population-based Asian study showed that patients still experience higher rates of cardiovascular events during long-term follow-up after IE, as compared with a propensity-matched control cohort [40]. The risk of readmission for heart failure was doubled (hazard ratio 2.2, 95% CI 2.0–2.4) in survivors of IE [40]. The excess risk was mainly observed during the first year following hospital discharge, underlining the need for a close follow-up after the acute phase of IE. In a single-centre study on 226 patients who survived more than 1 year after initial IE, heart failure and sudden death due to arrhythmias accounted for 19% of all deaths occurring during long-term follow-up, up to 20 years [16].

In conclusion, the frequency and prognostic impact of heart failure complications in IE highlight the need for prompt diagnosis and management, in particular the consideration of early surgery. Frequent difficulties in the diagnosis of heart failure and in risk-benefit analysis of early surgery highlight the need for multidisciplinary management in an endocarditis team before the occurrence of refractory heart failure or cardiogenic shock.

Table 9.2 Frequency of heart failure and valvular regurgitation during acute infective endocarditis in non-operated and operated patients

		Non-operated patients	Operated patients
Vikram et al.[25]	n=	283	230
	Congestive heart failure (%)	35	53
	New regurgitation (%)	53	74
Tornos et al. [14]	n=	77	82
	NYHA III–IV (%)	44	59
	Congestive heart failure (%)	31	41
Wang et al. [28]	n=	207	148
	Congestive heart failure (%)	28	53
Aksoy et al. [29]	n=	255	78
	NYHA III–IV (%)	10	37
	New AR (%)	15	36
	New MR (%)	38	45
Tleyjeh et al. [30]	n=	417	129
	NYHA III–IV (%)	20	39
	Severe regurgitation (%)	15	43
Sy et al. [31]	n=	161	62
	NYHA III–IV (%)	24	44
	Severe regurgitation (%)	40	73
Lalani et al. [32]	n=	832	720
	Congestive heart failure (%)	25	45
	Pulmonary edema (%)	15	28
	New regurgitation (%)	60	86
Bannay et al. [24]	n=	209	240
	Heart failure (%)	26	43
	Valvular regurgitation (%)	85	90
Galvez-Acebal et al. [33]	n=	602	417
	NYHA III–IV (%)	23	66
	Moderate-severe AR (%)	28	59
	Moderate-severe MR (%)	38	44
Martinez-Selles et al. [34]	n=	563	437
	Heart failure (%)	32	52
Chu et al. [35]	n=	552	733
	NYHA III–IV (%)	11	35
	New/worsening heart failure (%)	17	49
	Severe AR (%)	7	33
	Severe MR (%)	18	31

NYHA New York Heart Association

References

1. Stout KK, Verrier ED. Acute valvular regurgitation. Circulation. 2009;119(25):3232–41.
2. Zoghbi WA, Enriquez-Sarano M, Foster E, Grayburn PA, Kraft CD, Levine RA, Nihoyannopoulos P, Otto CM, Quinones MA, Rakowski H, Stewart WJ, Waggoner A, Weissman NJ. Recommendations for evaluation of the severity of native valvular regurgitation with two-dimensional and Doppler echocardiography. J Am Soc Echocardiogr. 2003;16(7): 777–802.
3. Nishimura RA, Otto CM, Bonow RO, Carabello BA, Erwin 3rd JP, Guyton RA, O'Gara PT, Ruiz CE, Skubas NJ, Sorajja P, Sundt 3rd TM, Thomas JD. 2014 AHA/ACC Guideline for the Management of Patients With Valvular Heart Disease: a report of the American College of Cardiology/American Heart Association Task Force on Practice Guidelines. Circulation. 2014;129(23):e521–643.
4. Gelsomino S, Maessen JG, van der Veen F, Livi U, Renzulli A, Luca F, Carella R, Crudeli E, Rubino A, Rostagno C, Russo C, Borghetti V, Beghi C, De Bonis M, Gensini GF, Lorusso R. Emergency surgery for native mitral valve endocarditis: the impact of septic and cardiogenic shock. Ann Thorac Surg. 2012;93(5):1469–76.
5. Olmos C, Vilacosta I, Fernandez C, Lopez J, Sarria C, Ferrera C, Revilla A, Silva J, Vivas D, Gonzalez I, San Roman JA. Contemporary epidemiology and prognosis of septic shock in infective endocarditis. Eur Heart J. 2013;34(26):1999–2006.
6. Kiefer T, Park L, Tribouilloy C, Cortes C, Casillo R, Chu V, Delahaye F, Durante-Mangoni E, Edathodu J, Falces C, Logar M, Miro JM, Naber C, Tripodi MF, Murdoch DR, Moreillon P, Utili R, Wang A. Association between valvular surgery and mortality among patients with infective endocarditis complicated by heart failure. JAMA. 2011;306(20):2239–47.
7. Habib G, Badano L, Tribouilloy C, Vilacosta I, Zamorano JL, Galderisi M, Voigt JU, Sicari R, Cosyns B, Fox K, Aakhus S. Recommendations for the practice of echocardiography in infective endocarditis. Eur J Echocardiogr. 2010;11(2):202–19.
8. Lancellotti P, Tribouilloy C, Hagendorff A, Popescu BA, Edvardsen T, Pierard LA, Badano L, Zamorano JL. Recommendations for the echocardiographic assessment of native valvular regurgitation: an executive summary from the European Association of Cardiovascular Imaging. Eur Heart J Cardiovasc Imaging. 2013;14(7):611–44.
9. Siciliano RF, Gualandro DM, Mueller C, Seguro LF, Goldstein PG, Strabelli TM, Arias V, Accorsi TA, Grinberg M, Mansur AJ, De Oliveira Jr MT. Incremental value of B-type natriuretic peptide for early risk prediction of infective endocarditis. Int J Infect Dis. 2014;29: 120–4.
10. Fernandez-Hidalgo N, Almirante B, Tornos P, Gonzalez-Alujas MT, Planes AM, Larrosa MN, Sambola A, Igual A, Pahissa A. Prognosis of left-sided infective endocarditis in patients transferred to a tertiary-care hospital--prospective analysis of referral bias and influence of inadequate antimicrobial treatment. Clin Microbiol Infect. 2011;17(5):769–75.
11. Hoen B, Alla F, Selton-Suty C, Beguinot I, Bouvet A, Briancon S, Casalta JP, Danchin N, Delahaye F, Etienne J, Le Moing V, Leport C, Mainardi JL, Ruimy R, Vandenesch F. Changing profile of infective endocarditis: results of a 1-year survey in France. JAMA. 2002;288(1): 75–81.
12. Sy RW, Kritharides L. Health care exposure and age in infective endocarditis: results of a contemporary population-based profile of 1536 patients in Australia. Eur Heart J. 2010;31(15): 1890–7.
13. Selton-Suty C, Celard M, Le Moing V, Doco-Lecompte T, Chirouze C, Iung B, Strady C, Revest M, Vandenesch F, Bouvet A, Delahaye F, Alla F, Duval X, Hoen B. Preeminence of Staphylococcus aureus in infective endocarditis: a 1-year population-based survey. Clin Infect Dis. 2012;54(9):1230–9.
14. Tornos P, Iung B, Permanyer-Miralda G, Baron G, Delahaye F, Gohlke-Barwolf C, Butchart EG, Ravaud P, Vahanian A. Infective endocarditis in Europe: lessons from the Euro heart survey. Heart. 2005;91(5):571–5.

15. Thuny F, Di Salvo G, Belliard O, Avierinos JF, Pergola V, Rosenberg V, Casalta JP, Gouvernet J, Derumeaux G, Iarussi D, Ambrosi P, Calabro R, Riberi A, Collart F, Metras D, Lepidi H, Raoult D, Harle JR, Weiller PJ, Cohen A, Habib G. Risk of embolism and death in infective endocarditis: prognostic value of echocardiography: a prospective multicenter study. Circulation. 2005;112(1):69–75.
16. Heiro M, Helenius H, Hurme S, Savunen T, Metsarinne K, Engblom E, Nikoskelainen J, Kotilainen P. Long-term outcome of infective endocarditis: a study on patients surviving over one year after the initial episode treated in a Finnish teaching hospital during 25 years. BMC Infect Dis. 2008;8:49.
17. Galvez-Acebal J, Rodriguez-Bano J, Martinez-Marcos FJ, Reguera JM, Plata A, Ruiz J, Marquez M, Lomas JM, de la Torre-Lima J, Hidalgo-Tenorio C, de Alarcon A. Prognostic factors in left-sided endocarditis: results from the Andalusian multicenter cohort. BMC Infect Dis. 2010;10:17.
18. Nadji G, Rusinaru D, Remadi JP, Jeu A, Sorel C, Tribouilloy C. Heart failure in left-sided native valve infective endocarditis: characteristics, prognosis, and results of surgical treatment. Eur J Heart Fail. 2009;11(7):668–75.
19. Hasbun R, Vikram HR, Barakat LA, Buenconsejo J, Quagliarello VJ. Complicated left-sided native valve endocarditis in adults: risk classification for mortality. JAMA. 2003;289(15): 1933–40.
20. Sy RW, Chawantanpipat C, Richmond DR, Kritharides L. Development and validation of a time-dependent risk model for predicting mortality in infective endocarditis. Eur Heart J. 2011;32(16):2016–26.
21. San Roman JA, Lopez J, Vilacosta I, Luaces M, Sarria C, Revilla A, Ronderos R, Stoermann W, Gomez I, Fernandez-Aviles F. Prognostic stratification of patients with left-sided endocarditis determined at admission. Am J Med. 2007;120(4):369 e1–7.
22. Lopez J, Fernandez-Hidalgo N, Revilla A, Vilacosta I, Tornos P, Almirante B, Sevilla T, Gomez I, Pozo E, Sarria C, San Roman JA. Internal and external validation of a model to predict adverse outcomes in patients with left-sided infective endocarditis. Heart. 2011;97(14): 1138–42.
23. Delahaye F. Is early surgery beneficial in infective endocarditis? A systematic review. Arch Cardiovasc Dis. 2011;104(1):35–44.
24. Bannay A, Hoen B, Duval X, Obadia JF, Selton-Suty C, Le Moing V, Tattevin P, Iung B, Delahaye F, Alla F. The impact of valve surgery on short- and long-term mortality in left-sided infective endocarditis: do differences in methodological approaches explain previous conflicting results? Eur Heart J. 2011;32(16):2003–15.
25. Vikram HR, Buenconsejo J, Hasbun R, Quagliarello VJ. Impact of valve surgery on 6-month mortality in adults with complicated, left-sided native valve endocarditis: a propensity analysis. JAMA. 2003;290(24):3207–14.
26. Habib G, Hoen B, Tornos P, Thuny F, Prendergast B, Vilacosta I, Moreillon P, de Jesus Antunes M, Thilen U, Lekakis J, Lengyel M, Muller L, Naber CK, Nihoyannopoulos P, Moritz A, Zamorano JL. Guidelines on the prevention, diagnosis, and treatment of infective endocarditis (new version 2009): the Task Force on the Prevention, Diagnosis, and Treatment of Infective Endocarditis of the European Society of Cardiology (ESC). Endorsed by the European Society of Clinical Microbiology and Infectious Diseases (ESCMID) and the International Society of Chemotherapy (ISC) for Infection and Cancer. Eur Heart J. 2009;30(19):2369–413.
27. Revilla A, Lopez J, Vilacosta I, Villacorta E, Rollan MJ, Echevarria JR, Carrascal Y, Di Stefano S, Fulquet E, Rodriguez E, Fiz L, San Roman JA. Clinical and prognostic profile of patients with infective endocarditis who need urgent surgery. Eur Heart J. 2007;28(1):65–71.
28. Wang A, Pappas P, Anstrom KJ, Abrutyn E, Fowler Jr VG, Hoen B, Miro JM, Corey GR, Olaison L, Stafford JA, Mestres CA, Cabell CH. The use and effect of surgical therapy for prosthetic valve infective endocarditis: a propensity analysis of a multicenter, international cohort. Am Heart J. 2005;150(5):1086–91.
29. Aksoy O, Sexton DJ, Wang A, Pappas PA, Kourany W, Chu V, Fowler Jr VG, Woods CW, Engemann JJ, Corey GR, Harding T, Cabell CH. Early surgery in patients with infective endocarditis: a propensity score analysis. Clin Infect Dis. 2007;44(3):364–72.

30. Tleyjeh IM, Ghomrawi HM, Steckelberg JM, Hoskin TL, Mirzoyev Z, Anavekar NS, Enders F, Moustafa S, Mookadam F, Huskins WC, Wilson WR, Baddour LM. The impact of valve surgery on 6-month mortality in left-sided infective endocarditis. Circulation. 2007;115(13): 1721–8.
31. Sy RW, Bannon PG, Bayfield MS, Brown C, Kritharides L. Survivor treatment selection bias and outcomes research: a case study of surgery in infective endocarditis. Circ Cardiovasc Qual Outcomes. 2009;2(5):469–74.
32. Lalani T, Cabell CH, Benjamin DK, Lasca O, Naber C, Fowler Jr VG, Corey GR, Chu VH, Fenely M, Pachirat O, Tan RS, Watkin R, Ionac A, Moreno A, Mestres CA, Casabe J, Chipigina N, Eisen DP, Spelman D, Delahaye F, Peterson G, Olaison L, Wang A. Analysis of the impact of early surgery on in-hospital mortality of native valve endocarditis: use of propensity score and instrumental variable methods to adjust for treatment-selection bias. Circulation. 2010;121(8):1005–13.
33. Galvez-Acebal J, Almendro-Delia M, Ruiz J, de Alarcon A, Martinez-Marcos FJ, Reguera JM, Ivanova-Georgieva R, Noureddine M, Plata A, Lomas JM, de la Torre-Lima J, Hidalgo-Tenorio C, Luque R, Rodriguez-Bano J. Influence of early surgical treatment on the prognosis of left-sided infective endocarditis: a multicenter cohort study. Mayo Clin Proc. 2014;89(10): 1397–405.
34. Martinez-Selles M, Munoz P, Arnaiz A, Moreno M, Galvez J, Rodriguez-Roda J, de Alarcon A, Garcia Cabrera E, Farinas MC, Miro JM, Montejo M, Moreno A, Ruiz-Morales J, Goenaga MA, Bouza E. Valve surgery in active infective endocarditis: a simple score to predict in-hospital prognosis. Int J Cardiol. 2014;175(1):133–7.
35. Chu VH, Park LP, Athan E, Delahaye F, Freiberger T, Lamas C, Miro JM, Mudrick DW, Strahilevitz J, Tribouilloy C, Durante-Mangoni E, Pericas JM, Fernandez-Hidalgo N, Nacinovich F, Rizk H, Krajinovic V, Giannitsioti E, Hurley JP, Hannan MM, Wang A. Association between surgical indications, operative risk, and clinical outcome in infective endocarditis: a prospective study from the International Collaboration on Endocarditis. Circulation. 2015;131(2):131–40.
36. Delahaye F, Rial MO, de Gevigney G, Ecochard R, Delaye J. A critical appraisal of the quality of the management of infective endocarditis. J Am Coll Cardiol. 1999;33(3):788–93.
37. Gaca JG, Sheng S, Daneshmand MA, O'Brien S, Rankin JS, Brennan JM, Hughes GC, Glower DD, Gammie JS, Smith PK. Outcomes for endocarditis surgery in North America: a simplified risk scoring system. J Thorac Cardiovasc Surg. 2011;141(1):98–106 e1–2.
38. Mirabel M, Sonneville R, Hajage D, Novy E, Tubach F, Vignon P, Perez P, Lavoue S, Kouatchet A, Pajot O, Mekontso-Dessap A, Tonnelier JM, Bollaert PE, Frat JP, Navellou JC, Hyvernat H, Hssain AA, Timsit JF, Megarbane B, Wolff M, Trouillet JL. Long-term outcomes and cardiac surgery in critically ill patients with infective endocarditis. Eur Heart J. 2014;35(18):1195–204.
39. The Joint Task Force on the Management of Valvular Heart Disease of the European Society of Cardiology (ESC), European Association for Cardio-Thoracic Surgery (EACTS), Vahanian A, Alfieri O, Andreotti F, Antunes MJ, Baron-Esquivias G, Baumgartner H, Borger MA, Carrel TP, De Bonis M, Evangelista A, Falk V, Iung B, Lancellotti P, Pierard L, Price S, Schafers HJ, Schuler G, Stepinska J, Swedberg K, Takkenberg J, Von Oppell UO, Windecker S, Zamorano JL, Zembala M, Bax JJ, Ceconi C, Dean V, Deaton C, Fagard R, Funck-Brentano C, Hasdai D, Hoes A, Kirchhof P, Knuuti J, Kolh P, McDonagh T, Moulin C, Popescu BA, Reiner Z, Sechtem U, Sirnes PA, Tendera M, Torbicki A, Von Segesser L, Badano LP, Bunc M, Claeys MJ, Drinkovic N, Filippatos G, Habib G, Kappetein AP, Kassab R, Lip GY, Moat N, Nickenig G, Otto CM, Pepper J, Piazza N, Pieper PG, Rosenhek R, Shuka N, Schwammenthal E, Schwitter J, Mas PT, Trindade PT, Walther T. Guidelines on the management of valvular heart disease (version, 2012). Eur Heart J. 2012;33(19):2451–96.
40. Shih CJ, Chu H, Chao PW, Lee YJ, Kuo SC, Li SY, Tarng DC, Yang CY, Yang WC, Ou SM, Chen YT. Long-term clinical outcome of major adverse cardiac events in survivors of infective endocarditis: a nationwide population-based study. Circulation. 2014;130(19):1684–91.

Chapter 10
Infectious Complications in Infective Endocarditis

Bradley Hayley and Kwan Leung Chan

Introduction

Infective endocarditis (IE) has intrigued the medical profession for many years because it mimics many diseases and a prompt diagnosis remains a challenge even in the present day. It is a serious medical condition with high in-hospital morbidity and mortality. In addition, the short term outcome is compromised after discharge from hospital [1]. Traditionally, the disease has been categorized into acute and subacute endocarditis based on the acuity of presentation and disease progression which are a result of the virulence of the infecting organism and the presence of pre-existing co-morbidities in the patient [2]. With advancement in the diagnosis and effective treatment, this categorization has become less clinically important and a greater focus should be on the early and comprehensive assessment of the destructive process of IE which will be crucial to the management such as the appropriateness and timing of early surgery. In this chapter our aims are to examine the myriad intracardiac complications due to endocarditis, and to discuss the risk factors and management issues in dealing with these complications.

Infective endocarditis can cause both acute and chronic impairment. Despite successful treatment with appropriate antimicrobial therapy, significant sequelae, both cardiac and non-cardiac, can develop. The major non-cardiac complications are listed in Table 10.1 and are discussed in other chapters of the book. The cardiac complications, in particular the valvular and perivalvular complications, are listed in Table 10.2. The acute complications tend to occur during the early days of the

B. Hayley, MD
Division of Cardiology, The Health Sciences Centre, Memorial University,
St. John's, Newfoundland and Labrador, Canada
e-mail: Brad.hayley@med.mun.ca

K. Leung Chan, MD, FRCPC, FAHA, FACC (✉)
Department of Cardiology, University of Ottawa Heart Institute, Ottawa, ON, Canada
e-mail: kchan@ottawaheart.ca

© Springer International Publishing Switzerland 2016
G. Habib (ed.), *Infective Endocarditis*, DOI 10.1007/978-3-319-32432-6_10

Table 10.1 Systemic sequelae of infective endocarditis

Neurological	Brain abscess, encephalitis, meningitis, embolic infarct, infective intracranial aneurysm, intracranial hemorrhage
Pulmonary	Diffuse alveolar damage, infarct, abscess, emphysema
Gastrointestinal	Hepatic or splenic infarct or abscess, hemorrhage, bowel ischemia from embolism or hypoperfusion, cholestasis
Renal	Glomerulonephritis, infarct, abscess
Others	Sepsis, vasculitis, osteomyelitis, immune complex pneumonia

Table 10.2 Valvular and perivalvular complications of infectious endocarditis

	Valvular	Perivalvular
Acute	Vegetations	Annular abscess
	Leaflet erosion or restriction	Myocardial abscess
	Leaflet or chordal tear	Conduction block
	Leaflet diverticulum or aneurysm	Erosion or compression of coronary arteries
	Perforation	Perivalvular regurgitation
		Pericarditis
		Hemopericardium
Chronic	Fibrosis	Perivalvular regurgitation
	Nodular calcification	Pseudoaneurysm
	Leaflet diverticulum or aneurysm	Fistula
	Perforation	

disease, while the chronic complications develop after the infection has been ongoing for some time, usually days to weeks, but can occur weeks to months after the infection has been treated or even after surgical intervention [3, 4]. Cardiac surgery in these patients not only has the up-front risks of a surgical procedure, but also carries potential long term complications such as reinfection, need for anticoagulation, recurrent regurgitation, and prosthetic device failure [4].

Valvular Complications

Anatomically normal cardiac structures are generally resistant to infectious colonization and do not allow microorganisms to adhere to their endothelium [5]. Pre-existent structural abnormalities may predispose to formation of sterile vegetations composed of fibrin and platelets that may be colonized by circulating microbes further compromising cardiac structures through release of inflammatory mediators. Bacteria such as Streptococci and Staphylocci are innately capable of adhering to vegetations and in some cases even to normal endothelium [5]. Approximately 75 % of patients diagnosed with bacterial endocarditis have a pre-existing cardiac abnormality [6]. Rheumatic heart disease is the most common anatomical condition

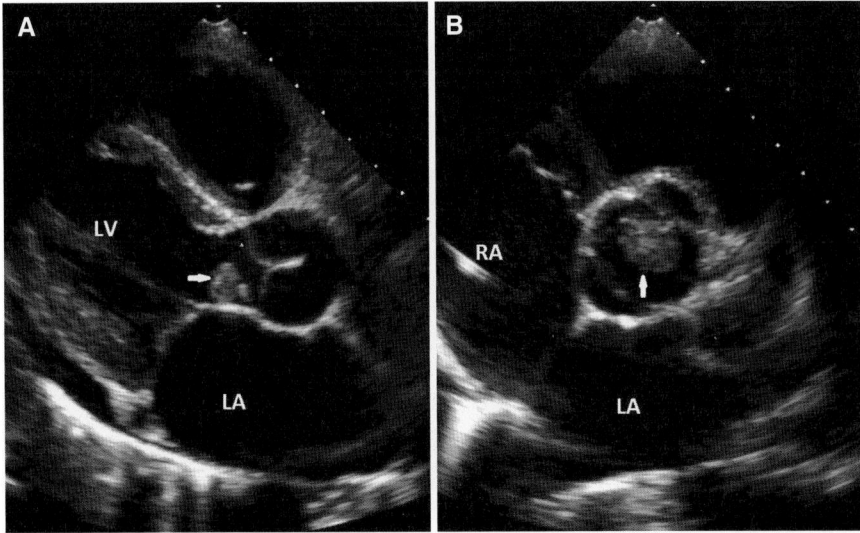

Fig. 10.1 A large vegetation (*arrow*) on the aortic valve in a patient with bicuspid aortic valve is demonstrated in both the transthoracic long-axis (**a**) and short-axis (**b**) views. *LA* left atrium, *LV* left ventricle, *RA* right atrium

in nonindustrial countries but only accounts for 10 % of cases in industrialized countries in which degenerative lesions predominate [1]. A vast array of structural complications may ensue and can result in significant hemodynamic consequences to the patient.

Vegetation

Vegetation is the hallmark of IE and should be recognized as the nidus of a destructive process that needs to be treated with prompt and appropriate antibiotic therapy (Fig. 10.1a, b). This process is dynamic and inflammatory responses are intimately involved. The valve leaflets are usually affected, but the other structures can also be involved including the chords, myocardium, perivalvular tissue and implanted leads or conduits. In the acute settings, vegetations lead to leaflet erosion or chordal rupture due to their predilection to the leaflet closure region resulting in valvular regurgitation. With proper medical treatment, vegetations generally regress with time and become more echodense, in tandem with a dramatic decrease in the embolic risk [3]. Nonetheless <10 % of the affected valves retains normal morphology and function, and the vast majority develop regurgitation due to the development of fibrosis, leaflet retraction and nodular calcification [7]. Valvular stenosis is uncommon, but can be present in patients with large vegetations usually caused by *Staphylococcus aureus* or fungi [8].

Fig. 10.2 The aneurysm (*arrow*) at the posterior mitral leaflet is demonstrated from the left atrial perspective by 3-D transesophageal echocardiography. There is a perforation at the belly of the aneurysm. *AML* anterior mitral leaflet, *AV* aortic valve, *PML* posterior mitral leaflet

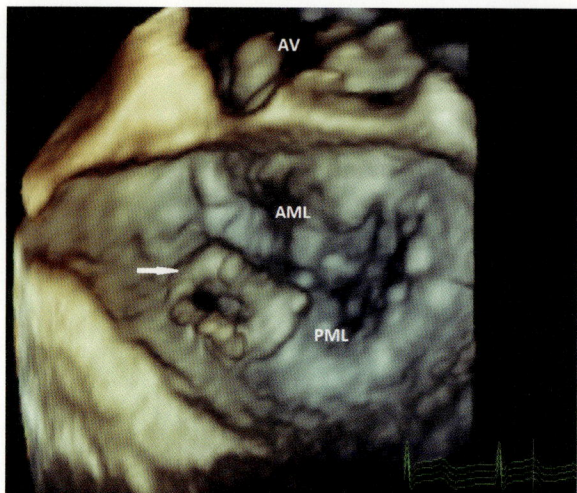

Leaflet Aneurysm and Perforation

Leaflet perforation is an important complication to recognize since it is frequently associated with significant regurgitation and heart failure [9]. Regurgitation in this setting is usually eccentric with the origin of the regurgitation jet away from the site of leaflet coaptation. Leaflet perforation particularly with the mitral valve occurs in the setting of valvular aneurysm or diverticulum (Figs. 10.2 and 10.3). Thus, if a leaflet aneurysm or diverticulum is present, perforation within the structure should be sought. Perforation of the anterior mitral leaflet should also raise the alert that aortic valve IE may be present with the aortic regurgitant jet impinging onto the anterior mitral leaflet resulting in aneurismal formation and perforation [9, 10]. In patients in whom the infection has responded to medical treatment, valvular perforation may be amenable to patch repair.

Valvular Regurgitation

Valvular regurgitation is a frequent complication of IE and when a new regurgitant murmur is recognized as a diagnostic criterion in the modified Duke criteria [11]. Left sided regurgitant lesion may result in signs of left heart failure and pulmonary congestion, which are negative prognosticators in patients with endocarditis [12, 13]. Regurgitation from IE is more likely to occur in the aortic valve than the mitral valve, perhaps due to its higher rate of infection [13]. Clinically, aortic regurgitation is more likely to result in findings of congestive failure than patients with mitral regurgitation due to IE [13]. Acute valvular insufficiency may present with signs of cardiogenic shock without a prominent murmur due to rapid equalization of pressure between the aorta and left ventricle in the case of aortic regurgitation and left ventricle and the left atrium in the case of mitral regurgitation.

Fig. 10.3 Photography of excised mitral leaflet with aneurysm formation and multiple perforations involving the anterior mitral leaflet

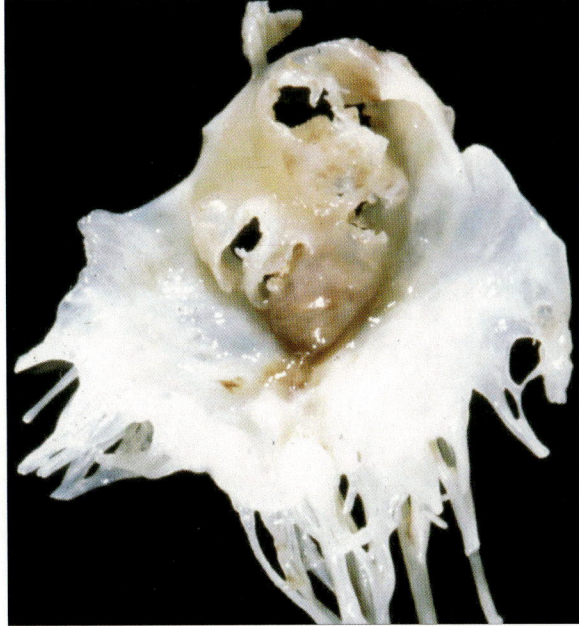

Right sided valve lesions often present more indolently even when acute severe regurgitation occurs. Tricuspid regurgitation is the most frequent right-sided valve lesion but rarely causes significant hemodynamic consequences by itself [14, 15]. Long standing severe tricuspid regurgitation may result in signs of right heart failure such as peripheral edema, pleural effusion and ascites. The pulmonic valve is relatively spared from infection with the exception of predisposing factors such as the tetralogy of Fallot or rheumatic heart disease [16].

Multiple mechanisms can be responsible for valvular regurgitation and often depend on the site of infection. Damage to supporting structures, such as chords, can result in chordal rupture with flail leaflet. Direct infection of the leaflet surface can result in the formation of diverticula that may predispose to leaflet perforation while damage to the leaflet tips may result in malcoaptation that can create a regurgitant orifice [12]. Although the mechanisms may differ, the clinical consequence is similar.

Valvular Stenosis

Endocarditis causing valvular stenosis is less frequently encountered than valvular regurgitation. In native valves, it occurs at <9 % of cases [8]. Prosthetic valves may become stenotic if large vegetations impact opening of the valve poppets and result in mechanical failure. Acute valve stenosis can result in heart failure or shock and could be accompanied by a systolic or diastolic murmur depending on the valve involved. Subacute stenosis may present with more gradual onset of symptoms with similar auscultatory findings.

Perivalvular Complications

Abscess

Perivalvular extension is a common complication in patients with IE and occurs in 10–40 % of patients with native valve IE, and the prevalence of perivalvular abscess is higher up to 56–100 % in prosthetic valve IE [17]. Baseline clinical characteristics such as sex, age, symptom duration and hemodynamic stability are similar in IE patients with and without perivalvular abscess. As well, IE patients with an abscess are not more likely to embolize once on antibiotic treatment [17]. However, severe valvular dysfunction and heart failure are more common in IE patients with perivalvular involvement. The risk factors associated with the development of perivalvular abscess are listed in Table 10.3 [17–19]. Abscess is more commonly seen in the aortic position and in intravenous drug users with left sided IE. The association with coagulase negative Staphyloccoci is mediated by the association with prosthetic valve IE, and the association with the presence of conduction block is a result of extension of the abscess to involve the conducting tissue.

Similar to vegetations, abscess is also a dynamic process. The periannular infection leads to necrosis and weakening of the adjacent tissue. Serial echocardiographic studies have demonstrated liquefaction and expansion of the perivalvular abscess, followed by cavitation and/or fistula communications or even drainage into the pericardial space [20, 21] (Fig. 10.4a–d).

We have reported on 43 consecutive patients with perivalvular abscess (native valve IE in 17 patients and prosthetic valve IE in 26 patients), 31 of whom underwent cardiac surgery and 12 received medical treatment alone due to prohibitive surgical risks. Transesophageal echocardiography was used to diagnose abscess and to follow-up the subsequent evolution of the perivalvular complications. Both groups had a high mortality in excess of 50 % at a mean follow-up of 4.8 years. Perivalvular complications such as pseudoaneurysms and fistulae developed in all the medically treated patients and in 10 of the 24 surgically treated patients [20]. Perivalvular complications were a predictor of reduced survival (hazard ratio 2.16) in spite of early surgery in the study by Aksoy et al. [22].

In summary, perivalvular abscess predicts a poor prognosis in patients with IE. These patients have a high incidence of perivalvular complication despite early

Table 10.3 Risk factors associated with development of perivalvular abscess

Risk factor	Relative risk	P value
Prosthetic valve	1.88	<0.01
Aortic position	1.81	< 0.01
Coagular negative staphylococci	1.77	< 0.05
Intravenous drug use	2.50	0.01
Heart block	2.66	< 0.01

Data from [17–19]

surgical intervention. They need to be closely monitored for evolution of the perivalvular infection process, even after surgical intervention. Furthermore, many of these patients would develop severe valvular regurgitation.

The microbiology of perivalvular abscess formation is diverse but largely similar to that for IE in general [17–19]. Many reports suggest that *Staphylococcus*

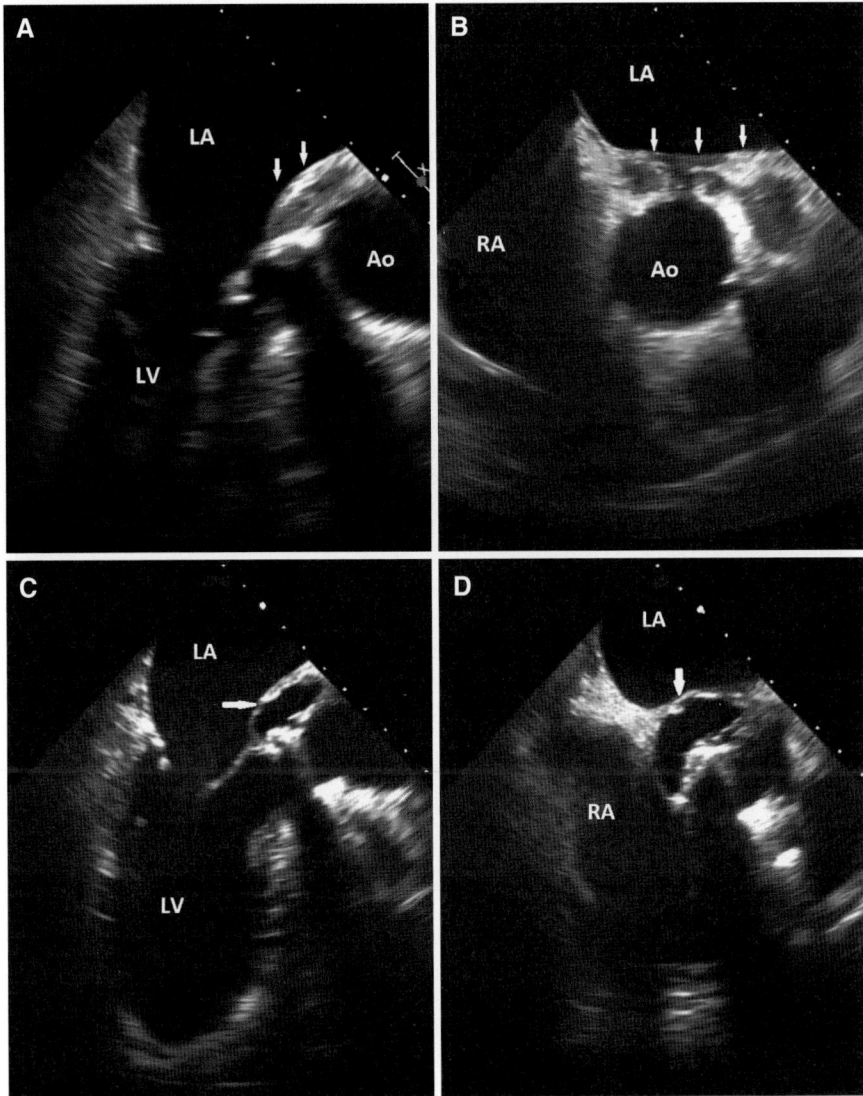

Fig. 10.4 An echolucent density (*arrows*) posterior to the aortic root consistent with a large abscess in the transesophageal echocardiogram long-axis (**a**) and short-axis (**b**) views. Two weeks later the long-axis (**c**) and short-axis (**d**) views show cavitation of the abscess to become a pseudoaneurysm (*arrow*) which communicates with the left ventricular outflow tract. *Ao* aorta, *LA* left atrium, *LV* left ventricle, *RA* right atrium

aureus is the most common organism in native valve IE complicated by perivalvular abscess, and coagulase negative staphylococci is a common pathogen in prosthetic valve IE with perivalvular abscess. Less frequent organisms include streptococci, enterococci and culture negative species such as the HACEK organisms. The diagnosis of fungi and less common microorganisms depends on astute clinical judgement and the result of serial blood cultures on specific media, although diagnostic imaging may occasionally gives clues to the etiologic agent.

Pseudoaneurysm

When an abscess begins to cavitate and expand, the weakened tissue may rupture and drain into the surrounding structures, resulting in the formation of pseudoaneurysm or fistula [20, 21] (Fig. 10.4a–d). In the case of periaortic abscess, communication with the aortic root is more likely than with the left ventricular outflow tract [20]. Fistula communication between the aorta and any of the four cardiac chambers can occur dependent on which of the aortic sinuses is involved by the abscess. We have observed that a perivalvular abscess can cavitate within 2 weeks and evolve into a pseudoaneurysm as early as 4 weeks following diagnosis [20]. Pseudoaneurysm is a pulsatile structure with an echolucent cavity that may contain debris associated with ongoing infection. It expands in systole and collapse in diastole when it communicates with the left ventricular outflow tract via the mitral-aortic intervalvular fibrosa (MAIVF), which is a relatively avascular structure situated between the aortic and mitral valves and is roofed by pericardium [22, 23]. In addition to direct extension of infection, MAIVF may be secondary traumatized and infected due to the impingement of an aortic regurgitant jet in the setting of aortic valve IE [4]. Pseudoaneurysm at MAIVF can also occur due to injury from valve implantation. Patients with bicuspid aortic valves may be more susceptible to develop pseudoaneurysm formation in the MAIVF because of intrinsic abnormalities of the connective tissue [24, 25].

Fistula

Fistula defines a communication between two cardiac chambers and is a serious complication of IE that can occur at multiple anatomic sites resulting in various hemodynamic effects [18, 26]. In patients with periaortic abscess, the central position of the aortic root enables fistula communication with any of the four cardiac chambers (Fig. 10.5a, b). Fistula formation is an indication of extensive tissue damage and not surprisingly half of the patients with aortic fistula would also have moderate or severe aortic regurgitation [26]. Patients with fistula have a higher incidence of congestive heart failure and a reduced survival, necessitating a greater need for surgical intervention [26, 27].

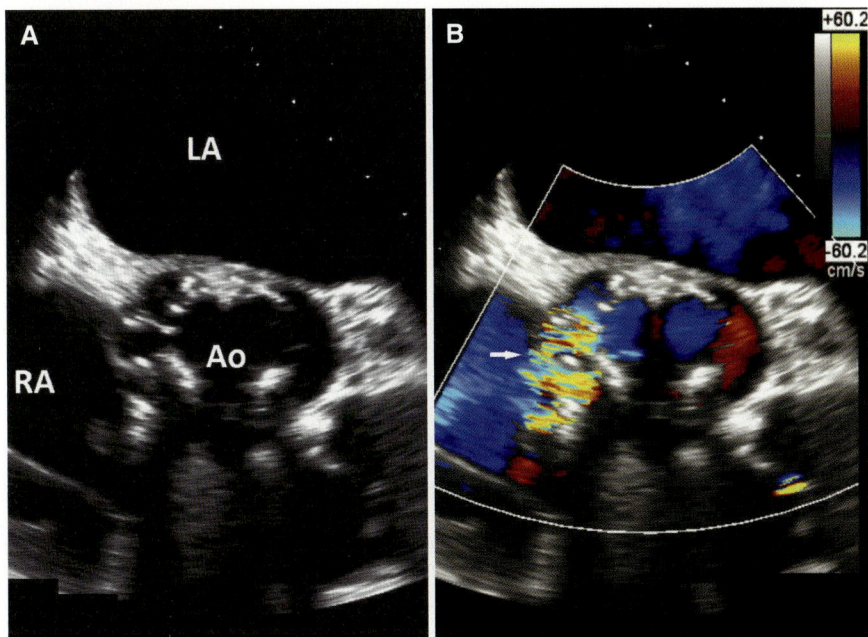

Fig. 10.5 (**a**) Transesophageal echocardiogram at the level of the aortic annulus in a patients with prosthetic aortic valve endocarditis. (**b**) Colour flow image shows a fistula (*arrow*) communicating the left ventricular outflow tract with the right atrium. *Ao* aorta, *LA* left atrium, *RA* right atrium

Valve Dehiscence

Valve dehiscence is a serious complication in patients with prosthetic valve IE. Destruction of the sewing ring may compromise the attachment of the prosthesis to the surrounding annulus. Perivalvular fistula may form in such situations and the patient's condition may range from clinically stable to cardiogenic shock from acute severe perivalvular insufficiency [28]. Dehiscence may also occur following valve implantation in IE patients with perivalvular complications. Reinfection is always a concern in this situation but non-infectious valve dehiscence is not uncommon in this clinical setting due to the friability of the annular tissue which does not allow secure anchoring of the sutures [29–32]. Although trivial or mild perivalvular regurgitation immediately post implant tends not to affect long term prognosis, significant leak may result in heart failure and the need for reoperation [29, 31].

Related Complications

Other serious complications may occur due to the perivalvular complications. The development of heart block is an indication of a periaortic abscess invading into the adjacent conduction system. Erosion and compression of the coronary arteries by a periaortic abscess can occur [33]. Extension or rupture into the pericardial space leading to cardiac tamponade is another rare but life threatening complication [34].

Imaging

Echocardiography

Echocardiography is a powerful tool for diagnosing perivalvular complications and 3-dimensional echocardiography has emerged as a promising imaging modality. Echocardiography is portable, relatively inexpensive and does not involve the use of ionizing radiation. Temporal and spatial resolution of ultrasound is high allowing visualization of small highly mobile vegetations. Transesophageal echocardiography (TEE) is superior to transthoracic echocardiography (TTE) in the detection of vegetation and abscess, but TEE is semi-invasive and has a small but definite risk (Table 10.3) [27, 30, 35–41].

Diagnosis of valvular vegetations by echocardiography relies on several important characteristics. Generally, vegetations are independently mobile echolucent masses located on valve surface adjacent to the closure region. The appearance may vary from serpiginous to sessile, making diagnosis challenging particular in the setting of suboptimal image quality, significant pre-existing valvular disease or artificial valves [35, 42]. Vegetations are small early in the disease course and can be missed on initial investigations [36, 37]. A high clinical suspicion of IE warrants repeat imaging in 7–10 days as progression of disease will become more evident over time [38].

A perivalvular abscess can often be detected by TTE or TEE based upon multiple imaging characteristics, many of which may be subtle. Annular thickening alone may be a clue to the presence of aortic root abscess with a value of 10 mm being reported as a specific but insensitive cut off. Echolucent areas adjacent to the valvular apparatus may signify abscess cavitation and increase the likelihood of the diagnosis [43] (Fig. 10.4a–d). TEE provides superior imaging of the perivalvular regions especially when prosthetic valves are implanted, although shielding from a prosthetic aortic valve may obscure the anterior aortic root which may be better visualized on TTE.

Pseudoaneurysm formation can often be visualized as an echo-lucent cavity communicating with the aorta or a cardiac chamber. Pulsatility of a cavity posterior to the aortic root adds to the diagnosis, as expansion during systole is indicative of connection with the left ventricular outflow tract and expansion in diastole is indicative of connection with the aortic root. Colour flow Doppler with the velocity scale reduced to detect low velocity flow can detect the communication even when it cannot be readily seen on 2D imaging [44] (Fig. 10.6a, b). An intracardiac fistula may

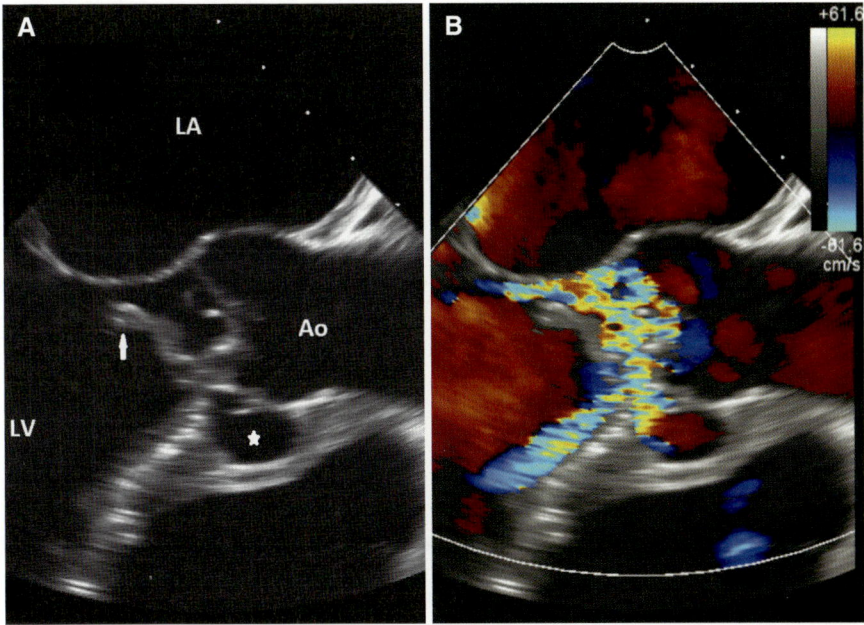

Fig. 10.6 (**a**) Aortic valve endocarditis with a large vegetation (*arrow*) and an echolucent cavity (*star*) anterior to the aortic root in the transesophageal long axis view. (**b**) Colour flow image shows severe perivalvular aortic regurgitation and communication between the aortic root and the aortic pseudoaneurysm. *Ao* aorta, *LA* left atrium, *LV* left ventricle

have similar appearance as a pseudoaneurysm which is now connecting two adjacent cardiac chambers [16]. Colour flow Doppler imaging will document a continuous flow from the high pressure chamber such as the left ventricle to a low pressure chamber such as the right atrium (Fig. 10.5a, b). A rocking motion of a prosthetic valve indicates valvular dehiscence [28]. Again, TEE imaging is superior to TTE in detecting the presence of a pseudoaneurysm and fistula (Table 10.4).

Computed Tomography (CT)

The spatial resolution of CT is excellent and thus CT may provide more detailed anatomical information regarding the structure of pseudoaneurysms, abscess cavities and fistulae [45]. Despite the advent of ultrafast scanners, CT still has limited temporal resolution compared to echocardiography, and has limited ability to detect valvular perforations and small intracardiac communications that are detectable by colour flow Doppler Imaging [45]. Other limitations of CT include the lack of portability, ionizing radiation and imaging artefacts from intracardiac devices and prosthetic valves.

Table 10.4 Sensitivities of transthoracic and transesophageal echocardiography in the detection of valvular and perivalvular involvement in infective endocarditis

	TTE	TEE
Native valve vegetation	44–63 %	87–100
Prosthetic valve vegetation	36–69 %	86–94 %
Fistula	53 %	97 %
Abscess	28–36 %	80–87 %
Pseudoaneurysm	43 %	90 %

TEE transesophageal echocardiogram, *TTE* transthoracic echocardiogram

Data from [27, 30, 35–40]

Treatment

The extent of tissue destruction and associated dysfunction has a crucial impact on the treatment of IE. Damage limited to valve leaflets with mild to moderate dysfunction can be treated medically provided the infecting microorganism is not resistant to the antibiotic therapy. Severe damage to the valve leaflet or the perivalvular structure usually leads to severe hemodynamic compromise requiring urgent surgical intervention [46]. In some situations, valve repair may be offered when the anatomy is favourable or the risk of re-infecting prosthetic material is high, such as in injection drug users. Prosthetic valve IEs are less likely to respond to antibiotic therapy alone and surgical intervention is frequently necessary, especially if valve dehiscence is present.

Most patients with severe perivalvular complications would require surgical intervention because of the aggressive nature of the infecting microorganism, the frequently associated hemodynamic derangement and the potential risk of rupture in the case of pseudoaneurysm and fistulae. Medical treatment alone may be effective in some of these patients, but they are likely the exception and no differentiating clinical features have been identified [20, 21].

The presence of perivalvular infection increases the complexity of any surgical treatment required to treat these patients. In addition to valve replacement, surgical drainage of perivalvular abscess, closure of fistula tracts and reconstruction using the pericardial patch may be necessary. Infection involving the origins of the coronary arteries may necessitate reimplantation or in some situations concurrent bypass surgery in conjunction with a root replacement procedure if debridement alone is not sufficient. The use of cryopreserved homografts with the accompanying aortomitral curtain and stentless valve conduits has been done when the tissue destruction is extensive [4].

References

1. Hoen B, Duval X. Clinical practice. Infective endocarditis. N Engl J Med. 2013;368(15): 1425–33.
2. Osler W. The principles and practice of medicine : designed for the use of practitioners and students of medicine. 14th ed. New York: Appletone; 1942.

3. Chan KL, Dumesnil JG, Cujec B, Sanfilippo AJ, Jue J, Turek MA, Robinson TI, Moher D. Investigators of the multicenter aspirin study in infective endocarditis a randomized trial of aspirin on the risk of embolic events in patients with infective endocarditis. J Am Coll Cardiol. 2003;42(5):775–80.
4. Kang N, Wan S, Ng CSH, Underwood MJ. Periannular extension of infective endocarditis. Ann Thorac Cardiovasc Surg. 2009;15(2):74–81.
5. Keynan Y, Rubinstein E. Pathophysiology of infective endocarditis. Curr Infect Dis Rep. 2013;15:342–6.
6. McKinsey DS, Ratts TE Bisno AL. Underlying cardiac lesions in adults with infective endocarditis the changing spectrum. Am J Med. 1987;82(4):681–8.
7. Rohmann S, Erbel R, Darius H, et al. Prediction of rapid versus prolonged healing of infective endocarditis by monitoring vegetation size. JASE. 1991;4:465–74.
8. Buchbinder NA, Roberts WC. Left-sided valvular active infective endocarditis. A study of forty-five necopsy patients. Am J Med. 1972;53(1):20–4.
9. Lester SJ, Wilansky S. Endocarditis and associated complications. Crit Care Med. 2007;35(8 Suppl):S384–91.
10. Anguera I, Miro JM, Evangelista A, Cabell CH, San Roman JA, et al. Periannular complications in infective endocarditis involving native aortic valves. Am J Cardiol. 2006;98:1254–60.
11. Li J, Sexton D, Mick N, et al. Proposed modifications of the duke criteria for the diagnosis of infective endocarditis. Clin Inf Dis. 2000;30:633–8.
12. Suty C, Celard M, Le Moing V, et al. Preeminence of staphylococcus aureus in infective endocarditis: a 1-year population-based survey. Clin Infect Dis. 2012;54(9):1230–9.
13. Hassine M, Boussada M, Tahar M, et al. Infective endocarditis complicated by heart failure: characteristics and prognosis. Arch Cardiovasc Dis Supp. 2015;7:44–57.
14. Chambers HF, Morris DL, Tauber MG, et al. Cocaine use and the risk for endocarditis in intravenous drug users. Ann Intern Med. 1987;106:833–6.
15. Moss R, Munt B. Injection drug use and right sided endocarditis. Heart. 2003;89:577–81.
16. Roberts WC, Buchbinder NA. Right-sided valvular infective endocarditis. A clinicopathologic study of twelve necopsy patients. Am J Med. 1972;53(1):7–19.
17. Graupner C, Vilacosta I, San Roman J, et al. Periannular extension of infective endocarditis. J Am Coll Cardiol. 2002;39(7):1204–11.
18. San Roman JA, Vilacosta I, Sarria C, et al. Clinical course, microbiologic profile, and diagnosis of periannular complications in prosthetic valve endocarditis. Am J Cardiol. 1999;83:1075–9.
19. Omani B, Shapiro S, Ginzton L, Robertson JM, Ward J, Nelson RJ, Bayer AS. Predictive risk factors for pericannular extension of native valve endocarditis. Clinical and echocardiographic analyses. Chest. 1989;96:1273–9.
20. Chan K. Early clinical and long-term outcomes of patients with infective endocarditis complicated by perivalvular abscess. CMAJ. 2002;167(1):19–24.
21. Byrd BF, Shelton ME, Wilson BH, Schillig S. Infective perivalvular abscess of the aortic ring: echocardiographic features and clinical course. Am J Cardiol. 1990;66:102–5.
22. Aksoy O, Sexton DJ, Wang A, Pappas PA, Kourany W, Chu V, Fowler Jr VG, Woods CW, Engemann JJ, Corey GR, Harding T, Cabell CH. Early surgery in patients with infective endocarditis: a propensity score analysis. Clin Infect Dis. 2007;44(3):364–72.
23. Pongratz G, Pohlmann M, Gehling G, Bachmann K. Images in cardiovascular medicine. Pseudoaneurysm in the intervalvular mitral-aortic region after endocarditis and prosthetic aortic valve replacement. Circulation. 1997;96:3241–2.
24. Xie M, Yuman L, Tsung O, et al. Pseudoaneurysm of the mitral-aortic intervalvular fibrosa. Int J Cardiol. 2013;166:2–7.
25. Bansal RC, Moloney PM, Marsa RJ, Jacobson JG. Echocardiographic features of a mycotic aneurysm of the left ventricular outflow tract caused by perforation of mitral-aortic intervalvular fibrosa. Circulation. 1983;67:930–4.
26. Tiwari KK, Murzi M, Mariani M, Glauber M. Giant pseudo-aneurysm of the left ventricle outflow tract after aortic root replacement for extensive endocarditis. Eur J Cardiothorac Surg. 2009;36:399.

27. Anguera I, Miro J, Vilacosta I, et al. Aorto-cavitary fistulous tract formation in infective endocarditis: clinical and echocardiographic features of 76 cases and risk factors for mortality. Eur Heart. 2005;26:288–97.
28. Krishna R, Casanova P, Larrauri-Reyes M, et al. Complete dehiscence and unseated prosthetic aortic valve causing severe aortic insufficiency: an unusual complication of prosthetic valve endocarditis. BMJ Case Rep. 2014; 206925.
29. Mullany CJ, Chua YL, Schaff HV, Steckelberg JM, Ilstrup DM, Orszulak TA, et al. Early and late survival after surgical treatment of culture-positive active endocarditis. Mayo Clin Proc. 1995;70:517–25.
30. Choussat R, Thomas D, Isnard R, Michel PL, Iung B, Hanania G, et al. Perivalvular abscesses associated with endocarditis: clinical features and prognostic factors of overall survival in a series of 233 cases. Eur Heart J. 1999;20:232–41.
31. Jault F, Gandjbakhch I, Chastre JC, Levasseur JP, Bors V, Gibert C, et al. Prosthetic valve endocarditis with ring abscesses: surgical management and long-term results. J Thorac Cardiovasc Surg. 1993;105:1106–13.
32. d'Udekem Y, David TE, Feindel CM, Armstrong S, Sun Z. Long-term results of surgery for active infective endocarditis. Eur J Cardiothorac Surg. 1997;11:46–52.
33. Allan R, Hynes M, Burwash IG, Veinot JP, Chan KL. Coronary artery complications in infective endocarditis. Ann Thorac Surg. 2008;86(4):1381.
34. Parashara DK, Jacobs LE, Kotler MN, Yazdanfar S, Speilman SR, et al. Angina caused by systolic compression of the left coronary artery as a result of pseudoaneurysm of the mitral-aortic intervalvular fibrosa. Am Heart J. 1995;129:417–21.
35. Rozich JD, Edwards WD, Hanna RD, et al. Mechanical prosthetic valve associated strands: pathologic correlates to transesophageal echocardiography. J Am Soc Echocardiogr. 2003;16:97–100.
36. Shapiro SM, Young E, De Guzman S, et al. Transesophageal echocardiography in diagnosis of infective endocarditis. Chest. 1994;105:377–82.
37. Erbel R, Rohmann S, Drexler M, et al. Improved diagnostic value of echocardiography in patients with infective endocarditis by transoesophageal approach. A prospective study. Eur Heart J. 1988;9:43–53.
38. Sochowski RA, Chan K-L. Implication of negative results on a monoplane transesophageal echocardiographic study in patients with suspected infective endocarditis. J Am Coll Cardiol. 1993;21:216–21.
39. Daniel WG, Mugge A, Martin RP, et al. Improvement in the diagnosis of abscess associated with endocarditis by transesophageal echocardiography. N Engl J Med. 1991;324:795–800.
40. Afridi I, Apostolidou MA, Saad RM, Zoghbi WA. Pseudoaneurysms of the mitral-aortic intervalvular fibrosa: dynamic characterization using transesophageal echocardiographic and doppler techniques. J Am Coll Cardiol. 1995;25:137–45.
41. Chan K, Cohen G, Sochowski R, Baird M. Complications of transesophageal echocardiography in ambulatory adult patients: analysis of 1500 consecutive patients. J Am Soc Echocardiogr. 1991;4:577–82.
42. Evangelista A, Gonzalez-Alujas M. Echocardiography in infective endocarditis. Heart. 2004;90:614–7.
43. Ellis S, Godstein J, Popp R. Detection of endocarditis-associated perivalvular abscesses by two-dimensional echocardiography. JACC. 1985;5(3):647–53.
44. Agirbasli M, Fadel B. Pseudoaneurysm of the mitral-aortic intervalvular fibrosa. Echocardiography. 1999;16(2):253–7.
45. Feuchtner G, Stolzmann P, Dichtl W, et al. Multislice computed tomography in infective endocarditis. J Am Coll Cardiol. 2009;53(5):436–44.
46. Nishimura R, Otto C, Bonow R, et al. AHA/ACC guidelines for the management of patients with valvular heart disease. Circulation. 2014;2014:129.

Chapter 11
Embolic Complications in Infective Endocarditits

Duk-Hyun Kang

Introduction

Embolic complications are caused by migration and embolization of vegetations. Systemic embolism is a frequent and life-threatening complication of infective endocarditis (IE) and most commonly involves the brain [1–5]. Cerebral embolism is the most serious complication with neurologic sequelae and the second most common cause of death after congestive heart failure in this patient population [2, 5]. Echocardiography plays a key role in assessing embolic risk as well as diagnosing IE and its complications, and patients with large vegetations have a higher risk of embolism [3, 6]. Early diagnosis of IE and prompt institution of antibiotic therapy is important in preventing embolic complications because the incidence of embolism is significantly reduced after initiation of antibiotic therapy [7–10]. Early surgical removal of vegetation during the first week of antibiotic therapy is also effective for decreasing embolic events [11, 12], but the decision to perform surgery in patients with IE has been a clinical dilemma. This chapter discusses clinical and echocardiographic factors related to risk of embolism, advances in medical and surgical treatment to decrease embolic events and the role of early surgery in preventing embolism in IE.

Risk of Embolism

Systemic embolization occurs in 22–50 % of patients with IE and involves the central nervous system in up to 65 % (Fig. 11.1a–d) [1–5]. Neurologic complications have a negative impact on outcome; overall mortality was 45 % in patients with

D.-H. Kang, MD, PhD
Department of Cardiology, University of Ulsan, Asan Medical Center, Seoul, South Korea
e-mail: dhkang@amc.seoul.kr

© Springer International Publishing Switzerland 2016
G. Habib (ed.), *Infective Endocarditis*, DOI 10.1007/978-3-319-32432-6_11

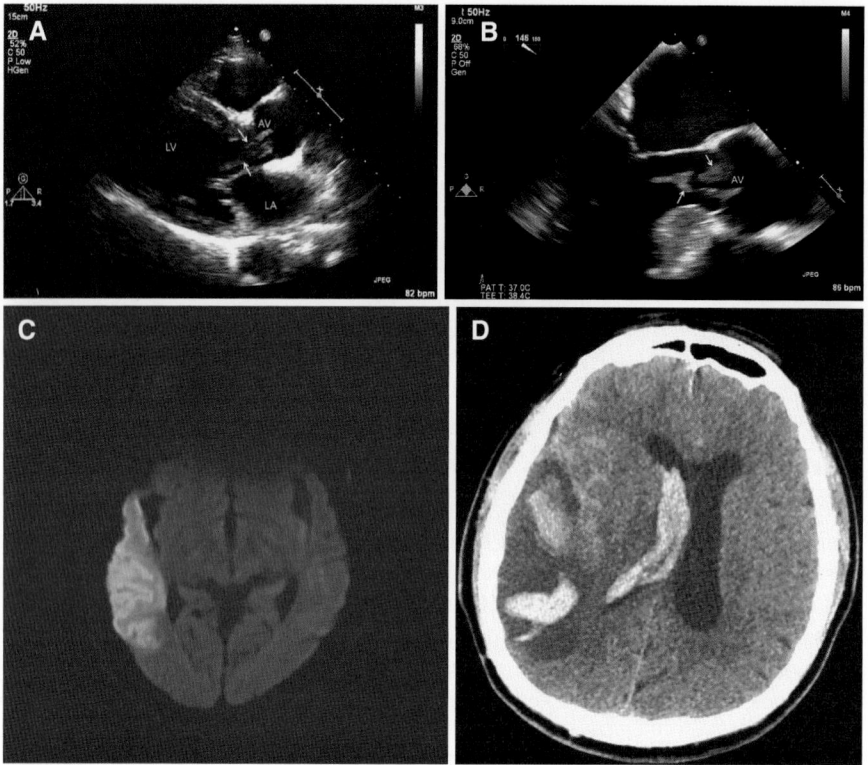

Fig. 11.1 Cerebral embolism in a patient with infective endocarditis. Transthoracic (**a**) and transesophageal (**b**) echocardiography showed multiple, large vegetations (*arrows*) on a native aortic valve, and acute cerebral embolic infarction in right temporal lobe was observed on magnetic resonance imaging (**c**). The cerebral computed tomography scan, performed 1 day later, demonstrated the development of intracerebral and intraventricular hemorrhage (**d**). *AV* aortic valve, *LA* left atrium, *LV* left ventricle

these complications and 24 % in those without [9]. Embolism also involve the coronary arteries, spleen, liver, kidney, bowel and peripheral vasculature in left-sided IE [13], while pulmonary embolism is frequent in right-sided and pacemaker IE [14]. Embolic complications may also be asymptomatic in about 20 % of patients and only be detected by systematic imaging [5].

Echocardiography plays a major role in predicting embolic risk. Several studies evaluated the value of echocardiography for predicting embolic events (Table 11.1). Di Salvo et al. [6] reported that *Staphylococcus* infection, right-side valve endocarditis and vegetation length and mobility were significantly associated with embolic events on univariate analysis, and vegetation length and mobility were the only predictors of embolism on multivariate analysis. Vilacosta et al. [15] investigated new embolic events occurring after institution of antibiotic therapy and concluded that an increase in vegetation size at echocardiographic follow-up might predict new embolic events. In a multicenter prospective study [3], vegetation length

Table 11.1 Clinical observational studies assessing embolic risk

Author (year)	Study design	No of subjects	Type of IE	Embolic events		Predictors
				Incidence	Type	
Di Salvo et al. [6] (2001)	Retrospective Single center	178	Left- and right-sided	37%	Total	Vegetation length, Vegetation mobility
Vilacosta et al. [15] (2002)	Prospective Multi-center	211	Left-sided IE	12.9%	New	Previous embolism, Increase in vegetation size, Large vegetations at mitral valve
Anderson et al. [16] (2003)	Retrospective single center	707	Left- and right-sided	9.6%	Stroke	Mitral valve IE
Thuny et al. [3] (2005)	Prospective multi-center	384	Left- and right-sided	34.1% 7.3%	Total New	S. bovis, S.aureus, Vegetation length, Vegetation mobility
Dickerman et al. [8] (2007)	Prospective multi-center	1437	Left-sided IE	15.2%	Stroke	S.aureus IE, Mitral valve vegetation
Thuny et al. [33] (2007)	Prospective Two center	496	Left- and right-sided	22%	Neurologic complication	Vegetation length, Mitral valve IE
Kim et al. [11] (2010)	Prospective Two center	68	Left-sided native valve IE	21%	New	Vegetation length
García-Cabrera et al. [9] (2013)	Retrospective Multi-center	1345	Left-sided IE	25%	Neurologic complication	Vegetation length, S. aureus IE, Mitral valve involvement, Anticoagulant therapy
Hubert et al. [10] (2013)	Prospective Two center	1022	Left- and right-sided	8.5%	New	Age, diabetes, atrial fibrillation, S. aureus, previous embolism, vegetation length

IE infective endocarditis

>10 mm and mobility of vegetation were predictors of new embolic events, and vegetation length >15 mm was a predictor of mortality in multivariable analysis. A recent multicenter cohort study also confirmed that vegetation length >10 mm was the most potent independent predictor of new embolic events [10].

Other factors associated with increased risk of embolism include previous embolism [15], infection with particular microorganism [3, 8, 9] and involvement of the mitral valve [8, 16] (Table 11.1). Hubert et al. [10] recently developed and validated a new prediction system for systemic embolism: the Embolic Risk French Calculator. Six variables associated with embolic risk were used to create the calculator: age, diabetes, atrial fibrillation, previous embolism, vegetation length >10 mm and *Staphylococcus aureus* infection. This risk calculator may be useful for assessing risk of embolism and facilitating management decisions in individual patients with IE.

Prevention of Embolism

Embolic events can occur before the diagnosis of IE and during antibiotic therapy after the diagnosis of IE. Delays in diagnosis have been related to increases of embolic events occurring before the diagnosis of IE, and echocardiography must be done rapidly for earlier diagnosis of IE as soon as IE is suspected. Rapid initiation of antibiotic therapy is also effective in preventing embolism [7–10], and several studies evaluated the effects of medical and surgical treatment on embolic complications (Table 11.2). In a multicenter cohort study [10], embolic events were 44.9 per 1000 patient-weeks in the first week and 21.3 in the second week after initiation of antibiotic therapy and then decreased rapidly to 2.4 in the sixth week (Fig. 11.2). In another multicenter cohort study [9], 86% of neurologic complications were observed before or during the first week of antibiotic therapy, with the incidence of neurologic complications markedly decreasing after appropriate antimicrobial therapy. An analysis from the International Collaboration on Endocarditis Prospective Cohort Study (ICE-PCS) [8] also showed that the incidence of stroke was 4.82 per 1000 patient-days in the first week of appropriate antimicrobial therapy and fell to 1.71 per 1000 patient-days in the second week, with further decreases thereafter. Because embolic risk decreases rapidly before vegetation size is significantly reduced, it is quite possible that the salutary effects of antibiotics on embolization may be related to their early effects on molecular and cellular milieu of the vegetation [8]. The diagnosis of IE must be made as soon as possible and empirical antibiotic therapy should be quickly introduced after blood cultures are obtained and modified based on antibiotic sensitivity data [17, 18]. Routine use of anticoagulant or antiplatelet agents is not recommended in patients with IE, and there is no evidence that use of aspirin or warfarin reduces the risk of embolism [19, 20].

Embolic events occurring during antibiotic therapy may be prevented by surgical removal of vegetation [10], but the decision to perform surgery on patients with IE has been a clinical dilemma. Early surgery is strongly indicated for patients with IE

Table 11.2 Clinical studies assessing the effect of treatment on embolic complications

Author (year)	Study design	No of subjects	Type of IE	Treatment	Summary of findings
Steckelberg et al. [7] (1991)	Retrospective single center	207	Left-sided native valve IE	Antibiotic therapy	Embolic event rate fell to 1.2 per 1000 patient-days after 2 weeks
Chan et al. [19] (2003)	Prospective multi-center randomized trial	115	Left-sided IE	Aspirin 325 mg/day	Embolic event rate was 28 % on aspirin and 20 % on placebo without a significant difference
Dickerman et al. [8] (2007)	Prospective multi-center cohort	1437	Left-sided IE	Antibiotic therapy	Stroke incidence was 4.82 per 1000 patient-days in the first week and fell to 1.71 in the second week with further decreases thereafter
Kim et al. [11] (2010)	Prospective two center cohort	132	Left-sided native valve IE	Early surgery within 7 days of diagnosis	Early surgery is associated with a decrease in embolic events
Kang et al. [12] (2012)	Prospective two center randomized trial	76	Left-sided native valve IE	Early surgery within 48 h of randomization	The rate of in-hospital death or embolic events was 3 % in the early surgery group and 23 % in the conventional treatment group (HR: 0.10; $p=0.03$)
García-Cabrera et al. [9] (2013)	Retrospective multi-center cohort	1345	Left-sided IE	Antibiotic therapy	Antimicrobial therapy reduced the risk of neurologic complications by 33–75 %
Hubert et al. [10] (2013)	Prospective two center cohort	1022	Left- and right-sided	Antibiotic therapy	The incidence of embolic events was highest during the first 2 weeks and then decreased rapidly

IE infective endocarditis

Fig. 11.2 Incidence of embolic events after initiation of antibiotic therapy. The incidence of embolic events was highest during the first 2 weeks after the initiation of antibiotic therapy (44.9 and 21.3 embolic events per 1000 patient-weeks in the first and second week) (From Hubert et al. [10]. With permission from Elsevier Limited)

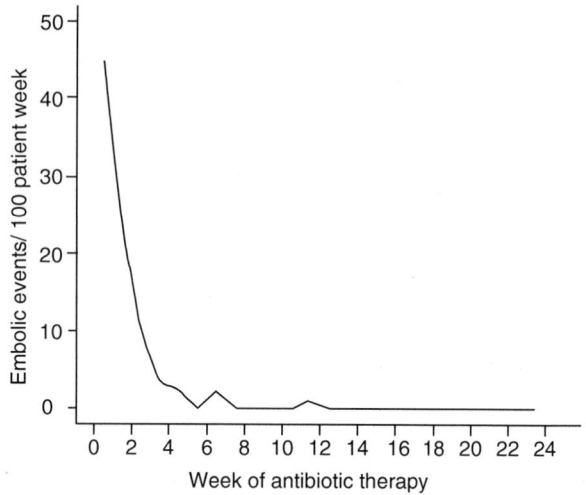

and congestive heart failure [13, 14, 18, 20], but indications for surgical intervention to prevent systemic embolism remain to be defined [14, 18]. Early identification of patients at high risk of embolism [3, 6], increased experience with complete excision of infected tissue and valve repair, and low operative mortality have raised arguments for early surgery [13, 21], but there have been concerns that such surgery may be more difficult to perform in the presence of active infection and inflammation, which leads to a high operative mortality and a high risk of postoperative valve dysfunction [22]. Consensus guidelines for performance of early surgery on the basis of vegetation were different (Fig. 11.3), and the 2006 American College of Cardiology/American Heart Association (ACC/AHA) guidelines recommended early surgery as a class IIa indication only in patients with recurrent emboli and persistent vegetation despite appropriate antibiotic therapy [23], and the 2009 European Society of Cardiology (ESC) guidelines recommend urgent surgery as a class I indication in patients with one or more embolic episodes and large vegetations (>10 mm in length) despite appropriate antibiotic therapy and urgent surgery as a class IIb indication in patients with isolated, very large vegetations (>15 mm) [14]. The recently revised 2014 AHA/ACC guidelines have added a class IIb indication for early surgery in patients with mobile, large vegetations (>10 mm) [18].

Early Surgery for Prevention of Systemic Embolism

As the risk of embolism is highest during the first few days after initiation of antibiotic therapy, the ESC guidelines clearly recommend that surgery to prevent embolism be performed very early on urgent (within a few days) basis [14]. By contrast, the 2014 AHA/ACC guidelines have not established the optimal timing of surgery

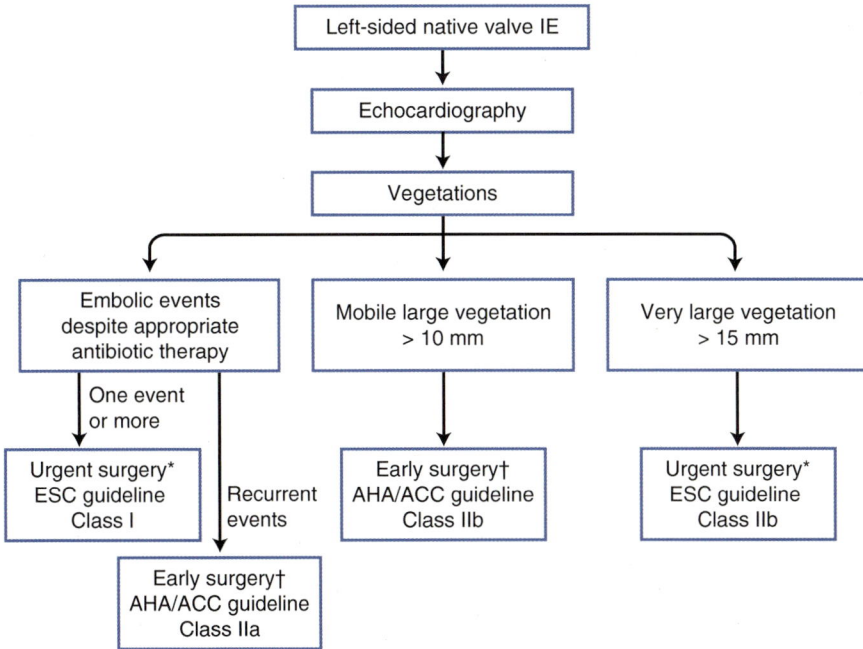

Fig. 11.3 Embolic indications and timing of surgery for patients with left-sided native valve infective endocarditis. Urgent surgery*: surgery performed within a few days; Early surgery†: surgery performed during initial hospitalization before completion of a full therapeutic course of antibiotics; *IE* infective endocarditis. *AHA/ACC guidelines* 2014 American Heart Association/American College of Cardiology guidelines, *ESC guidelines* 2009 European Society of Cardiology guidelines (Adapted from Habib et al. [14] and from Nishimura et al. [18])

for embolic indication and vaguely defined early surgery as surgery performed during initial hospitalization before completion of a full therapeutic course of antibiotics [18]. Since the benefits of surgery to prevent embolism are greatest during the first week of the diagnosis, deferring surgery after 1 to 2 weeks is of little value [8, 13]. With regard to the optimal timing of surgery, Thuny et al. [24] reported that the effect of early surgery (within 1 week) on mortality was not uniform, and surgery might be beneficial in patients with the most severe forms of IE including *Staphylococcus aureus* infection, heart failure, and larger vegetations, whereas early surgery was associated with increased risks of relapse and prosthetic valve dysfunction. In a multicenter observational study [11], clinical outcomes of early surgery were compared with conventional treatment in IE patients with embolic indications only. Patients in the early surgery group underwent surgery within 7 days of diagnosis (median interval, 2.5 days) because the benefits of surgery might be greatest if surgery was performed within that time, and patients in the conventional treatment group were referred for surgery only if they developed a surgical indication based on current guidelines. Mortality rates were similar in the two groups, but embolic events were significantly lower in the early surgery group without increase in recurrence of IE or prosthetic valve dysfunction. Previous observational studies comparing outcomes between surgery versus medical therapy were subject to the limitations of baseline differences, treatment selection and survivor biases [11, 24–28] and recent studies using propensity scoring models yielded conflicting results on the benefits of surgery [11, 24–27]. Although prospective, randomized trials may reduce differences in patient characteristics and these biases between treatment groups, ethical, logistical and financial constraints have deterred us from conducting a randomized trial.

Recently a randomized trial was conducted to compare clinical outcomes of early surgery with those of a conventional treatment strategy based on current guidelines in left-sided IE patients with high embolic risks [12]. The major hypothesis of this trial was that early surgery would decrease the rate of death or embolic events, as compared with conventional treatment.

Patients were eligible for enrollment if they were diagnosed as definite IE and had both severe mitral or aortic valve disease and maximal length of vegetation >10 mm, and were randomly assigned to early surgery (37 patients) or to conventional treatment (39 patients). All patients in the early surgery group underwent valve surgery within 48 h after randomization. Of the 39 patients in the conventional treatment group, 30 (77 %) patients underwent surgery during initial hospitalization ($n=27$) or during follow-up ($n=3$). The primary end point of in-hospital death and embolic events at 6 weeks occurred in 1 (3 %) patient in the early surgery group as compared with 9 (23 %) patients in the conventional treatment group (hazard ratio [HR], 0.10; 95 % confidence interval [CI], 0.01–0.82; P=0.03). There was no significant difference in all-cause mortality rate at 6 months (3 % vs 5 %; HR, 0.51; 95 % CI, 0.05–5.66; P=0.59) (Fig. 11.4a). The rate of the composite of death from any cause, embolic events, recurrence of IE, or repeat hospitalizations due to development of congestive heart failure at 6 months was 3 % in the early surgery group as compared with 28 % in the conventional management group (HR, 0.08; 95 % CI, 0.01–0.65; P=0.02) (Fig. 11.4b).

This randomized trial demonstrated that early surgery performed within 48 h after diagnosis reduced the primary endpoint (composite of in-hospital death and embolic events) by effectively decreasing systemic embolisms in patients with IE. Moreover, these improvements in clinical outcomes could be achieved without increases in operative mortality or recurrence of IE. Rapid diagnosis of IE, inclusion of patients with low operative risk and aggressive surgical approach may explain the substantially lower mortalities in both groups than that reported previously. However, this trial was limited in scope and excluded patients with major stroke, prosthetic valve endocarditis or aortic abscess and the incidence of *S. aureus* IE was lower than that in previous studies [2, 29]. Because IE is a highly variable disease and the risk-benefit ratio of early surgery over conventional treatment may differ according to the type of high risk situation and causative microorganism, additional randomized trials will be necessary to evaluate the efficacy and safety of early surgery in patients with complicated IE.

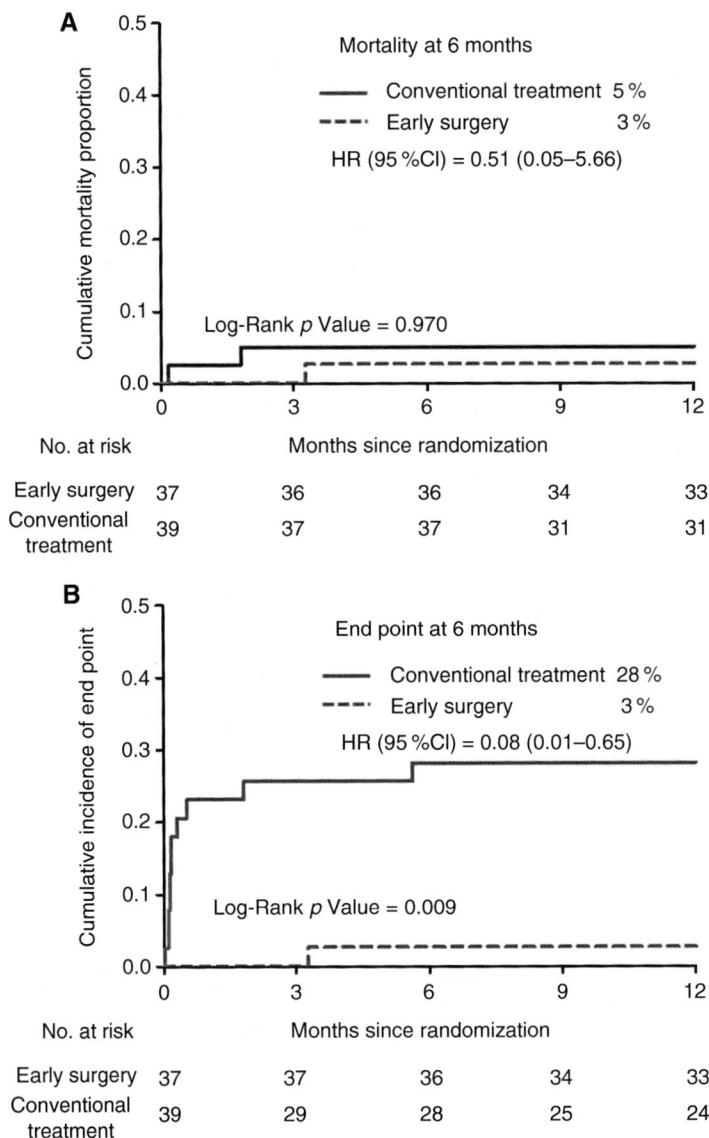

Fig. 11.4 Kaplan-Meier curve for the cumulative probabilities of death (**a**) and of the composite end point (**b**), according to treatment group. There was no significant between-group difference in all-cause mortality at 6 months (**a**). The rate of the composite of death from any cause, embolic events, recurrence of infective endocarditis, or repeat hospitalizations due to development of congestive heart failure at 6 months was 3 % in the early surgery group versus 28 % in the conventional management group (HR, 0.08; 95 % CI, 0.01–0.65; P=0.02) (**b**) (From Kang et al. [12]. With permission from NEJM)

Table 11.3 Characteristics favoring early surgery or watchful observation

Characteristics	Early surgery	Watchful observation
Embolic risk	**High**	**Low**
Vegetation size	Large	Small
Previous embolism	(+)	
Microorganism	*S aureus*	
Duration of antibiotic therapy	<1 week	>2 weeks
Operative risk	**Low**	**High**
EuroSCORE II, STS risk estimate	<4%	>8%
Valvular dysfunction	**Severe**	**Mild or moderate**
Likelihood of valve repair	**High**	**Low**
Other complications		
Heart failure	(+)	
Persistent infection	(+)	
Abscess	(+)	
Cerebral hemorrhage		(+)

EuroSCORE European system for cardiac operative risk evaluation, *STS* Society of Thoracic Surgeon

Multidisciplinary collaborations among the cardiologists, cardiac surgeons and infectious disease specialists are required for appropriate decisions about indication and timing of surgical intervention [13, 18], and these decisions should be based on individual risk-benefit analysis (Table 11.3). The potential benefits of surgery need to be weighed against its operative risks and long-term consequences. Operative mortality can be estimated from different scoring systems including the Society of Thoracic Surgeon (STS) risk estimate [30] or European system for cardiac operative risk evaluation (EuroSCORE) [31, 32]. Surgical option to prevent embolism is indicated when embolic risk exceeds operative risk of the individual patient and the benefit of surgery would be greater if conservative procedure preserving the native valve is likely or severe valvular regurgitation is associated.

Conclusion

Echocardiography plays a key role in assessing embolic risk and patients with large vegetations are at higher risk of embolism. Early diagnosis of IE and prompt initiation of antibiotic therapy is essential for preventing embolic complications of IE and early surgical removal of vegetation may reduce embolic events in patients at high embolic risk. The decision for surgery should be based on individual risk-benefit analysis, and early surgery is strongly indicated if embolic risk exceeds operative risk.

References

1. Mylonakis E, Calderwood SB. Infective endocarditis in adults. N Engl J Med. 2001;345:1318–30.
2. Hoen B, Duval X. Infective endocarditis. N Engl J Med. 2013;368:1425–33.
3. Thuny F, DiSalvo G, Belliard O, et al. Risk of embolism and death in infective endocarditis: prognostic value of echocardiography: a prospective multicenter study. Circulation. 2005;112(1):69–75.
4. Heiro M, Nikoskelainen J, Engbolm E, et al. Neurologic manifestations of infective endocarditis: a 17 year experience in a teaching hospital in Finland. Arch Intern Med. 2000;160:2781–7.
5. Habib G. Management of infective endocarditis. Heart. 2006;92(1):124–30.
6. Di Salvo G, Habib G, Pergola V, et al. Echocardiography predicts embolic events in infective endocarditis. J Am Coll Cardiol. 2001;37(4):1069–76.
7. Steckelberg JM, Murphy JG, Ballard D, et al. Emboli in infective endocarditis: the prognostic value of echocardiography. Ann Intern Med. 1991;114(8):635–40.
8. Dickerman SA, Abrutyn E, Barsic B, et al. The relationship between the initiation of antimicrobial therapy and the incidence of stroke in infective endocarditis: an analysis from the ICE Prospective Cohort Study (ICE-PCS). Am Heart J. 2007;154:1086–94.
9. García-Cabrera E, Fernández-Hidalgo N, Almirante B, et al. Neurologic complications of infective endocarditis. Risk factors, outcome and impact of cardiac surgery: a multicenter observational study. Circulation. 2013;127:2272–84.
10. Hubert S, Thuny F, Resseguier N, et al. Prediction of symptomatic embolism in infective endocarditis: construction and validation of a risk calculator in a multicenter cohort. J Am Coll Cardiol. 2013;62:1384–92.
11. Kim DH, Kang DH, Lee MZ, et al. Impact of early surgery on embolic events in patients with infective endocarditis. Circulation. 2010;122 Suppl 11:S17–22.
12. Kang DH, Kim YJ, Kim SH, et al. Early surgery versus conventional treatment for infective endocarditis. N Engl J Med. 2012;366:2466–73.
13. Prendergast BD, Tornos P. Surgery for infective endocarditis: who and when? Circulation. 2010;121(9):1141–52.
14. Habib G, Hoen B, Tornos P, et al. Guidelines on the prevention, diagnosis, and treatment of infective endocarditis (new version 2009): the Task Force on the Prevention, Diagnosis, and Treatment of Infective Endocarditis of the European Society of Cardiology (ESC). Eur Heart J. 2009;30(19):2369–413.
15. Vilacosta I, Graupner C, San Roman JA, et al. Risk of embolization after institution of antibiotic therapy for infective endocarditis. J Am Coll Cardiol. 2002;39:1489–95.
16. Anderson DJ, Goldstein LB, Wilkinson WE, et al. Stroke location, characterization, severity and outcome in mitral vs aortic valve endocarditis. Neurology. 2003;61:1341–6.
17. Thuny F, Grisoli D, Collart F, Habib G, Raoult D. Management of infective endocarditis: challenges and perspectives. Lancet. 2012;379:965–75.
18. Nishimura RA, Otto CM, Bonow RO, Carabello BA, Erwin III JP, Guyton RA, O'Gara PT, Ruiz CE, Skubas NJ, Sorajja P, Sundt III TM, Thomas JD. 2014 AHA/ACC guidelines for the management of patients with valvular heart disease: a report of the American College of Cardiology/American Heart Association Task Force on Practice Guidelines: developed in collaboration with the American Association for Thoracic Surgery, American Society of Echocardiography, Society for Cardiovascular Angiography and Interventions, Society of Cardiovascular Anesthesiologists, and the Society of Thoracic Surgeons. J Am Coll Cardiol. 2014;63:e57–185.
19. Chan KL, Dumesnil JG, Cujec B, et al. A randomized trial of aspirin on the risk of embolic events in patients with infective endocarditis. J Am Coll Cardiol. 2003;42:775–80.
20. Baddour LM, Wilson WR, Bayer AS, et al. Infective endocarditis: diagnosis, antimicrobial therapy, and management of complications: a statement for healthcare professionals from the

Committee on Rheumatic Fever, Endocarditis, and Kawasaki Disease, Council on Cardiovascular Disease in the Young, and the Councils on Clinical Cardiology, Stroke, and Cardiovascular Surgery and Anesthesia, American Heart Association: endorsed by the Infectious Diseases Society of America. Circulation. 2005;11(23):e394–433.

21. Tornos P, Iung B, Permanyer-Miralda G, et al. Infective endocarditis in Europe: lessons from the EuroHeart Survey. Heart. 2005;91(5):571–5.

22. Delahaye F. Is early surgery beneficial in infective endocarditis? A systematic review. Arch Cardiovasc Dis. 2011;104(1):35–44.

23. Bonow RO, Carabello B, Chatterjee K, et al. ACC/AHA 2006 guidelines for the management of patients with valvular heart disease: a report of the American College of Cardiology/American Heart Association Task Force on Practice Guidelines (Writing Committee to Revise the 1998 Guidelines for the Management of Patients with Valvular Heart Disease). Circulation. 2006;114(5):e84–231.

24. Thuny F, Beurtheret S, Mancini J, et al. The timing of surgery influences mortality and morbidity in adults with severe complicated infective endocarditis: a propensity analysis. Eur Heart J. 2011;32(16):2027–33.

25. Vikram HR, Buenconsejo J, Hasbun R, Quagliarello VJ. Impact of valve surgery on 6-month mortality in adults with complicated, left-sided native valve endocarditis: a propensity analysis. JAMA. 2003;290(24):3207–14.

26. Tleyjeh IM, Ghomrawi HM, Steckelberg JM, et al. The impact of valve surgery on 6-month mortality in left-sided infective endocarditis. Circulation. 2007;115(13):1721–8.

27. Lalani T, Cabell CH, Benjamin DK, et al. Analysis of the impact of early surgery on in-hospital mortality of native valve endocarditis: use of propensity score and instrumental variable methods to adjust for treatment-selection bias. Circulation. 2010;121(8):1005–13.

28. Tleyjeh IM, Steckelberg JM, Georgescu G, et al. The association between the timing of valve surgery and 6-month mortality in left-sided infective endocarditis. Heart. 2008;94(7):892–6.

29. Miro JM, Anguera I, Cabell CH, et al. Staphylococcus aureus native valve infective endocarditis: report of 566 episodes from the International Collaboration on Endocarditis Merged Database. Clin Infect Dis. 2005;41:507–14.

30. O'Brien SM, Shahian DM, Filardo G, Ferraris VA, Haan CK, Rich JB, Normand SL, DeLong ER, Shewan CM, Dokholyan RS, Peterson ED, Edwards FH, Anderson RP. Society of Thoracic Surgeons Quality Measurement Task Force. The Society of Thoracic Surgeons 2008 cardiac surgery risk model, part 2: isolated valve surgery. Ann Thorac Surg. 2009;88:S23–42.

31. Nashef SAM, Roques F, Michel P, Gauducheau E, Lemeshow S, Salamon R. European system for cardiac operative risk evaluation (EuroSCORE). Eur J Cardiothorac Surg. 1999;16:9–13.

32. Nashef SAM, Roques F, Sharples LD, et al. EuroSCORE II. Eur J Cardiothorac Surg. 2012;41:734–45.

33. Thuny F, Avierinos JF, Tribouilloy C, et al. Impact of cerebrovascular complications on mortality and neurologic outcome during infective endocarditis: a prospective multicenter study. Eur Heart J. 2007;28:1155–61.

Chapter 12
Neurological Complications in Infective Endocarditis

Ulrika Snygg-Martin

Introduction

Neurological complications in infective endocarditis (IE) are common but diverse in presentation and prognostic significance. The majority of these complications are established before IE is diagnosed [1–5] and the rate of new neurological events, mainly studied as incidence of ischaemic embolic episodes, has been shown to decrease rapidly after the initiation of effective antibiotic therapy [6, 7]. Several factors associated with higher risk of embolism or neurological complications have been identified including presence, size and mobility of vegetations on echocardiography, *S. aureus* aetiology, previous embolic event, mitral valve involvement, higher CRP levels, a procoagulant status and comorbid factors [8–16]. Most studies also reveal higher case fatality rates in IE episodes complicated by neurological events (Table 12.1).

Central nervous system (CNS) symptoms in IE are commonly divided into ischaemic lesions (infarction, transient ischaemic attack), haemorrhagic complications (intracerebral bleeding due to septic vasculitis, secondary bleeding into primary ischaemic infarctions, ruptured infectious aneurysms causing subarachoidal or intracerebral bleeding) or infectious manifestations (meningitis, brain abscess). More unspecific neurological symptoms described in IE are encephalopathy, seizures, headache and psychiatric manifestations [1, 2, 8] but the incidence of such events is not reported in studies based on diagnostic cerebral CT scans [3]. In modern studies with systematically performed MRI or careful clinical description of neurological symptomatology the clinical entity of encephalopathy has re-emerged [5, 17].

Cerebral involvement in IE is often multiple including ischaemic lesions in different vascular territories or concomitant ischaemic and haemorrhagic or infectious lesions. The clinical picture, however, is often is characterised by one type of neurological sign

U. Snygg-Martin, MD, PhD
Department of Infectious Diseases, Sahlgrenska University Hospital, Gothenburg, Sweden
e-mail: Ulrika.snygg-martin@infect.gu.se

© Springer International Publishing Switzerland 2016

149

G. Habib (ed.), *Infective Endocarditis*, DOI 10.1007/978-3-319-32432-6_12

Table 12.1 Incidence of symptomatic central nervous system complications in patients with infective endocarditis

Author	N	Symptomatic CNS complication (%)	Ischaemia (%)	Haemorrhage (%)	Meningitis (%)	Mortality ± CNS complication (%)
Harrison –67 [92]	116	28	22	–	19	67/44
Pruitt –78 [1]	218	39	28(17)	7	16	58/20
Hart –90 [18]	133	23	19	7	–	–
Kanter –91 [8]	166	35	20[a]		5	35/19
Pruitt –96 [57]	144	29	18		4	32/13
Heiro –00 [2]	218	25	11	2	4	24/10
Anderson –03 [93]	770	14	7	2	–	ns
Corral –07 [37]	550	13	8	3	2	34/11
Thuny –07 [3]	496	11 (22[b])	16[c]	4		1 year:25/19(ns)
Dickerman –07 [6]	1437	15	15[a]			–
Snygg-Martin –11 [4]	684	25	20[c]	2	6	27/10
Garcia-Cabrera –13 [5]	1345	25	14	5	6[d]	45/24

[a]Ischaemia-haemorrhage
[b]including silent CNS complications
[c]including TIA
[d]including encephalopathy

or even the absence of neurological symptoms, i.e. as a silent neurological complication [18–21]. In a carefully described material of 17 patients dying from IE in the 1930s, the fundamental pathological change in the brain was a diffuse embolic meningoencephalitis, from which various clinical manifestations arose [22]. Encephalopathy with impaired consciousness and meningism has also been argued to be of septic embolic origin [8, 19].

Incidence

Symptomatic neurological complications occur in 13–39 % of IE patients as summarized in Table 12.1, showing studies on cerebral complications in IE identified by clinical neurological symptoms during the last 50 years. The varying incidence reflects study population characteristics, diagnostic methods and used definitions, but a relatively stable incidence is seen despite mayor changes in IE epidemiology during this period [23]. Factors firmly correlated to an increased incidence of CNS complications, such as a high proportion of IE caused by S. aureus in a study population, are counteracted by a shorter delay to diagnosis in modern studies and a higher surgical rate. Embolic risk is reported to be age dependent by some authors [24], but results are conflicting and different risk estimates can be explained in a time-dependent manor with lower risk of embolic events in older patients in the prediagnostic and early treatment phase counteracted by higher risk in the late treatment and follow up period, relative to an age-dependent and comorbid related risk of stroke [13].

Studies not primarily focusing on neurological complications [25, 26] or with a narrow definition of neurological complications as strictly of embolic cerebrovascular origin, e.g. only regarding stroke with neurological deficit that lasts >24 h verified by cerebral imaging, have lower reported incidence of neurological complications, estimating 12–15 % [6, 27]. Higher numbers are reported in critically ill patients requiring intensive care admission [28]. Silent cerebral complications are even more common as shown by several studies using systematic CNS imaging [20, 29, 30].

However, it is important to stress that in the attempt to define true incidence or proportions of neurological complications in IE, the influence of referral and selection bias must be taken into account, apart from the patient, disease and diagnosis related characteristics discussed above.

Time Dependent Incidence

The majority of neurological complications are established before IE is diagnosed or even suspected and hence before the initiation of antibiotic treatment. Central nervous system symptoms are not infrequently what bring the IE patient to medical attention and in three out of four patients suffering neurological symptoms, these are evident at the time of presentation [5, 20, 31]. Lower numbers of pre-treatment neurological symptoms were reported in a large multicentre study from the ICE cohort [6] but by viewing stroke reported on the day of antibiotic initiation as pre-treatment events, the proportion is more in accord. In studies involving early neuro-imaging of the brain as an important diagnostic tool, giving a large proportion of silent and minor CNS complications found, a precise timing of cerebral lesions is not possible since neurological symptoms are missing or discrete.

What is repeatedly shown, however, is that the number of symptomatic neuro-logical complications rapidly decreases after initiation of antibiotic therapy [6, 7], thus making early diagnosis and treatment start the utmost important act to reduce number of neurological complications in IE patients. In the study by Dickerman et al. [6], the stroke rate during the first week of therapy was 4.8 per 1000 patient-days (not including strokes diagnosed on the first day of antibiotic treatment) and this rate fell in the second week of therapy to 1.7 of 1000 patient days ($P < 0.001$), a 65% reduction.

Although neurological complications with clinical symptoms are pre-treatment manifestations in most patients, new neurological symptoms, first time or recurrent, during antibiotic therapy occur in a substantial proportion of patients. Any type of clinically evident embolic manifestation is an important risk factor for a subsequent neurological complication, thus warranting close follow up with antibiotic optimi-sation if possible, new echocardiographic investigation and a surgical re-evaluation. Growing evidence also supports the predictive value of silent cerebral lesions to predict embolic risk [32]. The cerebral embolic risk beyond the first week is low, affecting less 1–3% of the total IE population [6], but embolic events are overrep-resented in IE patients during many months [13].

Clinical Manifestations

Ischemic Infarctions

Ischemic infarction is the most common symptomatic and asymptomatic neurologi-cal complication in IE. Neurological symptoms caused by ischaemic lesions are seen in 7–28% of all IE episodes, with a median incidence of 13.6% in a systematic review by the Global Burden of Disease (GOD) study group published in 2014 [27]. Regardless of type of neurological symptoms most abnormalities are small isch-aemic lesions being more frequent than large infarctions [29]. When asymptomatic lesions are regarded, a much higher proportion of IE episodes exhibit ischaemic complications, reaching 60–80% of all IE patients [20]. Ischaemic strokes account for approximately half of the symptomatic neurological complications in studies focusing on total neurological presentation in IE, but in many retrospective studies not involving a detailed symptom description or systematic MRI the proportion of ischaemic events of all neurological events is even higher.

Emboli from vegetations preferably involve the middle cerebral artery territory as a result of the high percentage of blood volume in these territories, resulting in hemiparetic syndrome of different degrees. Other symptoms described from ischaemic lesions in IE are hemianopsia, transient visual impairment, ataxia, aphasia, diplopia and minor motor impairment. Multifocal infarctions are also common and frequently involve the end arterial territories of cerebral vessels [2, 33, 34]. It is, however, surprisingly uncommon that these infected emboli give rise to intracerebral infections such as meningitis, infectious aneurysms or brain abscesses, possibly related to the effective protection the blood-brain barrier exhibits to haematogenous bacterial seeding. The clinical syndromes seen with punctuate cerebral infarctions are variable and often referred to as an altered level of consciousness or embolic encephalopathy without reported incidence of concomitant focal or multifocal neurological signs [35]. In one study describing 30 patients with neurological symptoms, 12 were characterized as having a clinical cerebrovascular event while 25 patients were showing ischaemic lesions on MRI [17]. About 20–40 % of IE episodes with cerebral embolism are described as having concomitant peripheral emboli, but numbers vary or is not reported [1, 36]. In studies describing embolic events overall the proportion of CNS embolic events account for approximately half but depends on mode of detection of embolic events i.e. the proportion of silent events included.

Transitory Ischaemic Attacks

Transitory ischaemic attacks (TIA) in IE patients are seen either as an isolated neurological event with good prognosis [2, 3] or as part of a more complex neurological symptomatology with concomitant MRI findings despite symptom remission [17]. Incidence of TIA is difficult to estimate due to the inherent transitory and often discrete nature of these complications, but TIA are reported in 2–6 % of IE episodes [2–4]. TIA more frequently is reported after initiation of antibiotic therapy compared to other neurological complications.

Intracranial Haemorrhage

Intracranial haemorrhage with neurological symptoms occurs in 2–7 % of patients with IE [1–3, 5, 18, 37] but the incidence is substantially higher in IE patients admitted to intensive care [28]. The three underlying mechanisms of haemorrhage are pyogenic arteritis and erosion of the arterial wall causing intracerebral bleeding, haemorrhagic transformation of an initially purely ischaemic infarction and rupture of infectious (mycotic) aneurysm with subarachnoidal and/or intracerebral bleeding [38, 39]. In studies detecting silent cerebral complications, the incidence of haemorrhagic complications is higher [21] and also in neurologically symptomatic patients with detected haemorrhage on CT or MRI the grade of symptoms may be discrete.

In several retrospective studies anticoagulant therapy has been associated with a higher risk of haemorrhagic complications in IE patients, especially in IE caused by S. aureus [5, 40–42], while other studies have failed to show this association [43]. Two cohort studies detected no increase in cerebral bleeding and a relative protective role of on-going well controlled anticoagulation against ischaemic infarctions in both staphylococcal IE [44] and in NVE patients on anticoagulation [45], but this has not been verified by others. However, when cerebral bleeding occurs in anticoagulated patients, the prognosis is poor also in contemporary studies [5, 42]. Intracranial haemorrhage can also rarely complicate bacterial meningitis with poor outcome and this is more often seen in anticoagulated patients [46].

Cerebral microbleeds, i.e., small perivascular intraparenchymal haemosidirin deposits only detectable by gradient echo T2-weighted MRI sequences, are increasingly acknowledged in IE as silent complications with potential as an additional diagnostic criterion for IE [30], and to predict intracerebral haemorrhage [47], but this requires further verification. Cerebral microbleeds are associated with small vessel disease in numerous cerebral and cerebrovascular conditions such as Alzheimer´s disease, TIA/infarction and hypertension, the underlying mechanism being microvasculopathy rather than haemorrhage [48].

Intracranial Infectious Aneurysms

Infectious aneurysm, also termed mycotic aneurysms, are rare complications of IE reported in 2–4 % of patients in studies based on detection in IE patients with neurological symptoms [49, 50]. Higher numbers are seen in MRI-based studies including angiographic sequences [30]. Out of all intracranial aneurysms, infectious aneurysms represent 0.7–6 %, and 80 % of intracranial infectious aneurysms are seen in the context of IE [51]. Intracranial infectious aneurysms are most commonly located in the distal branch points of the middle cerebral artery, while congenital aneurysms tend to be central [51, 52]. Infectious aneurysms arise from either septic microemboli to the vasa vasorum or bacterial escape from a septic embolus to the intraluminal arterial space, resulting in destruction of the vessel wall. Infectious aneurysms are actually pseudo-aneurysms in a pathological definition due to the involvement of the muscular arterial wall layer. Infectious aneurysms are thin-walled and friable, typically fusiform with a wide or absent neck, and are feared to exhibit a high tendency to rupture and haemorrhage. On the other hand, it is well known that these aneurysms may resolve with antibiotic therapy as documented in several case series [50, 53]. Consequently, when silent aneurysms are taken into account, the risk profile for rupture is less evident but probably smaller than when only symptomatic aneurysms are studied. The risk of late rupture after a completed full course of antibiotics for IE is low but still exists [54].

Diagnosis of intracranial infectious aneurysms is based on imaging by CT and/or MRI including angiographic sequences but conventional angiography can sometimes be needed and is always performed in endovascular treatment. Further technical development as well as availability and local expertise will influence the diagnostic algorithm in different centres.

Additional to rupture, which is the main risk and consequence of intracranial infectious aneurysms, these can cause minor focal deficits in combination with systemic infection related symptoms [1]. Severe headache in an IE patient can indicate the presence of an infectious aneurysm, and local expansion from an infectious aneurysm can cause cranial nerve palsy such as ophthalmoparesis, but these symptoms are unspecific, and an uncontrolled comparison showed no significant differences in neurological symptoms to distinguish patents who developed aneurysms [54]. However, the clinical presentation of an infectious aneurysm is related to rupture in 80 % of patients [51, 52]. Symptoms constitutes severe headaches with sudden onset, visual loss, seizures, impaired consciousness, hemiparesis or other focal neurological deficits related to subarachnoidal or intraparenchymal haemorrhage. Intraparenchymal haemorrhage is relatively more common after rupture of infectious aneurysms compared to after rupture of congenital intracranial aneurysm. Intracranial infectious aneurysms can also cause intraventricular haemorrhage.

The size of the infectious aneurysm does not reliably predict potential to rupture but can be used to guide treatment in unruptured aneurysms as described in one recent review, suggesting the use of antibiotics and serial imaging for stable, small (<10 mm) unruptured aneurysms and endovascular treatment for large, enlarging, or symptomatic unruptured aneurysms [50]. This recommendation has also been adopted in international endocarditis guidelines [55], but controversy remains and physicians will increasingly encounter this problem as improved imaging techniques visualize more asymptomatic unruptured aneurysms. If early cardiac surgery is required in patients with known intracranial aneurysms, preoperative endovascular intervention must be considered and is preferred to surgical intracranial intervention. Treatment of ruptured intracranial aneurysms requires immediate surgical or endovascular intervention, the choice of which depending on a large variation of factors not possible to cover algorithmically. Ruptured intracranial aneurysms with large intraparenchymal hematomas or those requiring occlusion of an artery supplying an eloquent territory should be treated with open microsurgery, the former to allow concomitant clot evacuation [51]. Surgical clipping can also be preferred in young, symptomatic patients without significant comorbidity who exhibit large and accessible aneurysms. In contemporary reviews endovascular techniques are favoured in a majority of patients but no specified endovascular approach (balloon occlusion, embolization, stent therapy) is shown to be superior [51]. The risks of procedure related complications and postoperative intracranial infections seem to be low. Given the heterogeneity of published studies, mostly case series or reviews [50–53], these conclusions are based low level evidence (Fig. 12.1a, b).

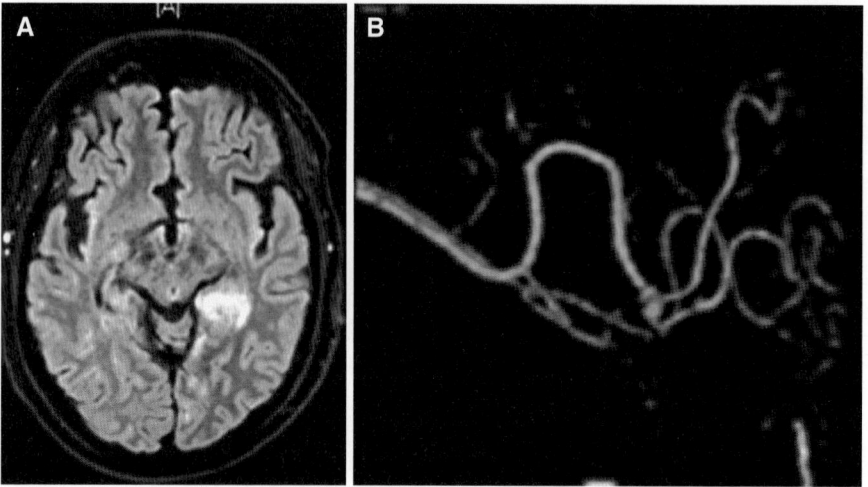

Fig. 12.1 Intracerebral haemorrhage and infectious aneurysm. 70-year-old man presenting with high fever and confusion but no focal signs or murmur. Initial CT scan shows ischaemic infarction that on day 6 has developed a haemorrhagic component. MRI shows a temporal infection with blood and a suspicion of infectious aneurysm (**a**) though the concomitant MRI angiography does not include the specific area. A conventional angiography verifies an intracranial infectious aneurysm on the left arteria cerebri media (**b**). The aneurysm is embolised in the same section

Meningitis

The incidence of meningitis in IE varies from 1 to 16 % in different studies and is, when it occurs, an early clinical manifestation of IE [19]. The detected rate of meningitis in different studies depends on the frequency of lumbar punctures performed in the specific study setting. The availability of non-invasive brain imaging methods have reduced this proportion, since meningism seldom is the only neurological symptom presented [19, 56]. This is illustrated by two studies including patients from different time periods by Pruitt et al., the first with IE patients from 1964 to 1973 when 85 % of the patients with neurological symptoms underwent lumbar puncture, the second with patients from 1988 to 1992, where the corresponding figure was 43 %. In the first study, the incidence of CSF anomalies indicative of meningitis was 16 % of all IE cases, in the second it was 4 % [1, 57].

Different types of IE associated meningitis are recognized, the most prevailing characterized by negative cerebrospinal fluid (CSF) culture and a relatively mild pleocytosis, thought to be caused by emboli to the brain or meninges from a primary cardiac focus without establishing bacterial growth in the CNS [2, 19, 28]. Culture-positive meningitis is more seldom seen in IE patients but has worse prognostic significance. Bacterial meningitis was caused (or complicated) by underlying IE in 2 % (24 patients) of 1025 meningitis identified from a nationwide cohort study of adults with community-acquired bacterial meningitis in the Netherlands performed from 2006 to 2012 [58]. Pneumococci and S. aureus were the most prevalent bacteria and the Osler triad (meningism endocarditis, pneumonia caused by pneumococci) was seen in five patients. While underlying endocarditis is uncommon in pneumococcal meningitis, the growth of S. aureus from CSF warrants a prompt and thorough diagnostic work up for IE, repeatedly performed if initial echocardiography is negative [5]. IE patients with meningitis as a concomitant finding with ischaemic cerebral lesions or with IE related meningitis carry a worse prognosis compared to patients without meningitis respectively compared to patients with meningitis without underlying IE [34, 58].

Brain Abscess

Bacterial brain abscesses are rare complications of endocarditis affecting 0.5–7 % of IE patients with the higher figure seen in IE patients admitted to intensive care [1, 5, 28], but in most studies regarding neurological or embolic complications in IE no brain abscesses at all are reported. Small multiple abscesses are more commonly detected than a single large abscess, which only occasionally is caused by underlying endocarditis. Silent brain microabscesses have also been found in studies where systematic MRI of the brain was performed, but in none of the patients as a single finding [21, 59]. Brain abscesses are defined as focal infection within the parenchyma starting in a localized area of cerebritis subsequently transformed to an encapsulated collection of pus. Presenting symptoms depend on stage, localization and size of the lesion. Brain abscesses can be detected by contrast enhanced CT scan with the typical finding of a hypodense lesion with a contrast-enhancing ring. MRI is a more sensitive modality for small lesions and to differentiate abscesses from necrotic neoplasms [60]. Treatment for brain abscesses in IE patients is usually conservative with antibiotics, the multifocal nature making surgical resection less feasible although it may be necessary in individual cases.

Silent Cerebral Embolism

Silent cerebral embolism is reported in 71 % of neurologically asymptomatic IE patients systematically investigated by brain MRI [21] and concomitant asymptomatic and symptomatic lesions are common [20, 29, 30]. Acute ischaemic lesions and cerebral microbleeds (if gradient echo T2-weighted MRI sequences are included in the study protocol) are most frequent but subarachnoidal and intracerebral bleeding, microabscesses and intracranial infectious aneurysm also appear. When systematic lumbar puncture is performed in IE patients, a high degree of CSF abnormalities indicating aseptic meningitis as well as parenchymal brain damage detected by specific markers are seen in both asymptomatic and neurologically symptomatic IE patients. Studies including IE patients with isolated MRI findings do not include a systematically investigated control group and only in one study a follow up MRI was performed [20] thus making over-diagnosis of IE related cerebral lesions a possibility. However, the commonly accepted principle of silent cerebral complications occurring in IE is substantiated as well as the additive information this provides in clinical decision making [61]. Evidence that detection of silent complications improve patient outcome is, however, still lacking.

Risk Factors for Neurological Complications

Several factors associated with a higher occurrence of neurological complications have been identified but the most consistent finding is that S. aureus IE carry a higher risk than IE from other aetiology, both correlating to overall incidence of neurological complications before and during IE therapy [14] and as an indicator of persistent embolic risk after insertion of antibiotic therapy [13]. Reservations must be made for less common IE pathogens such as candida and non-viridians streptococci [12], where case reports and clinical experience also indicate high embolic risk but incidence not is reported separately in larger studies. The presence and size of valvular vegetations is also associated to risk of CNS complications and embolic events to other organs and plays a key role in predicating new embolic events [6, 9, 62]. Vegetation mobility is investigator dependent but has been shown to be an independent indicator of embolic risk in several setting [9, 12, 31]. Vegetation on the mitral valve also carries a higher tendency to embolize in some studies although this is a less uniform finding [63]. A previous embolic event is a risk factor for a new embolic event and is used in surgical algorithms as a factor favouring early surgery. High CRP levels as well as younger age may correlate to embolic risk but is probably a surrogate marker of the high embolic risk in S. aureus IE [10]. Other laboratory findings may be associated with enhanced embolic tendency in IE patients but play little or no role in the practical IE management today.

While a prospective randomised study has ruled out the role of initiating antiplatelet therapy to reduce the risk of embolic events in IE [64], the effect of ongoing antiplatelet therapy on incidence of embolic and neurological events in IE patients is debated. Some retrospective studies indicate a lower embolic occurrence of embolic events in patients already on aspirin when IE is diagnosed or a lower likelihood of vegetation formation in patients with cardiovascular implantable electronic device infections [65, 66]. Other relatively large studies with a prospective inclusion of patients but a retrospective analysis of antiplatelet effect on embolic tendency cannot reproduce these findings [4, 67]. From what we know today, antiplatelet therapy does not play a role in the development and management of IE but a more specific interaction between S. aureus and aspirin is plausible based on clinical and experimental studies [68, 69]. Regarding on-going oral anticoagulants of warfarin-type when IE is diagnosed, two cohort studies have found a lower risk of ischaemic infarctions in anticoagulated patients compared to non-anticoagulated patients [44, 45] but this has not been reproduced and the main concern is still the increased individual risk of cerebral haemorrhage seen in warfarin-treated patients with S. aureus IE in other studies [5, 41, 42]. Oral anticoagulation in septic patients is difficult to manage and supratherapeutic levels of International Normalized Ratio (INR) risks increasing serious cerebral bleeding, even though this has been difficult to verify in specific studies [42]. No experience of novel direct acting anticoagulants in IE patients with neurological complications has been published so far.

Reflecting optimal patient management, an important distinction is between variables associated with a high number of neurological complications in IE patients and risk factors that are possible to influence. The two areas where individual patient care is paramount is the time to institution of adequate antibiotic therapy, i.e. diagnostic delay, since neurological risk decrease rapidly after antibiotics are started, and a judicious decision regarding surgical removal of vegetations. This has to be balanced to operative risk in the individual patient also taking previous embolic events and coexisting cerebral lesions, vegetation characteristics, duration of antibiotic therapy and additional surgical indications or likelihood of progressive structural damage in the heart with predicted later need for surgery into account. A prospective randomized trial from South Korea has influenced the level of evidence but areas of controversy remain. In this study, 76 patients with large (>10 mm) vegetations and severe valvular regurgitation on the mitral or aortic valve but without urgent indication for valve surgery were randomised to early (<48 h) surgery to prevent embolism or treatment according to international guidelines [70]. The risk of embolic events was reduced significantly from 21 % (all within 6 weeks of randomisation) in the conventional treatment group (half including the CNS) to no embolic events after randomization in the early surgery group. In-hospital and 6 month mortality was not influenced and the surgical rate in the conventional treatment group was also high (77 %). Limitations of study applicability in other IE populations include low surgical risk among study patients, few S. aureus IE, and inclusion exclusively of patients with severe mitral or aortic valve regurgitation, thus making extrapolation to patients with large vegetations as sole surgical indication hypothetical

Prognosis in IE with Neurological Complications

The occurrence of symptomatic neurological complications is associated with a higher case fatality rate in most studies (Table 12.1) while asymptomatic lesions are considered not to influence prognosis based on a prospective studies although not uniformly found [3, 29, 71]. Conclusions regarding prognostic importance of neurological events are biased by several factors influencing outcome in IE, such as S. aureus aetiology, age, comorbidity and referral bias, but in spite of these reservations an increased mortality in IE patients suffering symptomatic neurological complications is credible. In one study where 44 patients with native valve IE had a symptomatic ischaemic infarctions verified by CT or MRI, 9 patients (20 %) died during index hospitalization, 8 (18 %) had major sequelae (hemiparesis, aphasia) and 11 (25 %) minor sequelae (minor weakness, dysphasia, cognitive impairment) at hospital discharge [45]. Studies on neurological recovery in IE patients are scarce but in surgically treated IE patients, 30 % having neurological complications prior to cardiac surgery, in-hospital mortality was 17 % in patients with preoperative cerebral while 54 % of patients achieved full neurological recovery. A worse prognosis was seen in patients with large cerebral infarctions and patients with multiple types of neurological complications. Stroke in IE patients is considered to have a favourable prognosis as compared with stroke resulting from other causes [34].

Management

Several aspects on the management of IE patients with symptomatic and asymptomatic neurological complications are not studied, or even possible to study, in a unobjectionable way and recommendations are in general based on low level evidence though some prospective randomised studies have been performed in this area [64, 72]. The main issues are how to reduce the risk of neurological complications, how to diagnose and handle established complications and how to manage associated medical and surgical questions such as the need for cardiac surgery and on-going anticoagulant therapy. The question regarding how to minimize the risk of neurological complications is addressed above in the risk factor section and is shortly summarized as early detection and institution of antibiotic therapy and cardiac surgery in selected patients, the latter based on assumed risk for new embolic events, surgical risk and presence of concomitant surgical indications. The diagnostic possibilities include clinical neurological examination, radiological investigation by CT, MRI and occasionally conventional angiography and lumbar puncture to detect pleocytosis, positive culture and the presence of brain damage markers in CSF. The remaining issues regarding handling are addressed below.

Management of Established Neurological Complications

In ischaemic lesions no specific medical or endovascular intervention is indicated apart from initiation or optimisation of antibiotic therapy. A prospective randomised study has ruled out the role of initiating antiplatelet therapy in patients after IE diagnosis to reduce the risk of future embolic events [64]. On-going antiplatelet therapy should only be interrupted in the presence of major bleeding but is elsewise continued. Though not shown in a prospective randomised study, IE per se is not an indication to start anticoagulation. The effectiveness of anticoagulation to prevent cerebral embolism is documented in patients with mechanical valve prosthesis and atrial fibrillation but not in the initial IE phase when embolic risk is high but quickly reduced by antibiotic induced infection control. Anticoagulation in IE patients have the same indications as in other patients but regarding on-going anticoagulation in IE patients with neurological complications special considerations must be made.

In ischaemic stroke without haemorrhage, replacement of oral anticoagulant therapy by unfractionated or low-molecular heparin for 1–2 weeks should be considered to get a more controllable situation. In the absence of stroke, replacement of oral anticoagulant therapy should also be considered in S. aureus IE [55]. Only single reports regarding IE in patients using the new direct acting oral anticoagulants have been published [73] and so far nothing is known about specific risks related to neurological complications in these patients.

Thrombolysis is contraindicated in IE patients due to increased intracranial haemorrhage risk but since large trials of thrombolytic therapy of acute ischemic stroke excluded patients with septic embolization this is based on risk assumption. Published systematic reviews do not address the role of thrombolytic therapy in the setting of septic embolization to the brain such as in infective endocarditis [74]. The haemorrhagic risk is documented in published case reports [75–78] although thrombolysis has been effective and safe in individual patients [78, 79]. However, since IE diagnosis is not always obvious or considered at initial patient presentation [80] and the standard of care in acute ischaemic stroke has become treatment with thrombolysis within 3–6 h of symptom onset, a subset of IE patients with ischaemic infarctions will probably be treated with thrombolysis in the future despite the existing contraindication and thus more information will become available. An alternative to thrombolysis is mechanical thrombectomy with lower risk of complicating intracerebral bleeding in a few published successful cases [81–84]. Although an interventional approach for treatment of acute ischaemic stroke related to IE is a promising option, it is controversial and a cautious clinical decision should be made on a case-by-case basis (Fig. 12.2a–d).

Intracerebral haemorrhages of all types, possibly with the exception of small silent haemorrhages found on MRI screening and ruptured intracranial infectious aneurysms treated with endovascular methods and without large intraparenchymal bleeding, contraindicate cardiac surgery for at least 4 weeks [33, 85, 86]. However, shorter delay and successful outcome has been reported in one study when cerebral hematoma is small (<1–2 cm) [86]. Underlying intracranial infectious aneurysms should be looked for in IE patients with neurological symptoms and verified intracerebral bleeding by use of non-invasive techniques such as CT or MRI angiography, but if these investigations are negative and suspicion remains high conventional four-vessel angiography should be considered. The handling of intracranial infectious aneurysms is outlined in the section above. Ongoing anticoagulation must be stopped and reversed in all cases of significant intracerebral bleeding regardless of indication for anticoagulation, but the demand and tempo of reinstitution differ according to anticoagulation indication. Some authors favour 10–14 days without anticoagulation [87] but the decision is preferably made on an individual basis following a multidisciplinary discussion. Reinitiation of anticoagulation should be started with unfractionated or low-molecular weight heparin.

Meningitis and cerebral abscesses in IE are treated with antibiotics according to guidelines for both IE and CNS infections implicating the use of antibiotics with good CNS penetration as well as documented IE effect, such as cephalosporins or penicillins with good CNS penetration. Isoxazolyl-penicillins, i.e., cloxacillin,

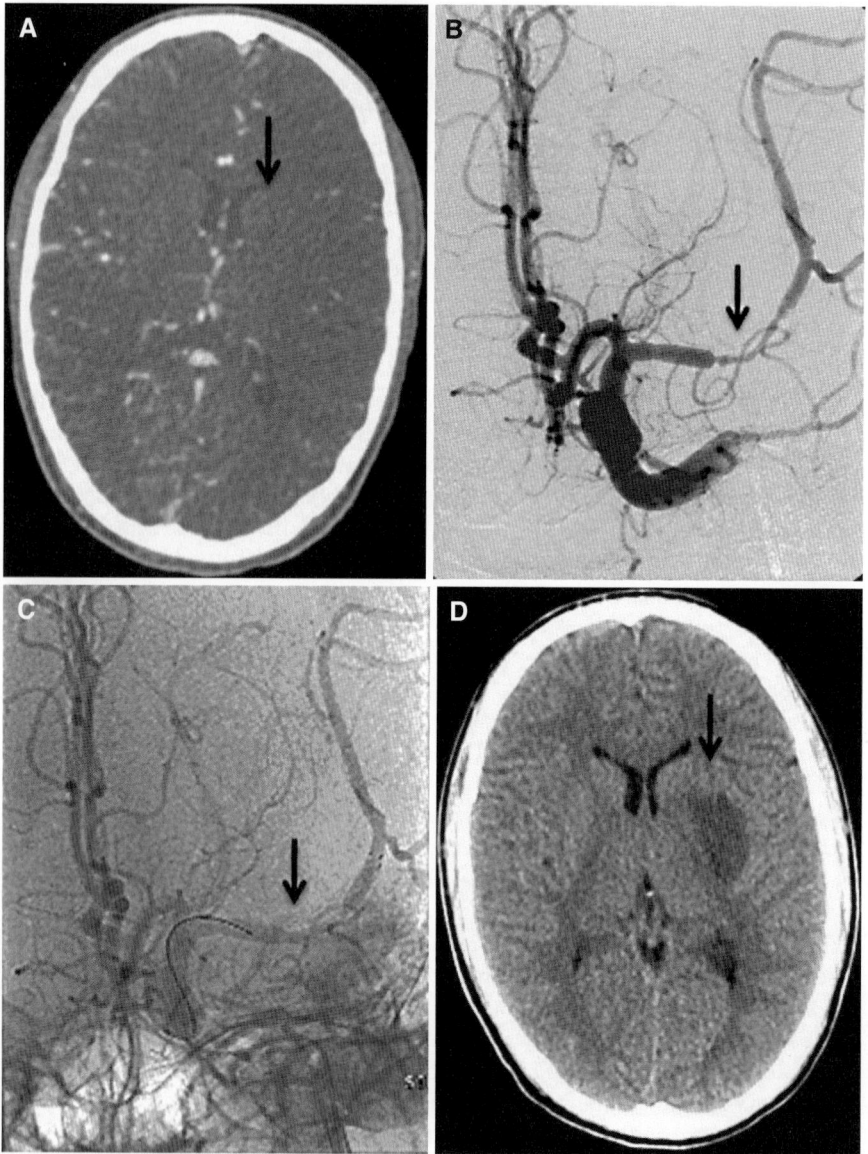

Fig. 12.2 Thrombectomy. 16 year old boy presenting with fever, headache, no initial murmur. Sudden onset of right-sided hemiparesis. Acute CT shows early signs of lower left temporal ischaemic infarction (**a**). Four-vessel angiography shows proximal occlusion in the left arteria cerebri media (**b**). Thrombectomy is performed (**c**). Follow up CT shows infarction without haemorrhagic transformation (**d**). Underlying S. aureus mitral valve endocarditis is confirmed by TEE

should not be used as long as significant intracerebral infections remain, due to high serum albumin binding and low CNS penetration [88]. In large cerebral abscesses, drainage may be necessary and oedema surrounding an abscess frequently motivates the addition of steroids. Surgical decisions can typically be taken regardless of coexisting meningitis or small abscesses while large abscesses needing neurosurgical intervention may influence surgical timing on an individual basis.

Surgical Considerations

Successful management of IE requires a combined medical and surgical approach in 30–60 % of patients. The safety of cardiac surgery and cardiopulmonary bypass in patients with acute CNS complications is, however, unclear and highly individualized due to type of IE and neurological complication, comorbidity, timing and local expertise among other factors. Neurological deficits can exacerbate due to heparinization and subsequent haemorrhagic conversion, while hypotension during surgery and anaesthesia might worsen cerebral ischemia and increase parenchymal damage. No large prospective studies have directly assessed whether and when to undertake valve repair in IE patients, though one prospective study has addressed the question of early surgery with vegectomy within 48 h to prevent embolism in IE patients with large vegetations and severe mitral or aortic valve regurgitation [72]. Propensity score analyses and other statistical modifications have been used to compensate for methodological flaws in different study populations, and a relatively uniform approach to surgical indications is seen in international guidelines [55, 70], but issues regarding timing in the setting of preoperative cerebral complications add a further angle to the problem.

The risk of neurological deterioration when cardiac surgery is performed after a silent cerebral emboli without haemorrhagic components or a TIA is considered low although not uniformly so [3, 29, 71] and surgery should proceed without delay if indication remains. After a clinically relevant ischaemic stroke, recent guidelines based recommendation is not to postpone urgently indicated cardiac surgery for heart failure, uncontrolled infection, abscess or persistent high embolic risk unless neurological symptoms are severe (i.e., coma) as long as cerebral haemorrhage has been excluded by cranial CT or MRI. If urgent surgery is not necessary praxis is to wait 1 week or more after an ischemic stroke, since several studies indicate worse in-hospital outcome in patients with preceding ischaemic lesions undergoing cardiac surgery for IE, which must be balanced to short- and long-term beneficial effects from early surgery seen in many, but not all, patients [33, 89]. Some authors have suggested correlating the size of the cerebral infarction to timing of surgery but this has not been done in most studies [90]. Following intracranial haemorrhage surgery should in general be delayed for 1 month or more as outlined above. Recommendations are not based on high level evidence but are balanced conclusions drawn from observational studies and meta-analyses [34, 86, 89–91] and will probably be subject to modifications as more information and advanced treatment options become available.

References

1. Pruitt AA, Rubin RH, Karchmer AW, Duncan GW. Neurologic complications of bacterial endocarditis. Medicine (Baltimore). 1978;57(4):329–43.
2. Heiro M, Nikoskelainen J, Engblom E, Kotilainen E, Marttila R, Kotilainen P. Neurologic manifestations of infective endocarditis: a 17-year experience in a teaching hospital in Finland. Arch Intern Med. 2000;160(18):2781–7.
3. Thuny F, Avierinos JF, Tribouilloy C, Giorgi R, Casalta JP, Milandre L, et al. Impact of cerebrovascular complications on mortality and neurologic outcome during infective endocarditis: a prospective multicentre study. Eur Heart J. 2007;28(9):1155–61.
4. Snygg-Martin U, Rasmussen RV, Hassager C, Bruun NE, Andersson R, Olaison L. The relationship between cerebrovascular complications and previously established use of antiplatelet therapy in left-sided infective endocarditis. Scand J Infect Dis. 2011;43(11–12):899–904.
5. Garcia-Cabrera E, Fernandez-Hidalgo N, Almirante B, Ivanova-Georgieva R, Noureddine M, Plata A, et al. Neurological complications of infective endocarditis: risk factors, outcome, and impact of cardiac surgery: a multicenter observational study. Circulation. 2013;127(23):2272–84.
6. Dickerman SA, Abrutyn E, Barsic B, Bouza E, Cecchi E, Moreno A, et al. The relationship between the initiation of antimicrobial therapy and the incidence of stroke in infective endocarditis: an analysis from the ICE Prospective Cohort Study (ICE-PCS). Am Heart J. 2007;154(6):1086–94.
7. Paschalis C, Pugsley W, John R, Harrison MJ. Rate of cerebral embolic events in relation to antibiotic and anticoagulant therapy in patients with bacterial endocarditis. Eur Neurol. 1990;30(2):87–9.
8. Kanter MC, Hart RG. Neurologic complications of infective endocarditis. Neurology. 1991;41(7):1015–20.
9. Di Salvo G, Habib G, Pergola V, Avierinos JF, Philip E, Casalta JP, et al. Echocardiography predicts embolic events in infective endocarditis. J Am Coll Cardiol. 2001;37(4):1069–76.
10. Durante Mangoni E, Adinolfi LE, Tripodi MF, Andreana A, Gambardella M, Ragone E, et al. Risk factors for "major" embolic events in hospitalized patients with infective endocarditis. Am Heart J. 2003;146(2):311–6.
11. Buyukasyk NS, Ileri M, Alper A, Senen K, Atak R, Hisar I, et al. Increased blood coagulation and platelet activation in patients with infective endocarditis and embolic events. Clin Cardiol. 2004;27(3):154–8.
12. Hill EE, Herijgers P, Claus P, Vanderschueren S, Peetermans WE, Herregods MC. Clinical and echocardiographic risk factors for embolism and mortality in infective endocarditis. Eur J Clin Microbiol Infect Dis. 2008;16:16.
13. Hubert S, Thuny F, Resseguier N, Giorgi R, Tribouilloy C, Le Dolley Y, et al. Prediction of symptomatic embolism in infective endocarditis: construction and validation of a risk calculator in a multicenter cohort. J Am Coll Cardiol. 2013;62(15):1384–92.
14. Miro JM, Anguera I, Cabell CH, Chen AY, Stafford JA, Corey GR, et al. Staphylococcus aureus native valve infective endocarditis: report of 566 episodes from the International Collaboration on Endocarditis Merged Database. Clin Infect Dis. 2005;41(4):507–14.
15. Habib G. Embolic risk in subacute bacterial endocarditis: determinants and role of transesophageal echocardiography. Curr Infect Dis Rep. 2005;7(4):264–71.
16. Tischler MD, Vaitkus PT. The ability of vegetation size on echocardiography to predict clinical complications: a meta-analysis. J Am Soc Echocardiogr. 1997;10(5):562–8.
17. Goulenok T, Klein I, Mazighi M, Messika-Zeitoun D, Alexandra JF, Mourvillier B, et al. Infective endocarditis with symptomatic cerebral complications: contribution of cerebral magnetic resonance imaging. Cerebrovasc Dis. 2013;35(4):327–36.
18. Hart RG, Foster JW, Luther MF, Kanter MC. Stroke in infective endocarditis. Stroke. 1990;21(5):695–700.

19. Roder BL, Wandall DA, Espersen F, Frimodt-Moller N, Skinhoj P, Rosdahl VT. Neurologic manifestations in Staphylococcus aureus endocarditis: a review of 260 bacteremic cases in nondrug addicts. Am J Med. 1997;102(4):379–86.
20. Snygg-Martin U, Gustafsson L, Rosengren L, Alsio A, Ackerholm P, Andersson R, et al. Cerebrovascular complications in patients with left-sided infective endocarditis are common: a prospective study using magnetic resonance imaging and neurochemical brain damage markers. Clin Infect Dis. 2008;47(1):23–30.
21. Hess A, Klein I, Iung B, Lavallee P, Ilic-Habensus E, Dornic Q, et al. Brain MRI findings in neurologically asymptomatic patients with infective endocarditis. AJNR Am J Neuroradiol. 2013;34(8):1579–84.
22. Toone CE. Cerebral manifestations of bacterial endocarditis. Ann Intern Med. 1941;14: 1551–74.
23. Murdoch DR, Corey GR, Hoen B, Miro JM, Fowler Jr VG, Bayer AS, et al. Clinical presentation, etiology, and outcome of infective endocarditis in the 21st century: the International Collaboration on Endocarditis-Prospective Cohort Study. Arch Intern Med. 2009;169 (5):463–73.
24. Durante-Mangoni E, Bradley S, Selton-Suty C, Tripodi MF, Barsic B, Bouza E, et al. Current features of infective endocarditis in elderly patients: results of the International Collaboration on Endocarditis Prospective Cohort Study. Arch Intern Med. 2008; 168(19):2095–103.
25. Sunder S, Grammatico-Guillon L, Baron S, Gaborit C, Bernard-Brunet A, Garot D, et al. Clinical and economic outcomes of infective endocarditis. Infect Dis (Lond). 2015;47 (2):80–7.
26. Leone S, Ravasio V, Durante-Mangoni E, Crapis M, Carosi G, Scotton PG, et al. Epidemiology, characteristics, and outcome of infective endocarditis in Italy: the Italian Study on Endocarditis. Infection. 2012;40(5):527–35.
27. Bin Abdulhak AA, Baddour LM, Erwin PJ, Hoen B, Chu VH, Mensah GA, et al. Global and regional burden of infective endocarditis, 1990–2010: a systematic review of the literature. Glob Heart. 2014;9(1):131–43.
28. Sonneville R, Mirabel M, Hajage D, Tubach F, Vignon P, Perez P, et al. Neurologic complications and outcomes of infective endocarditis in critically ill patients: the ENDOcardite en REAnimation prospective multicenter study. Crit Care Med. 2011;39(6):1474–81.
29. Cooper HA, Thompson EC, Laureno R, Fuisz A, Mark AS, Lin M, et al. Subclinical brain embolization in left-sided infective endocarditis: results from the evaluation by MRI of the brains of patients with left-sided intracardiac solid masses (EMBOLISM) pilot study. Circulation. 2009;120(7):585–91.
30. Duval X, Iung B, Klein I, Brochet E, Thabut G, Arnoult F, et al. Effect of early cerebral magnetic resonance imaging on clinical decisions in infective endocarditis: a prospective study. Ann Intern Med. 2010;152(8):497–504. W175.
31. Thuny F, Di Salvo G, Belliard O, Avierinos JF, Pergola V, Rosenberg V, et al. Risk of embolism and death in infective endocarditis: prognostic value of echocardiography: a prospective multicenter study. Circulation. 2005;112(1):69–75.
32. Iung B, Tubiana S, Klein I, Messika-Zeitoun D, Brochet E, Lepage L, et al. Determinants of cerebral lesions in endocarditis on systematic cerebral magnetic resonance imaging: a prospective study. Stroke. 2013;44(11):3056–62.
33. Eishi K, Kawazoe K, Kuriyama Y, Kitoh Y, Kawashima Y, Omae T. Surgical management of infective endocarditis associated with cerebral complications. Multi-center retrospective study in Japan. J Thorac Cardiovasc Surg. 1995;110(6):1745–55.
34. Ruttmann E, Willeit J, Ulmer H, Chevtchik O, Hofer D, Poewe W, et al. Neurological outcome of septic cardioembolic stroke after infective endocarditis. Stroke. 2006;37(8):2094–9.
35. Singhal AB, Topcuoglu MA, Buonanno FS. Acute ischemic stroke patterns in infective and nonbacterial thrombotic endocarditis: a diffusion-weighted magnetic resonance imaging study. Stroke. 2002;33(5):1267–73.

36. Fabri Jr J, Issa VS, Pomerantzeff PM, Grinberg M, Barretto AC, Mansur AJ. Time-related distribution, risk factors and prognostic influence of embolism in patients with left-sided infective endocarditis. Int J Cardiol. 2006;110(3):334–9.
37. Corral I, Martin-Davila P, Fortun J, Navas E, Centella T, Moya JL, et al. Trends in neurological complications of endocarditis. J Neurol. 2007;27:27.
38. Hart RG, Kagan-Hallet K, Joerns SE. Mechanisms of intracranial hemorrhage in infective endocarditis. Stroke. 1987;18(6):1048–56.
39. Masuda J, Yutani C, Waki R, Ogata J, Kuriyama Y, Yamaguchi T. Histopathological analysis of the mechanisms of intracranial hemorrhage complicating infective endocarditis. Stroke. 1992;23(6):843–50.
40. Delahaye JP, Poncet P, Malquarti V, Beaune J, Gare JP, Mann JM. Cerebrovascular accidents in infective endocarditis: role of anticoagulation. Eur Heart J. 1990;11(12):1074–8.
41. Tornos P, Almirante B, Mirabet S, Permanyer G, Pahissa A, Soler-Soler J. Infective endocarditis due to Staphylococcus aureus: deleterious effect of anticoagulant therapy. Arch Intern Med. 1999;159(5):473–5.
42. Cho IJ, Kim JS, Chang HJ, Kim YJ, Lee SC, Choi JH, et al. Prediction of hemorrhagic transformation following embolic stroke in patients with prosthetic valve endocarditis. J Cardiovasc Ultrasound. 2013;21(3):123–9.
43. Leport C, Vilde JL, Bricaire F, Cohen A, Pangon B, Gaudebout C, et al. Fifty cases of late prosthetic valve endocarditis: improvement in prognosis over a 15 year period. Br Heart J. 1987;58(1):66–71.
44. Rasmussen RV, Snygg-Martin U, Olaison L, Buchholtz K, Larsen CT, Hassager C, et al. Major cerebral events in Staphylococcus aureus infective endocarditis: is anticoagulant therapy safe? Cardiology. 2009;114(4):284–91.
45. Snygg-Martin U, Rasmussen RV, Hassager C, Bruun NE, Andersson R, Olaison L. Warfarin therapy and incidence of cerebrovascular complications in left-sided native valve endocarditis. Eur J Clin Microbiol Infect Dis. 2010;30(2):151–7.
46. Mook-Kanamori BB, Fritz D, Brouwer MC, van der Ende A, van de Beek D. Intracerebral hemorrhages in adults with community associated bacterial meningitis in adults: should we reconsider anticoagulant therapy? PLoS One. 2012;7(9), e45271.
47. Okazaki S, Sakaguchi M, Hyun B, Nagano K, Tagaya M, Sakata Y, et al. Cerebral microbleeds predict impending intracranial hemorrhage in infective endocarditis. Cerebrovasc Dis. 2011;32(5):483–8.
48. Schrag M, Greer DM. Clinical associations of cerebral microbleeds on magnetic resonance neuroimaging. J Stroke Cerebrovasc Dis. 2014;23(10):2489–97.
49. Gonzalez I, Sarria C, Lopez J, Vilacosta I, San Roman A, Olmos C, et al. Symptomatic peripheral mycotic aneurysms due to infective endocarditis: a contemporary profile. Medicine (Baltimore). 2014;93(1):42–52.
50. Peters PJ, Harrison T, Lennox JL. A dangerous dilemma: management of infectious intracranial aneurysms complicating endocarditis. Lancet Infect Dis. 2006;6(11):742–8.
51. Gross BA, Puri AS. Endovascular treatment of infectious intracranial aneurysms. Neurosurg Rev. 2013;36(1):11–9. discussion 9.
52. Ducruet AF, Hickman ZL, Zacharia BE, Narula R, Grobelny BT, Gorski J, et al. Intracranial infectious aneurysms: a comprehensive review. Neurosurg Rev. 2010;33(1):37–46.
53. Corr P, Wright M, Handler LC. Endocarditis-related cerebral aneurysms: radiologic changes with treatment. AJNR Am J Neuroradiol. 1995;16(4):745–8.
54. Salgado AV, Furlan AJ, Keys TF. Mycotic aneurysm, subarachnoid hemorrhage, and indications for cerebral angiography in infective endocarditis. Stroke. 1987;18(6):1057–60.
55. Habib G, Hoen B, Tornos P, Thuny F, Prendergast B, Vilacosta I, et al. Guidelines on the prevention, diagnosis, and treatment of infective endocarditis (new version 2009): the Task Force on the Prevention, Diagnosis, and Treatment of Infective Endocarditis of the European Society of Cardiology (ESC). Eur Heart J. 2009;30(19):2369–413.
56. Angstwurm K, Halle E, Wetzel K, Schultze J, Schielke E, Weber JR. Isolated bacterial meningitis as the key syndrome of infective endocarditis. Infection. 2004;32(1):47–50.

57. Pruitt AA. Neurological complications of infective endocarditis: a review of an evolving disease and its management issues in the 1990s. Infect Dis Clin Pract. 1996;5:101–13.
58. Lucas MJ, Brouwer MC, van der Ende A, van de Beek D. Endocarditis in adults with bacterial meningitis. Circulation. 2013;127(20):2056–62.
59. Ferreyra MC, Chavarria ER, Ponieman DA, Olavegogeascoechea PA. Silent brain abscess in patients with infective endocarditis. Mayo Clin Proc. 2013;88(4):422–3.
60. Alvis Miranda H, Castellar-Leones SM, Elzain MA, Moscote-Salazar LR. Brain abscess: current management. J Neurosci Rural Pract. 2013;4 Suppl 1:S67–81.
61. Iung B, Klein I, Mourvillier B, Olivot JM, Detaint D, Longuet P, et al. Respective effects of early cerebral and abdominal magnetic resonance imaging on clinical decisions in infective endocarditis. Eur Heart J Cardiovasc Imaging. 2012;13(8):703–10.
62. Thuny F, Beurtheret S, Mancini J, Gariboldi V, Casalta JP, Riberi A, et al. The timing of surgery influences mortality and morbidity in adults with severe complicated infective endocarditis: a propensity analysis. Eur Heart J. 2011;32(16):2027–33.
63. Vilacosta I, Graupner C, San Roman JA, Sarria C, Ronderos R, Fernandez C, et al. Risk of embolization after institution of antibiotic therapy for infective endocarditis. J Am Coll Cardiol. 2002;39(9):1489–95.
64. Chan KL, Dumesnil JG, Cujec B, Sanfilippo AJ, Jue J, Turek MA, et al. A randomized trial of aspirin on the risk of embolic events in patients with infective endocarditis. J Am Coll Cardiol. 2003;42(5):775–80.
65. Anavekar NS, Tleyjeh IM, Anavekar NS, Mirzoyev Z, Steckelberg JM, Haddad C, et al. Impact of prior antiplatelet therapy on risk of embolism in infective endocarditis. Clin Infect Dis. 2007;44(9):1180–6.
66. Habib A, Baddour LM, Sohail MR. Impact of antiplatelet therapy on clinical manifestations and outcomes of cardiovascular infections. Curr Infect Dis Rep. 2013;15(4):347–52.
67. Chan KL, Tam J, Dumesnil JG, Cujec B, Sanfilippo AJ, Jue J, et al. Effect of long-term aspirin use on embolic events in infective endocarditis. Clin Infect Dis. 2008;46(1):37–41.
68. Sedlacek M, Gemery JM, Cheung AL, Bayer AS, Remillard BD. Aspirin treatment is associated with a significantly decreased risk of Staphylococcus aureus bacteremia in hemodialysis patients with tunneled catheters. Am J Kidney Dis. 2007;49(3):401–8.
69. Kupferwasser LI, Yeaman MR, Shapiro SM, Nast CC, Sullam PM, Filler SG, et al. Acetylsalicylic acid reduces vegetation bacterial density, hematogenous bacterial dissemination, and frequency of embolic events in experimental Staphylococcus aureus endocarditis through antiplatelet and antibacterial effects. Circulation. 1999;99(21):2791–7.
70. Baddour LM, Wilson WR, Bayer AS, Fowler Jr VG, Bolger AF, Levison ME, et al. Infective endocarditis: diagnosis, antimicrobial therapy, and management of complications: a statement for healthcare professionals from the Committee on Rheumatic Fever, Endocarditis, and Kawasaki Disease, Council on Cardiovascular Disease in the Young, and the Councils on Clinical Cardiology, Stroke, and Cardiovascular Surgery and Anesthesia, American Heart Association: endorsed by the Infectious Diseases Society of America. Circulation. 2005;111(23):e394–434.
71. Misfeld M, Girrbach F, Etz CD, Binner C, Aspern KV, Dohmen PM, et al. Surgery for infective endocarditis complicated by cerebral embolism: a consecutive series of 375 patients. J Thorac Cardiovasc Surg. 2014;147(6):1837–46.
72. Kang DH, Kim YJ, Kim SH, Sun BJ, Kim DH, Yun SC, et al. Early surgery versus conventional treatment for infective endocarditis. N Engl J Med. 2012;366(26):2466–73.
73. Stollberger C, Bonner E, Finsterer J. Enterococcus faecalis bacteremia and mitral valve endocarditis under dabigatran for stroke prevention. Int J Cardiol. 2014;174(3):836–8.
74. Furlan A, Higashida R, Wechsler L, Gent M, Rowley H, Kase C, et al. Intra-arterial prourokinase for acute ischemic stroke. The PROACT II study: a randomized controlled trial. Prolyse in Acute Cerebral Thromboembolism. JAMA. 1999;282(21):2003–11.
75. Walker KA, Sampson JB, Skalabrin EJ, Majersik JJ. Clinical characteristics and thrombolytic outcomes of infective endocarditis-associated stroke. Neurohospitalist. 2012;2(3):87–91.
76. Bhuva P, Kuo SH, Claude Hemphill J, Lopez GA. Intracranial hemorrhage following thrombolytic use for stroke caused by infective endocarditis. Neurocrit Care. 2009;12(1):79–82.

77. Junna M, Lin CC, Espinosa RE, Rabinstein AA. Successful intravenous thrombolysis in isch-emic stroke caused by infective endocarditis. Neurocrit Care. 2007;6(2):117–20.
78. Ong E, Mechtouff L, Bernard E, Cho TH, Diallo LL, Nighoghossian N, et al. Thrombolysis for stroke caused by infective endocarditis: an illustrative case and review of the literature. J Neurol. 2013;260(5):1339–42.
79. Siccoli M, Benninger D, Schuknecht B, Jenni R, Valavanis A, Bassetti C. Successful intra-arterial thrombolysis in basilar thrombosis secondary to infectious endocarditis. Cerebrovasc Dis. 2003;16(3):295–7.
80. Epaulard O, Roch N, Potton L, Pavese P, Brion JP, Stahl JP. Infective endocarditis-related stroke: diagnostic delay and prognostic factors. Scand J Infect Dis. 2009;15:1–5.
81. Toeg HD, Al-Atassi T, Kalidindi N, Iancu D, Zamani D, Giaccone R, et al. Endovascular treat-ment for cerebral septic embolic stroke. J Stroke Cerebrovasc Dis. 2014;23(5):e375–7.
82. Dababneh H, Hedna VS, Ford J, Taimeh Z, Peters K, Mocco J, et al. Endovascular intervention for acute stroke due to infective endocarditis: case report. Neurosurg Focus. 2012;32(2), E1.
83. Sontineni SP, Mooss AN, Andukuri VG, Schima SM, Esterbrooks D. Effectiveness of throm-bolytic therapy in acute embolic stroke due to infective endocarditis. Stroke Res Treat. 2010; 2010(10):9.
84. Kang G, Yang TK, Choi JH, Heo ST. Effectiveness of mechanical embolectomy for septic embolus in the cerebral artery complicated with infective endocarditis. J Korean Med Sci. 2013;28(8):1244–7.
85. Wilbring M, Irmscher L, Alexiou K, Matschke K, Tugtekin SM. The impact of preoperative neurological events in patients suffering from native infective valve endocarditis. Interact Cardiovasc Thorac Surg. 2014;18(6):740–7.
86. Shang E, Forrest GN, Chizmar T, Chim J, Brown JM, Zhan M, et al. Mitral valve infective endocarditis: benefit of early operation and aggressive use of repair. Ann Thorac Surg. 2009;87(6):1728–33. discussion 34.
87. Morris NA, Matiello M, Lyons JL, Samuels MA. Neurologic complications in infective endo-carditis: identification, management, and impact on cardiac surgery. Neurohospitalist. 2014;4(4):213–22.
88. Norgaard M, Gudmundsdottir G, Larsen CS, Schonheyder HC. Staphylococcus aureus menin-gitis: experience with cefuroxime treatment during a 16 year period in a Danish region. Scand J Infect Dis. 2003;35(5):311–4.
89. Barsic B, Dickerman S, Krajinovic V, Pappas P, Altclas J, Carosi G, et al. Influence of the tim-ing of cardiac surgery on the outcome of patients with infective endocarditis and stroke. Clin Infect Dis. 2013;56(2):209–17.
90. Hosono M, Sasaki Y, Hirai H, Sakaguchi M, Nakahira A, Seo H, et al. Considerations in tim-ing of surgical intervention for infective endocarditis with cerebrovascular complications. J Heart Valve Dis. 2010;19(3):321–5.
91. Rossi M, Gallo A, Joseph De Silva R, Sayeed R. What is the optimal timing for surgery in infective endocarditis with cerebrovascular complications? Interact Cardiovasc Thorac Surg. 2011;14(1):72–80.
92. Harrison MJ, Hampton JR. Neurological presentation of bacterial endocarditis. Br Med J. 1967;2(5545):148–51.
93. Anderson DJ, Goldstein LB, Wilkinson WE, Corey GR, Cabell CH, Sanders LL, et al. Stroke location, characterization, severity, and outcome in mitral vs aortic valve endocarditis. Neurology. 2003;61(10):1341–6.

Part VI
Specific Situations

Chapter 13
Prosthetic Valve Endocarditis

Sylvestre Marechaux and Christophe Tribouilloy

Introduction

Although relatively rare (1–6 % of patients with valve prosthesis), infective endo-carditis (IE) is a severe complication of valve replacement [1]. All types of valve prostheses can be involved, including bioprosthesis, mechanical prosthesis, homo-grafts and xenografts or transcatheter aortic valve replacement (TAVR). The diag-nosis and management of prosthetic valve infective endocarditis (PVE) are more challenging than in the case of native valve IE. The prognosis of PVE remains poorer than that of native valve IE despite improvements in surgical and medical management [1].

Epidemiology

Prosthetic valve endocarditis has been reported to occur with an incidence of 0.3–1.2 % per patient-year [2, 3]. It accounts for around 20 % of all cases of IE in recent reports [4, 5]. The early PVE (<2 months) rate was 14 % in the multicentre ICE study [5] and 22 % (<1 year) in a French report [4]. Risk factors for PVE are

Electronic supplementary material The online version of this chapter (doi:10.1007/978-3-319-32432-6_13) contains supplementary material, which is available to authorized users.

S. Marechaux, MD, PhD
Département de Cardiologie, Groupement des Hôpitaux de l'Institut Catholique de Lille,
Hôpital Saint Philibert, Lomme, France
e-mail: Sylvestre.marechaux@gmail.com

C. Tribouilloy, MD, PhD (✉)
Service de Cardiologie, Centre Hospitalier Universitaire d'Amiens, Hôpital Sud,
Amiens, France
e-mail: Tribouilloy.christophe@chu-amiens.fr

advanced age, multivalvular interventions, and a history of IE responsible for prosthetic valve replacement [6].

Both mechanical and bioprosthetic valves can be involved by the infection, with similar 5-year infection rates (5.7 %). However, mechanical prosthetic valves seem to be at higher risk of infection during the first 3 months [7]. The risk of IE seems to be slightly higher for aortic valves compared to mitral valves. The IE rate after TAVR was 1.5 % at 2-year follow-up in the PARTNER registry and has been reported to be 3.4 % at 1 year [8]. In a recent multicentre registry, IE occurred in 29 out of 2579 patients (1.13 %) after TAVR [9]. The incidence of TAVR-related PVE was 1.1 % (23 out of 2133 patients), 1.98 % (6 out of 303 patents) after transfemoral and transapical TAVR, respectively, and 1.93 % (23 out of 1191 patients) and 0.45 % (6 out of 1343 patients) after balloon-expandable and self-expandable TAVR implantation, respectively. TAVR-PVE was diagnosed as early-onset in 28 % of cases, intermediate-onset in 52 % of cases and late-onset in 20 % of cases, resulting in a higher incidence within the first 12 months after TAVR (80 %) and lower rates of late-onset PVE (20 %) in contrast with surgical prosthetic valve endocarditis [9, 10]. In another multicentre registry, the incidence of IE 1 year after TAVR was 0.50 % and orotracheal intubation (hazard ratio: 3.9; P=0.004) and the self-expandable CoreValve system (hazard ratio: 3.12; P=0.007) were independently associated with IE [11].

The Bentall procedure seems to be at higher risk of IE compared to conservative procedures such as the David procedure [12, 13]. IE after mitral valve repair is rare (1.5 % at 20-year follow-up) [14]. IE after Mitraclip procedure also seems to be uncommon [15, 16].

Microbiology

Classically, the interval between the diagnosis of PVE and cardiac surgery is used to differentiate early PVE (<2 months), intermediate PVE between 2 months and 1 year, and late PVE (>1 year). Because of significant differences between the microbiology of PVE observed within 1 year of operation and later, the cut-off between early/intermediate and late PVE could be 1 year [17].

Staphylococcal infection is the most common form of PVE; *Staphylococcus aureus* is the most common causative microorganism, closely followed by coagulase-negative staphylococci, especially in the context of healthcare-related infection. *Staphylococci* (frequently methicillin-resistant), fungi, and gram-negative bacilli are the main causes of early/intermediate PVE, suggesting perioperative nosocomial infection or infection related to greater exposure to healthcare contact during a period when the prosthetic valve is not completely endothelialized [5]. One half of all cases of coagulase-negative staphylococcal IE (16 % of all cases of PVE) occurs during the 2 months to one year postoperative period and are associated with a high rate of intracardiac abscess and mortality [18, 19]. Culture results can remain negative during the first 2 months in almost 17 % of cases [5]. Blood culture-negative early PVE is due to specific aetiologies, as fungi are the most common pathogens identified in blood culture-negative early PVE (16 %) [20], while *Candida* spp. and *Histoplasma capsulatum* are the species most frequently isolated. The microbiology of late PVE more closely resembles that of native valve IE. Staphylococci, oral streptococci, *Streptococcus bovis*, and enterococci are the most common organisms most likely related to community-acquired infections. *Enterococcus*-PVE is associated with a high risk of recurrence when managed conservatively [21]. Culture results are negative in approximately 10 % of cases of late PVE.

According to a recent multicentre study, the most common causes of PVE after TAVR were staphylococci (31 %), enterococci (21 %) and streptococci (14 %) [9]. *Staphylococcus aureus* and coagulase-negative staphylococci were the most prevalent organisms (50 %) in the early-onset group. Staphylococcal, enterococcal, and nonviridans streptococcal species each accounted for 20 % of intermediate-onset IE. Staphylococci (33 %) and enterococci (33 %) were the most common causes of late PVE.

Pathophysiology

Circulating microorganisms responsible for PVE colonise thrombotic material encountered on or around the prosthesis. Because microorganisms cannot adhere to the leaflets of mechanical prosthetic valves provided they are free of thrombotic material [2], the pathogenesis of mechanical PVE involved a periannular site with frequent abscess formation. Conversely, infection is more frequently located on the leaflets in bioprosthetic PVE, leading to cusp rupture, perforation, and vegetations. In early PVE, the infection usually involves the junction between the sewing ring and the annulus, leading to perivalvular abscess, dehiscence, pseudoaneurysms, and fistula regardless of the type of prosthesis (bioprosthesis or mechanical prosthesis) [2, 7, 22]. Early PVE (< postoperative 6 months) and aortic valve involvement were both associated with an increased risk of periannular complications, with a 17 % risk of LV-aorta fistula in the case of aortic PVE in the retrospective ICE cohort [23]. The risk of fistula is twofold higher in patients with PVE compared to patients with native valve IE (1.8 % vs 3.5 %). Perivalvular abscess was diagnosed by either echocardiography or surgery in 35 % of patients with PVE [4].

Diagnosis

Clinical Presentation

Early PVE often presents clinically with fever or inflammatory syndrome, which are nonspecific during the early postoperative period. Similarly, fever is the main clinical sign in late PVE. Unexplained fever in a patient with a cardiac device should raise the suspicion of infective endocarditis. Heart failure may be present in

30 % of patients with PVE, similar to the rate observed in native valve IE [4, 5]. However, despite a similar frequency of embolic events, the frequency of cerebro-vascular haemorrhage is higher in patients with PVE compared to patients with native valve IE, probably due to the need for anticoagulation with mechanical prostheses.

Echocardiography

As for native valve IE, echocardiography remains the cornerstone of (1) the positive diagnosis of PVE and its complication; (2) the decision–making process; and (3) the follow-up of patients with PVE. The diagnosis of endocarditis is more difficult in the presence of a prosthetic valve compared to a native valve due to reverbera-tions and high reflectance leading to shadowing behind the prosthesis. Transoesophageal echocardiography is mandatory for the assessment of PVE, because of its better sensitivity and specificity for the detection of vegetations and abscesses. Perivalvular lesions are more frequent than vegetations in patients with PVE. Perivalvular abscesses are frequently observed at the aortic annulus with ini-tially echo-free parietal thickening with no circulating flow on colour Doppler imaging (Fig. 13.1a, b, Video 13.1) then usually progressing to pseudoaneurysms with circulating flow on colour Doppler imaging (Fig. 13.2a–c, Video 13.2) or into fistula (Fig. 13.3, Video 13.3). In addition, these abnormalities are frequently responsible for *de novo* regurgitation which is a major Duke criterion of IE. It is frequently difficult to assess the site of these regurgitations compared with the post-operative echocardiogram. These regurgitations may be either intraprosthetic or periprosthetic. Quantification of regurgitation must be based on a multiparametric approach, as recommended by current guidelines. The combination of TTE and TEE provides the most complete assessment of the prosthesis, by using all available windows to establish the diagnosis, as vegetations can be easily obscured in the case of PVE. TEE allows better visualization of the atrial surface of mitral valve prosthe-ses; TTE allows better visualization of the anterior surface, while TEE allows better visualization of the posterior portion of the aortic annulus and the aorta. Three dimensional real-time TEE combined with Doppler colour imaging (Fig. 13.4a–f, Video 13.4) allows assessment of the entire circumference of mitral valve prosthe-ses to facilitate the detection of periprosthetic regurgitation or lesions. In addition, small vegetations can be missed even with TEE. Suture material can be confused with small vegetations and may be responsible for false-positive findings. In addi-tion, the distinction between vegetations and thrombus is nearly impossible using echocardiography. Abscess may be difficult to diagnose by echocardiography in the presence of PVE with small abscesses, at the early phase of aortic abscesses pre-senting only thickening of the aortic root, and after a Bentall procedure. Consequently, although TEE provides more reliable imaging than TTE in both PVE and native valve IE, the combined value of TTE and TEE is lower in PVE than in

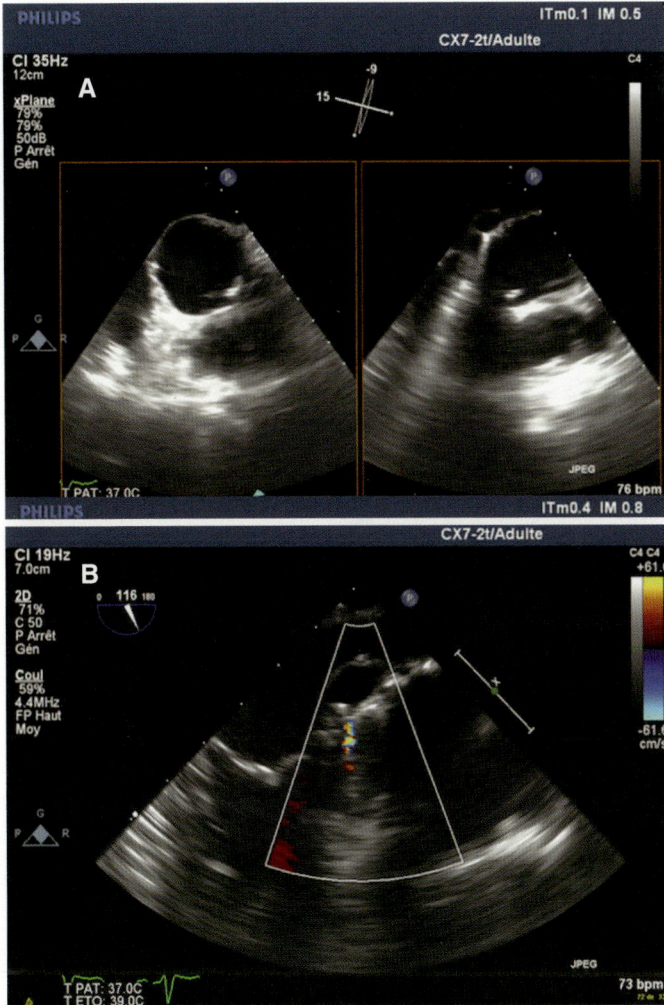

Fig. 13.1 Posterior perivalvular abscess of the aortic annulus (aortic bioprosthesis) without circulating flow using colour Doppler imaging (transoesophageal orthogonal short and long axis views (**a**) and Video 13.1) and colour Doppler imaging (**b**))

native valve IE [24]. TTE and TEE may initially give false-negative results in the presence of true PVE and must be repeated in the case of a high level of clinical suspicion. In a recent multicentre registry of TAVR-related PVE, vegetations were present in 77 % of patients (transcatheter valve leaflets: 39 %; stent frame: 17 %; mitral valve: 21 %) [11]. The Duke criteria have been shown to be less helpful in prosthetic valve endocarditis because of their lower sensitivity in this setting [25–27].

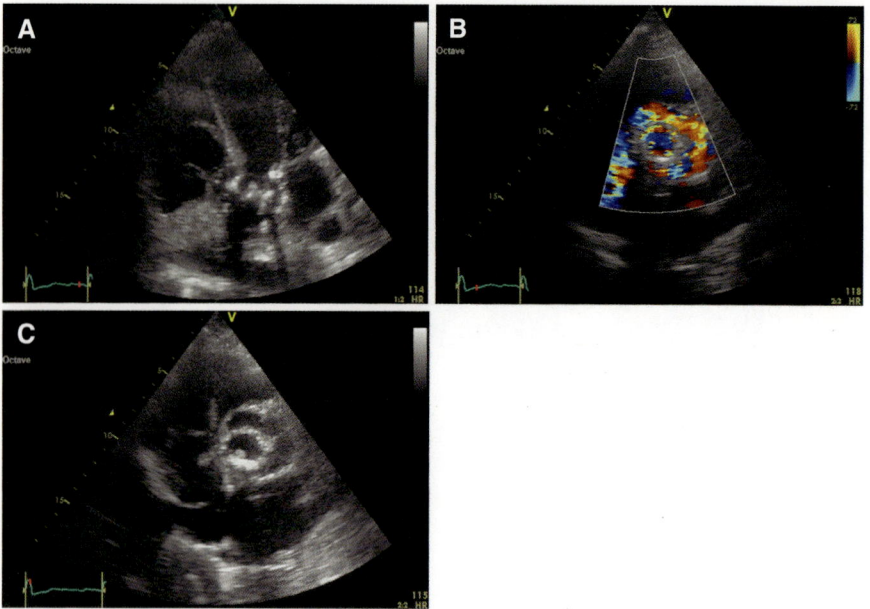

Fig. 13.2 Circumferential perivalvular (aortic bioprosthesis) circulating abcess of the aortic annulus (**a**, apical long axis view, short axis view with (**b** and Video 13.2) and without (**c**) Doppler colour flow mapping)

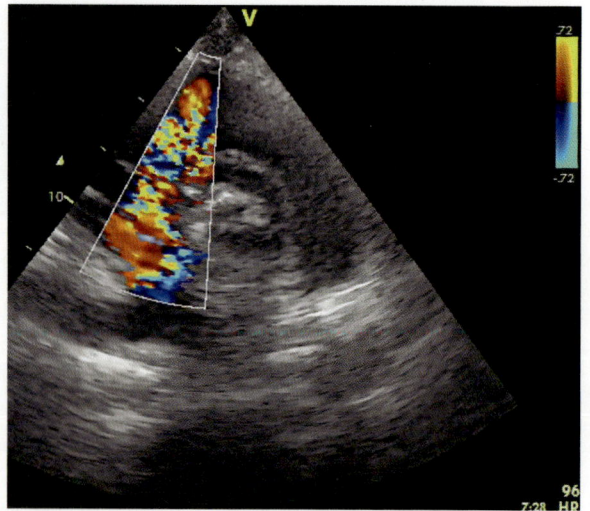

Fig. 13.3 Circumferential perivalvular (aortic bioprosthesis) circulating abcess of the aortic annulus with aorto-pulmonary fistula (Video 13.3)

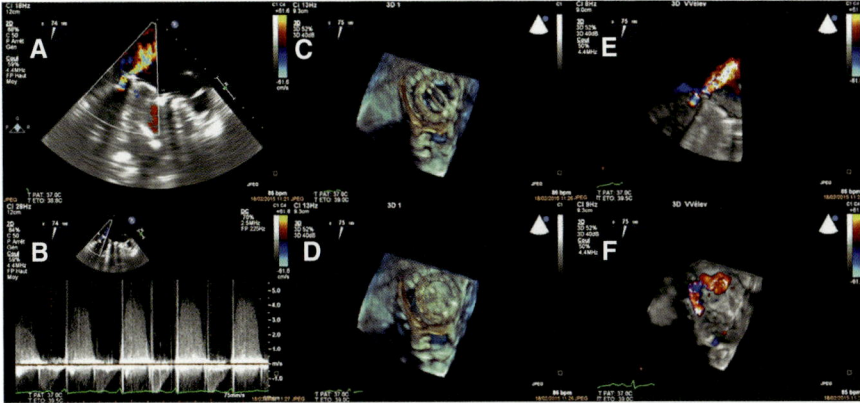

Fig. 13.4 Paraprosthetic severe mitral regurgitation with prosthetic dehiscence in a patient with staphylococcal endocarditis 10 months after mitral valve replacement. Real time TEE with and without Doppler colour flow mapping allows the accurate identification of perivalvular lesions. (**a**): 70° long mid-oesophageal view, (**b**): continuous Doppler waveform of the regurgitant jet, (**c**): Saint Jude prosthesis in diastole and (**d**): systole, (**e**) and (**f**): extent of the regurgitant jet by 3D Doppler colour flow mapping (Video 13.4)

Other Imaging Modalities

The use of ^{18}F-fluorodeoxyglucose (^{18}F-FDG) PET-CT allows the detection of enhanced glucose metabolism within organs. Although classically used for diagnosis and staging of cancer, ^{18}F-FDG PET-CT has been shown to be useful for the diagnosis and monitoring of inflammatory and infectious conditions. Several reports, mostly concerning PVE, have shown important results of ^{18}F-FDG PET-CT imaging in IE [28–30]. Abnormal FDG uptake around a prosthetic valve constitutes a new major criterion in the 2015 version of ESC guidelines that increases the sensitivity of modified Duke criteria at admission from 70 to 97 % [31–33]. In addition, whole-body imaging is also useful to detect emboli, metastatic infections and primary tumours. However, ^{18}F-FDG PET-CT presents a number of limitations. Issues such as the limit of detection of small oscillating vegetations in the presence of high glucose metabolism and heart muscle movements, timing of ^{18}F-FDG PET-CT in relation to the start of antibiotic therapy, and the reliability of ^{18}F-FDG PET-CT in slowly evolving infections and poorly controlled diabetic patients have not been clarified. Due to the high glucose metabolism in brain tissue, ^{18}F-FDG PET-CT is less suitable for detection of infectious embolic events in the brain. Lastly, caution must be exercised when interpreting ^{18}F-FDG PET-CT in patients who have recently undergone cardiac surgery, as false-positive results may be observed during the postoperative period. Consequently, patients in whom cardiac surgery had been performed during the previous 1 month were not included in the major reports on the value of ^{18}F-FDG PET-CT in PVE [31]. Figure 13.5 illustrates the case of a patient with intermittent fever and skin lesions of vasculitis 6 months after bioprosthetic aortic valve replacement. Despite 3 normal

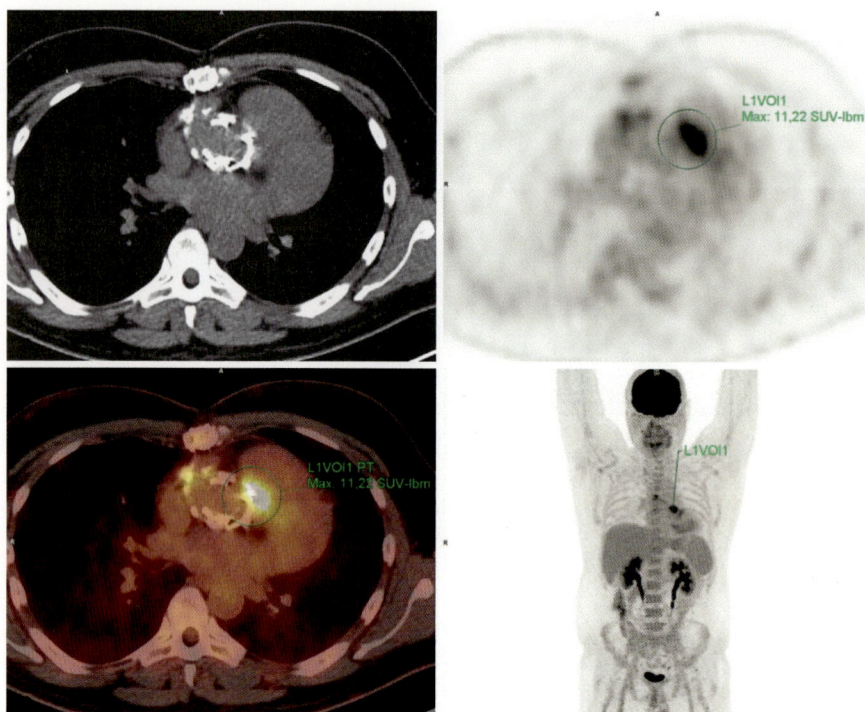

Fig. 13.5 18F-FDG PET-CT in a patient with suspected PVE 6 months after aortic valve replacement by a bioprosthesis. An abnormal FDG uptake around a prosthetic valve was found (SUV max 11.2). Blood cultures were positive at Propionebacterium acnes and the final diagnosis of endocarditis was retained despite normal TEE

TEE examinations performed at 10-day intervals, blood cultures revealed the presence of *Propionibacterium acnes*, leading to a diagnosis of infective endocarditis. Early ^{18}F-FDG PET-CT was positive (Fig. 13.5).

Fagman et al. recently investigated the role of ECG-gated 64-slice CT in the diagnosis of aortic prosthetic valve IE [33]. Low-dose CT performed in the context of ^{18}F-FDG PET is neither electrocardiogram-gated nor contrast-enhanced, and therefore unable to detect vegetations. In a series of 27 patients, these authors showed that the strength of agreement between ECG-gated CT and TEE was good for abscess and dehiscence, and moderate for vegetations. In comparison with intraoperative findings, CT detected three additional valvular pseudoaneurysms that were not detected by TEE. In two of these cases, the pseudoaneurysm was located close to the right coronary cusp, a location that is difficult to investigate by TEE. In a recent report, CT resulted in a major diagnostic change in 21 % of patients with suspected PVE compared with TTE and TEE, also mainly driven by the novel detection of valvular pseudoaneurysms by CT [34]. Importantly, CT offers the possibility to rapidly image not only the heart and other organs but also to identify both cardiac lesions and extracardiac complications, such as embolic events, infectious aneurysms, haemorrhages and septic metastases. In addition, CT can allow preop-

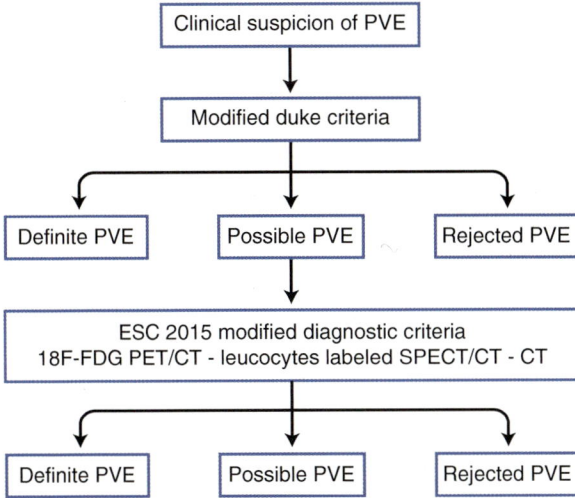

```
              ┌──────────────────────────┐
              │  Clinical suspicion of PVE │
              └──────────────────────────┘
                           │
              ┌──────────────────────────┐
              │    Modified duke criteria  │
              └──────────────────────────┘
```

┌──────────────┐   ┌──────────────┐   ┌──────────────┐
│ Definite PVE │   │ Possible PVE │   │ Rejected PVE │
└──────────────┘   └──────────────┘   └──────────────┘

┌──┐
│   ESC 2015 modified diagnostic criteria   │
│ 18F-FDG PET/CT - leucocytes labeled SPECT/CT - CT   │
└──┘

┌──────────────┐   ┌──────────────┐   ┌──────────────┐
│ Definite PVE │   │ Possible PVE │   │ Rejected PVE │
└──────────────┘   └──────────────┘   └──────────────┘

Fig. 13.6 Algorithm of evaluation of patients with suspected prosthetic valve endocarditis (*PVE*) using PET/CT or leucocytes labeled SPECT/CT (From Authors/Task Force [32]. With permission of Oxford University Press)

erative anatomical assessment of the coronary bed [35]. The main limitation of widespread use of this technique in comparison with ^{18}F-FDG PET-CT is that contrast agents may be harmful in frail patients with renal failure or haemodynamic instability because of the risk of worsening renal impairment in combination with antibiotic nephrotoxicity. In some cases, the indications for CT scan may be limited to the brain and its arteries. Specific guidelines are needed to clearly define the appropriate situations in which this modality should be used. Interestingly, it has been suggested that fusion of CT angiography and ^{18}F-FDG-PET may refine the diagnostic value of each of these diagnostic tools in the setting of PVE [36].

The results of leukocyte SPECT/CT in IE patients are discordant, but few case reports have shown SPECT/CT to be helpful in patients with PVE [37]. Leukocyte SPECT/CT is more specific for the detection of infectious foci than ^{18}F-FDG PET-CT, but also much more time-consuming. Moreover, ^{18}F-FDG PET-CT seems to have a better spatial resolution and photon detection efficiency.

Figure 13.6 presents the algorithm for assessment of patients with suspected PVE, taking into account both classical modified Duke criteria and ^{18}F-FDG PET-CT/leucocytes labeled SPECT/CT and CT findings [32].

Prognosis

The prognosis of PVE remains poor with an in-hospital mortality of 20–25 %, and a higher mortality than in case of native valve IE [4, 5]. Early PVE is classically associated with a very high mortality rate (40 to 75 %). However, in the recent ICE study, in-hospital mortality was higher during the intermediate period (>2 months) than at the early period (<2 months, 23 vs 47%) [5]. A major factor associated with in-hospital mortality is *Staphylococcus aureus* infection [38], as the in-hospital mortality rate was particularly high (36%) in the case of *Staphylococcus aureus*, followed by coagulase-negative *Staphylococcus* spp. (24%) and oral streptococci (9%) [18]. In a series of 122 cases of PVE, the 4-month mortality rate was 34%, and *S. aureus* was identified as the main predictor of death (75% vs 15% with other pathogens) [39].

Complications of PVE are clearly associated with a higher mortality rate [40, 41]. In the landmark report by Calderwood et al. [40], a 23% mortality rate was reported in the presence of PVE. Patients with complicated prosthetic valve endocarditis (new or changing heart murmur, new or worsening heart failure, new or progressive cardiac conduction abnormalities, or prolonged fever during therapy) had a higher mortality than patients with uncomplicated infection (Odds Ratio: 6.4, p=0.0009) [40]. In 104 patients with PVE, severe heart failure (Odds Ratio 5.5) and *S. aureus* infection (Odds Ratio: 6.1) were the only independent predictors of in-hospital death, which occurred in 22 (21%) patients [42]. In the ICE report, factors associated with in-hospital mortality were advanced age, healthcare–associated infection, severe comorbidity, persistent bacteraemia, septic shock, intravascular device source, congestive heart failure, renal failure, mediastinitis and intracardiac abscess [5]. These results therefore suggest that a subset of patients with PVE, i.e. patients with staphylococcal PVE and patients with complicated PVE, should be managed more aggressively.

Few studies have reported the medium-term and long-term outcome of patients with PVE [43]. The 32-month mortality of patients who survived the in-hospital period is high, around 25%, and is associated with early PVE, comorbidities, severe heart failure, *Staphylococcus* infection, and new prosthetic valve dehiscence [42]. However, four-year event-free survival in survivors to the active phase was not different between patients with early and late PVE in another report (74% and 82%, respectively) [44]. Ten-year survival has been reported at 28% in medically managed patients compared with 58% in surgically managed patients (p=0.04) [43]. It is noteworthy that redo surgery for PVE is associated with an increased risk of mortality compared to redo surgery for another cause (5-year survival 37 vs 63% and 10-year survival 31 vs 56%) [45]. Freedom from re-operation due to recurrent endocarditis at 10 years has been reported to be 86% for early PVE compared to 92% for late PVE patients (p=0.17) [46]. A 5-year survival rate of 75% was reported in complex prosthetic valve endocarditis (PVE) involving the aortic root in patients undergoing root replacement based on the Cabrol or Bentall procedures [47].

PVE after TAVR appears to be associated with very high mortality, with a 62% mortality rate with a median follow-up of 393 days in a multicentre registry of IE after TAVR. The only predictor of all-cause mortality in this report was the presence of chronic kidney disease (hazard ratio: 3.7; 95% CI: 1.2–11.2; p=0.023) [9]. Complications of IE are frequent in these patients, the most frequent being heart failure. However, most patients do not undergo valve intervention, resulting in high in-hospital and 1-year follow-up mortality rates [11]. However, the results of a another recent pooled analysis of data from the literature suggest that this condition is not inevitably fatal in these fragile patients and that aggressive treatment may be justified by a 6-month survival of 60 % [48].

Treatment

Surgery

The indication for valve surgery in the case of PVE remains a subject of debate in the absence of randomized controlled trials conducted in patients with PVE. In clinical practice, surgery is performed more frequently in the case of PVE in younger patients with intracardiac abscess, coagulase-negative *Staphylococcus* PVE, and congestive heart failure [38]. After adjustment for these determinants, in-hospital mortality was associated with brain embolization (OR: 11.12, 95 % CI: 4.16–29.73) and *Staphylococcus aureus* infection (OR: 3.67, 95 % CI: 1.29–9.74), with a trend toward a benefit of surgery (OR: 0.56, 95 % CI: 0.23–1.36) in Wang's report [38].

Some studies, limited by their small sample size and their single-centre design, have reported a benefit of surgery in PVE. In addition, a selection bias in favour of surgery is frequently observed, as some patients are denied surgery despite a surgical indication due to their comorbidities or the presence of septic shock [49]. In a recent large multicentre study involving 1025 patients with PVE [50], which tried to adjust for survival bias and timing of surgery, early valve replacement was not associated with lower in-hospital and 1-year mortality compared with medical therapy [50]. Similarly, in a prospective, multinational cohort of patients with *Staphylococcal aureus* PVE, early valve surgery, defined as replacement of the infected prosthetic valve within the first 60 days after admission for PVE, was not associated with reduced 1-year mortality [51]. In addition, a minimal follow-up of 188 days is required to find an overall survival advantage of early surgery [52]. However, both in-hospital and long-term mortality appeared to be reduced by a surgical approach in high-risk subgroups of patients with staphylococcal PVE and complicated PVE [42]. In contrast, a subset of medically treated patients characterized by age less than 50 years, ASA score III, and without cardiac, central nervous system, or systemic complications, could be cured without surgical intervention [32, 53]. It is noteworthy that the decision to operate should be based on a consensus from a heart team involving cardiologists, infectiologists and surgeons. In the absence of randomized controlled trials, this decision depends on the presence of poor prognosis factors described in PVE, including staphylococcal PVE and complicated PVE (haemodynamic and embolic complications). Indications for surgery in cases of PVE proposed by the 2015 ESC guidelines on prevention, diagnosis and treatment of infective endocarditis are detailed in Table 13.1 [32] and more extensively in Chap. 22 [32]. In summary, complicated PVE, staphylococcal PVE, and early PVE are associated with a poorer prognosis, if treated without surgery, and must be managed aggressively. Patients with non-complicated, non-staphylococcal late PVE can be managed conservatively with close follow-up.

Table 13.1 Indications and timing of surgery in PVE according to the 2015 ESC guidelines on prevention, diagnosis and treatment of infective endocarditis

Indications for surgery	Timing	Class	Level
1. Heart failure			
Aortic or mitral PVE with severe acute regurgitation, obstruction or fistula causing refractory pulmonary oedema or cardiogenic shock	Emergency	I	B
Aortic or mitral PVE with severe acute regurgitation, obstruction or fistula causing symptoms of heart failure or echocardiographic signs of poor haemodynamic tolerance	Urgent	I	B
2. Uncontrolled infection			
Locally uncontrolled infection (abscess, false aneurysm, fistula, enlarging vegetation)	Urgent	I	B
Infection caused by fungi or multiresistant organisms	Urgent/Elective	I	C
Persisting positive blood cultures despite appropriate antibiotic therapy and adequate control of septic metastatic foci	Urgent	IIa	B
PVE caused by staphylococci or non-HACK gram-negative bacteria (most cases of early PVE)	Urgent/Elective	IIa	C
3. Prevention of embolism			
Aortic or mitral PVE with persistant vegetations >10 mm after one or more embolic episode despite appropriate antibiotic therapy	Urgent	I	B
Aortic or mitral PVE with isolated very large vegetations (>30 mm)	Urgent	IIa	B
Aortic or mitral PVE with isolated large vegetations (>15 mm) and no other indication for surgery	Urgent	IIb	C

From Authors/Task Force et al. [32]. With permission of Oxford University Press

The surgical treatment of PVE remains a challenge [54] because of the complexity of the operation, and because PVE is frequently associated with perivalvular abscess [23]. The main objectives of surgery are to control infection by debridement with removal of infected and necrotic tissue and reconstruction of cardiac morphology including replacement of the prosthesis. The choice of the optimal substitute after PVE remains controversial in this setting. In mitral PVE, prosthetic valve replacement using either mechanical or biological prosthesis is usually performed. In aortic PVE, homografts have been believed to be the best substitute, particularly in the presence of aortic abscess [55–57]. However, some authors consider that the benefit of homograft surgery is related more to the surgeon's ability to extirpate all infected tissues than to the type of valve used for replacement [54], as Avierinos et al found that in-hospital mortality, ten-year survival and risk of recurrence were not influenced by the type of prosthesis implanted (homograft vs conventional prosthesis) [58]. However, an advantage of homograft tissue is that it can be potentially extended into the distal ascending and transverse aortic arch when necessary [59].

Ross procedure is usually not considered in the particular setting of PVE, although it has already been used for the treatment of active endocarditis with extensive involvement of the aortic root with encouraging results [60].

Medical Treatment

Recommendations for antimicrobial therapy do not differ from those of native IE except for *Staphylococcus aureus* infections [32]. An oxacillin/cloxacillin, gentamicin and rifampin triple combination is commonly used, with more prolonged antibiotic therapy (particularly including gentamicin) than in native valve IE [32]. Vancomycin should be used in addition to rifampin and gentamicine methicillin-resistant *Staphylococcus aureus* PVE. Daptomycin is used only in the presence of a contraindication to vancomycin. This vancomycin – gentamicin – rifampin triple combination should be used empirically in the case of negative blood cultures or while waiting for blood culture results for "first year" PVE, because of the high likelihood of methicillin-resistant *Staphylococcus aureus*. The treatment of fungal endocarditis consists of valve replacement associated with intravenous amphotericin B and azole. In a very recent ICE report involving Candida IE patients, 46 % of whom had PVE (32/70 patients), echinocandin-based therapy seemed to be as effective as amphotericin B-based therapy, although this preliminary report needs to be confirmed [61]. For mechanical prostheses, vitamin K antagonists should be stopped and replaced by heparin until the need for invasive procedures and neurological complications appears unlikely [62].

References

1. Vongpatanasin W, Hillis LD, Lange RA. Prosthetic heart valves. N Engl J Med. 1996; 335:407–16.
2. Piper C, Korfer R, Horstkotte D. Prosthetic valve endocarditis. Heart. 2001;85:590–3.
3. Mylonakis E, Calderwood SB. Infective endocarditis in adults. N Engl J Med. 2001; 345:1318–30.
4. Selton-Suty C, Celard CM, Le Moing V, et al. Preeminence of *Staphylococcus aureus* in infective endocarditis: a 1-year population-based survey. Clin Infect Dis. 2012;54:1230–9.
5. Wang A, Athan E, Pappas PA, et al. Contemporary clinical profile and outcome of prosthetic valve endocarditis. JAMA. 2007;297:1354–61.
6. Farinas MC, Perez-Vazquez A, Farinas-Alvarez C, et al. Risk factors of prosthetic valve endocarditis: a case-control study. Ann Thorac Surg. 2006;81:1284–90.
7. Blackstone EH, Kirklin JW. Death and other time-related events after valve replacement. Circulation. 1985;72:753–67.
8. Kodali SK, Williams MR, Smith CR, et al. Two-year outcomes after transcatheter or surgical aortic-valve replacement. N Engl J Med. 2012;366:1686–95.
9. Latib A, Naim C, De Bonis M, et al. TAVR-associated prosthetic valve infective endocarditis: results of a large, multicenter registry. J Am Coll Cardiol. 2014;64:2176–8.

10. Martinez-Selles M, Bouza E, Diez-Villanueva P, et al. Incidence and clinical impact of infective endocarditis after transcatheter aortic valve implantation. EuroIntervention. 2016;11(10):1180–7.
11. Amat-Santos IJ, Messika-Zeitoun D, Eltchaninoff H, et al. Infective endocarditis after transcatheter aortic valve implantation: results from a large multicenter registry. Circulation. 2015;131:1566–74.
12. Hagl C, Strauch JT, Spielvogel D, et al. Is the Bentall procedure for ascending aorta or aortic valve replacement the best approach for long-term event-free survival? Ann Thorac Surg. 2003;76:698–703; discussion 703.
13. Liebrich M, Kruszynski MK, Roser D, et al. The David procedure in different valve pathologies: a single-center experience in 236 patients. Ann Thorac Surg. 2013;95:71–6.
14. David TE, Armstrong S, McCrindle BW, Manlhiot C. Late outcomes of mitral valve repair for mitral regurgitation due to degenerative disease. Circulation. 2013;127:1485–92.
15. Kluge JG, Hagendorff A, Pfeiffer D, Jurisch D, Tarr A. Active infective prosthetic endocarditis after percutaneous edge-to-edge mitral valve repair. Eur J Echocardiogr. 2011;12:710.
16. Frerker C, Kuck HH, Schmidt T, et al. Severe infective endocarditis after MitraClip implantation treated by cardiac surgery. EuroIntervention. 2015;11(3):351–4.
17. Lopez J, Revilla A, Vilacosta I, et al. Definition, clinical profile, microbiological spectrum, and prognostic factors of early-onset prosthetic valve endocarditis. Eur Heart J. 2007;28:760–5.
18. Chu VH, Miro JM, Hoen B, et al. Coagulase-negative staphylococcal prosthetic valve endocarditis – a contemporary update based on the International Collaboration on Endocarditis: prospective cohort study. Heart. 2009;95:570–6.
19. San Martin J, Sarria C, de las Cueva C, Duarte J, Gamallo C. Relevance of clinical presentation and period of diagnosis in prosthetic valve endocarditis. J Heart Valve Dis. 2010;19:131–8.
20. Thuny F, Fournier PE, Casalta J, et al. Investigation of blood culture-negative early prosthetic valve endocarditis reveals high prevalence of fungi. Heart. 2010;96:743–7.
21. Anderson DJ, Olaison L, McDonald JR, et al. Enterococcal prosthetic valve infective endocarditis: report of 45 episodes from the International Collaboration on Endocarditis-merged database. Eur J Clin Microbiol Infect Dis. 2005;24:665–70.
22. Moreillon P, Que YA. Infective endocarditis. Lancet. 2004;363:139–49.
23. Anguera I, Miro JM, San Roman JA, et al. Periannular complications in infective endocarditis involving prosthetic aortic valves. Am J Cardiol. 2006;98:1261–8.
24. Habib G, Thuny F, Avierinos JF. Prosthetic valve endocarditis: current approach and therapeutic options. Prog Cardiovasc Dis. 2008;50:274–81.
25. Lamas CC, Eykyn SJ. Suggested modifications to the Duke criteria for the clinical diagnosis of native valve and prosthetic valve endocarditis: analysis of 118 pathologically proven cases. Clin Infect Dis. 1997;25:713–9.
26. Pedersen WR, Walker M, Olson JD, et al. Value of transesophageal echocardiography as an adjunct to transthoracic echocardiography in evaluation of native and prosthetic valve endocarditis. Chest. 1991;100:351–6.
27. Perez-Vazquez A, Farinas MC, Garcia-Palomo JD, et al. Evaluation of the Duke criteria in 93 episodes of prosthetic valve endocarditis: could sensitivity be improved? Arch Intern Med. 2000;160:1185–91.
28. Bertagna F, Bisleri G, Motta F, et al. Possible role of F18-FDG-PET/CT in the diagnosis of endocarditis: preliminary evidence from a review of the literature. Int J Cardiovasc Imaging. 2012;28:1417–25.
29. Millar BC, Prendergast BD, Alavi A, Moore JE. 18FDG-positron emission tomography (PET) has a role to play in the diagnosis and therapy of infective endocarditis and cardiac device infection. Int J Cardiol. 2013;167:1724–36.
30. Saby L, Le Dolley Y, Laas O, et al. Early diagnosis of abscess in aortic bioprosthetic valve by 18F-fluorodeoxyglucose positron emission tomography-computed tomography. Circulation. 2012;126:e217–20.
31. Saby L, Laas O, Habib G, et al. Positron emission tomography/computed tomography for diagnosis of prosthetic valve endocarditis: increased valvular 18F-fluorodeoxyglucose uptake as a novel major criterion. J Am Coll Cardiol. 2013;61:2374–82.

32. Authors/Task Force M, Habib G, Lancellotti P, Antunes MJ, Bongiorni MG, Casalta JP, et al. 2015 ESC Guidelines for the management of infective endocarditis: The Task Force for the Management of Infective Endocarditis of the European Society of Cardiology (ESC)Endorsed by: European Association for Cardio-Thoracic Surgery (EACTS), the European Association of Nuclear Medicine (EANM). Eur Heart J. 2015;36(44):3075–128.
33. Fagman E, Perrotta S, Bech-Hanssen O, Flinck A, Lamm C, Olaison L, et al. ECG-gated computed tomography: a new role for patients with suspected aortic prosthetic valve endocarditis. Eur Radiol. 2012;22(11):2407–14.
34. Habets J, Tanis W, van Herwerden LA, et al. Cardiac computed tomography angiography results in diagnostic and therapeutic change in prosthetic heart valve endocarditis. Int J Cardiovasc Imaging. 2014;30:377–87.
35. Feuchtner GM, Stolzmann P, Dichtl W, et al. Multislice computed tomography in infective endocarditis: comparison with transesophageal echocardiography and intraoperative findings. J Am Coll Cardiol. 2009;53:436–44.
36. Tanis W, Scholtens A, Habets J, et al. CT angiography and (1)(8)F-FDG-PET fusion imaging for prosthetic heart valve endocarditis. JACC Cardiovasc Imaging. 2013;6:1008–13.
37. Thomson LE, Goodman MP, Naqvi TZ, et al. Aortic root infection in a prosthetic valve demonstrated by gallium-67 citrate SPECT. Clin Nucl Med. 2005;30:265–8.
38. Wang A, Pappas P, Anstrom KJ, et al. The use and effect of surgical therapy for prosthetic valve infective endocarditis: a propensity analysis of a multicenter, international cohort. Am Heart J. 2005;150:1086–91.
39. Wolff M, Witchitz S, Chastang C, Regnier B, Vachon F. Prosthetic valve endocarditis in the ICU. Prognostic factors of overall survival in a series of 122 cases and consequences for treatment decision. Chest. 1995;108:688–94.
40. Calderwood SB, Swinski LA, Karchmer AW, Waternaux CM, Buckley MW. Prosthetic valve endocarditis. Analysis of factors affecting outcome of therapy. J Thorac Cardiovasc Surg. 1986;92:776–83.
41. John MD, Hibberd PL, Karchmer AW, Sleeper LA, Calderwood SB. Staphylococcus aureus prosthetic valve endocarditis: optimal management and risk factors for death. Clin Infect Dis. 1998;26:1302–9.
42. Habib G, Tribouilloy C, Thuny F, et al. Prosthetic valve endocarditis: who needs surgery? A multicentre study of 104 cases. Heart. 2005;91:954–9.
43. Akowuah EF, Davies W, Oliver S, et al. Prosthetic valve endocarditis: early and late outcome following medical or surgical treatment. Heart. 2003;89:269–72.
44. Castillo JC, Anguita MP, Torres F, et al. Long-term prognosis of early and late prosthetic valve endocarditis. Am J Cardiol. 2004;93:1185–7.
45. Leontyev S, Borger MA, Modi P, et al. Redo aortic valve surgery: influence of prosthetic valve endocarditis on outcomes. J Thorac Cardiovasc Surg. 2011;142:99–105.
46. Musci M, Hubler M, Amiri A, et al. Surgical treatment for active infective prosthetic valve endocarditis: 22-year single-centre experience. Eur J Cardiothorac Surg. 2010;38:528–38.
47. Wilbring M, Tugtekin SM, Alexiou K, Matschke K, Kappert U. Composite aortic root replacement for complex prosthetic valve endocarditis: initial clinical results and long-term follow-up of high-risk patients. Ann Thorac Surg. 2012;94:1967–74.
48. Loverix L, Juvonen T, Biancari F. Prosthetic endocarditis after transcatheter aortic valve implantation: pooled individual patient outcome. Int J Cardiol. 2015;178:67–8.
49. Habib G. Management of infective endocarditis. Heart. 2006;92:124–30.
50. Lalani T, Chu VH, Park LP, et al. In-hospital and 1-year mortality in patients undergoing early surgery for prosthetic valve endocarditis. JAMA Intern Med. 2013;173:1495–504.
51. Chirouze C, Alla F, Fowler Jr VG, et al. Impact of early valve surgery on outcome of Staphylococcus aureus prosthetic valve infective endocarditis: analysis in the International Collaboration of Endocarditis-Prospective Cohort study. Clin Infect Dis. 2015;60:741–9.
52. Bannay A, Hoen B, Duval X, et al. The impact of valve surgery on short- and long-term mortality in left-sided infective endocarditis: do differences in methodological approaches explain previous conflicting results? Eur Heart J. 2011;32:2003–15.

53. Sohail MR, Martin KR, Wilson WR, et al. Medical versus surgical management of *Staphylococcus aureus* prosthetic valve endocarditis. Am J Med. 2006;119:147–54.
54. David TE, Gavra G, Feindel CM, et al. Surgical treatment of active infective endocarditis: a continued challenge. J Thorac Cardiovasc Surg. 2007;133:144–9.
55. Glazier JJ, Verwilghen J, Donaldson RM, Ross DN. Treatment of complicated prosthetic aortic valve endocarditis with annular abscess formation by homograft aortic root replacement. J Am Coll Cardiol. 1991;17:1177–82.
56. Grinda JM, Mainardi JL, D'Attellis N, et al. Cryopreserved aortic viable homograft for active aortic endocarditis. Ann Thorac Surg. 2005;79:767–71.
57. Lopes S, Calvinho P, de Oliveira F, Antunes M. Allograft aortic root replacement in complex prosthetic endocarditis. Eur J Cardiothorac Surg. 2007;32:126–30; discussion 131–2.
58. Avierinos JF, Thuny F, Chalvignac V, et al. Surgical treatment of active aortic endocarditis: homografts are not the cornerstone of outcome. Ann Thorac Surg. 2007;84:1935–42.
59. Preventza O, Mohamed AS, Cooley DA, et al. Homograft use in reoperative aortic root and proximal aortic surgery for endocarditis: a 12-year experience in high-risk patients. J Thorac Cardiovasc Surg. 2014;148:989–94.
60. Prat A, Saez de Ibarra JI, Vincentelli A, et al. Ross operation for active culture-positive aortic valve endocarditis with extensive paravalvular involvement. Ann Thorac Surg. 2001;72:1492–5; discussion 1495–6.
61. Arnold CJ, Johnson M, Bayer AS, et al. Candida infective endocarditis: an observational cohort study with a focus on therapy. Antimicrob Agents Chemother. 2015;59(4):2365–73.
62. Whitlock RP, Sun JC, Fremes SE, Rubens FD, Teoh KH. Antithrombotic and thrombolytic therapy for valvular disease: antithrombotic therapy and prevention of thrombosis, 9th ed: American College of Chest Physicians Evidence-Based Clinical Practice Guidelines. Chest. 2012;141:e576S–600.

Chapter 14
Cardiac Device Related Endocarditis

Sana Arif, Larry M. Baddour, and M. Rizwan Sohail

Introduction

Indications for cardiac implantable electronic device (CIED) therapy have gradually expanded [1], and consequently we are witnessing an increase in rate of cardiac device implantation [2, 3]. However, epidemiologic studies suggest that the increase in the rate of CIED related infections has outpaced the increase in implantation rate. Data from the National Hospital Discharge Survey [4] show that between 1996 and 2003, there was a 49 % rise in the number of new cardiac devices being implanted in the United States. While patient demographics remain unchanged, the number of hospitalizations from CIED infections increased by 3.1-fold [4]. Similar findings were noted in a study by Cabell et al. [5] on Medicare beneficiaries between 1990 and 1999. Trend analysis revealed that while the rate of CIED implantation increased by 42 %, during the same time period the rate of device infections increased by 124 % (from 0.94 to 2.11 cases per 1000 beneficiaries). It was also noted that the rate of device infections was two-fold higher in the African American population in comparison to Caucasians [5]. The reasons for the rising rate of CIED infection, disproportionate to implantation rate, are not completely understood. It may be partly due to aging population and frequent comorbid conditions in the device recipients [6]. Moreover, as patients receiving device therapy are living longer, they are more likely to undergo device exchanges or develop infections. Greater physician awareness and increased availability of better imaging techniques to detect the underlying lead infection may also contribute to higher rate of CIED infection diagnosis.

S. Arif, MB, BS
Department of Internal Medicine, Duke University Medical Center, Durham, NC, USA
e-mail: sana.arif@dm.kuke.edu

L.M. Baddour, MD • M.R. Sohail, MD (⊠)
Department of Infectious Diseases and Cardiovascular Diseases, Mayo Clinic College of Medicine, Rochester, MN, USA
e-mail: Baddour.larry@mayo.edu; Sohail.muhammad@mayo.edu

© Springer International Publishing Switzerland 2016
G. Habib (ed.), *Infective Endocarditis*, DOI 10.1007/978-3-319-32432-6_14

Table 14.1 Risk factors for cardiac implantable electronic device (CIED) infections

Host factors
Oral anticoagulation use
Long term corticosteroid therapy
Fever within 24 h of implantation
Presence of a permanent central venous catheter (example dialysis catheter)
Renal insufficiency or hemodialysis
Diabetes mellitus
Congestive heart failure
Malignancy or immunocompromised host status
Longer duration of CIED therapy
Male gender
History of prior CIED infection
Device factors
Presence of more than two electrode leads
Temporary pacing before permanent device placement
Recent device manipulation
History of multiple device-related procedures
Procedure related factors
No antibiotic prophylaxis before device implantation
Operator inexperience
Placement of device generator
Replacement or revision procedure

The estimated incidence rate of CIED infections varies from is ~ 1–7 % [7–10]. Infections are more common during revision procedures than primary device implantation [10]. CIED related infective endocarditis (CIED-IE) accounts for approximately 10–23 % of all device infections [11, 12]. This wide variation in estimates is primarily due to varying definitions used for CIED-IE in published literature and different rates of transesophageal echocardiography (TEE) to detect CIED lead vegetation in various studies.

Risk Factors

Risk factors for device infection and CIED-IE can be broadly categorized into host-related, device-related and procedure-related factors (Table 14.1). Several investigations have explored risk factors for CIED infection with varying results. The Prospective Evaluation of Pacemaker Lead Endocarditis (PEOPLE) study was a nationwide, multicenter prospective survey of the incidence and risks factors of cardiac device-related infections in France. Overall, 6319 patients were enrolled at 44 medical centers and followed for a year. Forty-two patients developed device-related infectious complications during the 12-month follow-up period. Early re-intervention, for instance to evacuate a pocket hematoma or lead revision, was found to be a leading risk factor for infection. The presence of fever 24 h prior to implantation was also associated with an increased risk for subsequent device infection. No significant difference was seen in the infection rate between single versus dual chamber devices. Interestingly, patients who had a temporary pacing wire prior to insertion of a permanent device were twice as likely to develop device infection when compared to those who did not have a temporary pacing system. Pre-operative antibiotics were shown to have a preventive role [8].

A review of Danish registry of 46,299 patients who underwent pacemaker implantation reported 596 cases of infection. In this analysis, patients who underwent device replacement procedures were at a higher risk for infection as compared to patients with their initial pacemaker implantation. Additional risk factors, which were found to be significant in multivariable analysis, were male sex, younger age of patient at time of implantation (longer time living with a device), and absence of perioperative antimicrobial prophylaxis. Dual chamber pacing mode, though significant in the univariate analysis, was not statistically significant in the multivariate model [13].

A retrospective study which compared 93 patients with CIED-IE to 323 patients with CIED pocket infection showed that patients with CIED-IE were more likely to have been on chronic corticosteroid therapy, receiving chronic immunomodulator therapy, were on hemodialysis or had a history of a remote infection [14]. In another retrospective case–control study from Mayo Clinic, prolonged corticosteroid therapy, presence of >2 pacing leads (>2 leads versus 2 leads) and lack of pre-operative antibiotic prophylaxis were independent predictors of CIED infection in multivariable analysis [15].

Association of comorbid conditions with higher rate of CIED infection has been demonstrated in multiple studies. In a retrospective, single center case–control study, patients with device infections were more likely to be diabetic, had congestive heart failure, were on oral anticoagulation therapy and had prior device manipulation. Renal insufficiency was associated with much higher rate of infection (42 % among infected patients compared to 13 % in control patients) [16]. Similarly, increased risk of infection in patients with moderate to severe chronic kidney disease (CKD) was also observed in a study by Tompkin et al. [17].

Procedure related factors also influence the risk of subsequent CIED infection. Operator inexperience was linked to a higher rate of CIED infection in an analysis of Medicare Provider database by Al-Khatib et al. [18]. A retrospective review of ICD infections from 1983 to 1999 from Massachusetts General Hospital revealed that patients who received a pectoral device were less likely to have infectious complications when compared to placement of an abdominal device [19].

Pathogenesis

Patients can develop CIED-IE via two potential mechanisms:

1. Device generator pocket infection with microorganism tracking along the transvenous leads to involve intra-cardiac portion of the electrode.
2. Hematogenous seeding of the transvenous leads or device generator pocket from bloodstream infection from a remote focus.

Infection of the generator pocket could occur at the time of device implantation or during device manipulation (generator exchange/upgrade or lead revision/manipulation). Device pocket can also get contaminated and infected if the generator or leads erode through the skin. Occasionally it may not be possible to distinguish whether indolent device infection is the cause of skin erosion or the result of generator or lead erosion. Possibility of bacterial contamination of the device generator at the time of implantation was studied in an investigation by Da Costa et al. where serial skin and pocket samples were taken on 103 patients, before and after device insertion. The patients were followed for a mean duration of 16.5 months, during which four patients developed infection. In 2 of the cases Staphylococcus schleiferi was isolated, which was molecularly identical to the strain initially found in the pacemaker pocket, suggesting that pocket contamination occurred at the time of implantation [20].

Risk of hematogenous seeding of the device lead and subsequent CIED-IE depends on the type of organism and the duration of bloodstream infection. In a recent study from Mayo Clinic [21], investigators reviewed 131 patients with CIED who presented with *S. aureus* bacteremia (SAB) and had no clinical signs of device pocket infection. Forty-five (34 %) of these patients were found to have underlying CIED infection based on clinical or echocardiographic criteria. The presence of a pacemaker rather than an ICD, history of >1 device-related procedure, and longer duration of SAB were independently associated with an increased risk of CIED infection in multivariable model analysis. Based on the risk scores, authors proposed a prediction model that suggests that patients who had none of these high-risk features had a very low risk of underlying CIED infection and could be monitored closely without immediate device extraction. In another investigation from the same institution [22], investigators studied the rate, risk factors, and outcomes of CIED infection in 74 consecutive patients with bacteremia caused by Gram-positive cocci (GPC) other than *S. aureus*. Twenty-two (30 %) of 74 patients with non–*S. aureus* GPC bacteremia had underlying CIED infections. Coagulase-negative staphylococci (CoNS) accounted for 73 % of CIED infections. The number of leads, the presence of abandoned leads, and prior generator replacement were associated with CIED infection. Based on these data, gram positive cocci have a high propensity for hematogenous seeding of CIED leads and TEE should be performed in all of these cases to evaluate for any evidence of underlying CIED infection.

Unlike staphylococci, gram-negative bloodstream infections typically do not result in hematogenous seeding of the device leads. In a retrospective cohort study by Uslan et al. [23] of 49 patients who underwent CIED placement and subsequently developed gram negative bacteremia, only three patients (two definite and one probable case) had evidence of CIED infection. Both the confirmed cases had a generator site infection, suggesting that device was the source of bloodstream infection. There were no cases of hematogenous seeding of leads by gram-negative bacteremia from a distant focus.

Pathogen Related Factors

These are the most important factors that influence the risk of device infection and are the least modifiable. Various bacteria have different virulence factors that enable them to attach to a foreign device. *S. epidermidis* initially attaches to foreign surfaces using non-specific factors such as surface tension, hydrophobicity and adhesins. The organisms then attach to one another using polysaccharide intracellular adhesins (PIA) and form a biofilm [24, 25]. *S. aureus* on the other hand relies more on interaction with host-tissue ligands (fibronectin, collagen, fibrinogen which are part of the extracellular matrix) instead of adhesins. It attaches to these ligands with the help of surface proteins that are termed MSCRAMM (microbial surface components recognizing adhesive matrix molecules) [24, 26].

Once bound to prosthesis surfaces, staphylococci establish a biofilm (slime layer) which is a surface-associated community of one or more microbial species that are firmly attached to each other and the solid surface. They are encased in an extracellular polymeric matrix that holds the biofilm together [25]. Organisms in a biofilm are more resistant to antimicrobial therapy possibly due to the physical protection from the layer of matrix which encases them [27]. Moreover, low metabolic activity and slower rate of replication of bacteria encased in the biofilm makes them more resistant to killing by cell-wall active agents (beta-lactams and glycolopeptides) that primarily target rapidly replicating bacteria. Consequently, it is almost impossible to cure these device infections by anti-microbial therapy alone and CIED removal is recommended for all cases of proven device infection.

Device Related Factors

Physical and biochemical properties of the polymer used to make the device generator shell, lead insulation material and electrode tips can play a vital role in allowing or inhibiting bacterial adhesion. One of the main parameters that predict bacterial adhesion is the degree of hydrophobicity of the device surface. The higher the hydrophobicity of surface material, the greater the bacterial adhesion [25, 28]. An irregular surface or the shapes of the surface can affect adhesion as well. The impact of choice of device materials on the risk of infection is not well characterized and should be explored.

Microbiology

Staphylococci are the most common cause of CIED infections and CIED related endocarditis. A retrospective review of 189 cases of CIED infections, between 1991 and 2003, showed that 29 % of the cases were caused by *S. aureus* and 42 % of the infections were caused by coagulase negative staphylococci (CoNS). Only 9 % of the cases were due to gram-negative bacilli. Polymicrobial infection was identified in 7 % of the cases [29]. Up to 7 % of the cultures were negative, primarily due to prior exposure to antibiotics. Other commensal pathogens such as streptococci, corynebacterium sp. and propionibacterium sp. are less common causes. Cases of coxiella, candida species and non-tuberculous mycobacteria causing CIED infections are rare and are usually the subject of case reports [30].

Microbiology of CIED infection varies based on the timing of onset of infection after device implantation (Fig. 14.1) [31]. In the first few weeks after implantation, device infections are predominantly due to *S. aureus* [30]. Non-staphylococcal infections tend to occur much later after implantation of CIED [32]. The prevalence of methicillin resistance among the staphylococci species causing device infections varies based on the geographical location and various studies have shown different rates [30, 33]. *S. aureus* bloodstream infections seen early (<3 months after implantation) are usually associated with the implantation procedure. However, *S. aureus* related CIED infections which occur later in the course (>1 year after insertion of device) are usually due to hematogenous seeding from a secondary source of infection [30]. While a temporal relationship has been described in *S. aureus* infections, with generator pocket infections occurring in the first year and endovascular

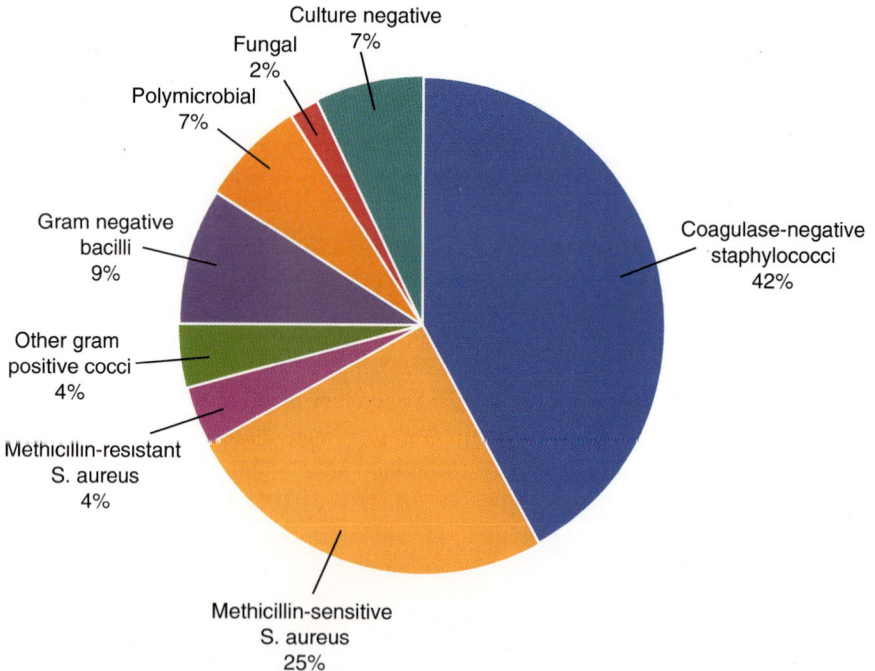

Fig. 14.1 Microbiology of CIED infections (From Sohail et al. [29]. Reprinted with permission from Elsevier Limited)

infections presenting much later, no similar association has been reported for CoNS infections [34].

Clinical Manifestations

Generator pocket infection is the most common manifestation of CIED infection. Patients with pocket site infections typically present with pain, erythema, drainage, swelling, tenderness or dehiscence at the site of the generator. Patients with CIED lead infections typically present with systemic signs like fever, chills, rigors, malaise, or signs of severe sepsis. As device leads are in close proximity to tricuspid valve, right-sided endocarditis can develop with septic emboli to lungs. However, valvular infection in CIED infections is not limited to right-side and aortic and mitral infection may occur with systemic embolization to brain, bones, joints, liver, spleen or kidneys. Other manifestations of CIED-IE vary based on the causative pathogen and may include cutaneous lesions, heart failure or immunologic phenomenon such as glomerulonephritis. Occasionally, cases of CIED-IE may present as a fever of unknown origin with few to no other symptoms.

A multi-center study that used data from the International Collaboration on Endocarditis (ICE) registry, which span 61 centers across 28 countries, reported clinical manifestation and outcome of 177 patients with CIED-IE [35]. Majority (81 %) of the patients presented with fever and 149 (84 %) had positive blood cultures. Overall, 159 patients that were classified as having CIED-IE had vegetations on echocardiography and 76 % of these had a vegetation on the intra-cardiac portion of the device lead. Concomitant heart valve involvement was seen in 63 patients. The tricuspid valve was most frequently involved (43 cases) and the pulmonic valve being the least affected (one case only).

In a retrospectively study that included 60 patients with CIED-IE, more than 30 % of the cases occurred within 1 year of the implantation procedure. An elevated C-reactive protein (CRP) or sedimentation rate (ESR) was present in 58 cases (96.6 %) but leukocytosis (>10,000/mm^3) was observed in only 29 cases (48 %). A positive culture (either blood or lead culture) was obtained in 53 out of 60 cases (88 %). Pulmonary embolism was diagnosed in 16 cases (27 %). CIED lead infection was complicated by upper extremity deep vein thrombosis at the side of the device leads in five cases [36].

Symptoms of CIED-IE can be very non-specific. In a retrospective study from Sweden that included 44 episodes of pacemaker endocarditis, 38 patients presented with fever without any other focal signs of device infection. Signs of pacemaker pocket infection were only seen in six cases. Fourteen percent of the cases had systemic embolic phenomenon, with lungs being the most common site [22]. In one study that compared 323 cases of CIED infection to 93 cases of CIED-IE, presence of fever and leukocytosis in patients with suspected device infection were independent predictors of device-related endocarditis in multivariable analysis [14]. Patients undergoing hemodialysis were more likely to have CIED-IE compared to those in the non-HD group (41 % versus 21 %) in a report from Mayo Clinic [37]. All the patients undergoing routine hemodialysis presented with bloodstream infections in this series and 77 % of the patients had fever and leukocytosis on presentation.

Diagnosis

CIED infections can present with very diverse manifestations. While patients with pocket infection tend to have local signs at the generator site, fever may be the only manifestation of CIED-IE. Therefore, any patient receiving CIED therapy who presents with fever should have at least two sets of Blood cultures drawn prior to starting antimicrobial therapy [33]. If the patient is found to have a bloodstream infection, particularly with staphylococcal species, a TEE should be performed to evaluate for underlying endocarditis [33]. While transthoracic echocardiography (TTE) is very good at defining ventricular dysfunction and pulmonary vascular pressures, it is not very sensitive in picking up vegetations for endocarditis. In a prospective study done by Victor et al. [38] on 23 patients with pacemaker lead infection, only seven patients (30%) were found to have vegetations by TTE. However, vegetations were seen in 21 cases on TEE (91 %). It was felt that on TTE it is difficult to differentiate between the valve, the lead and possible lesion, partly because echoes induced by the leads interfere with the imaging of small sized structures.

A prospective study by Narducci et al. [39] showed that intra-cardiac echocardiography (ICE) was more sensitive in comparison to TEE in picking up IE in patients with cardiac devices. TEE frequently failed to detect lesions on leads in the right ventricle, close to the tricuspid valve, possibly due to the TEE transducer being further away from the right ventricle. ICE provided better visualization of the right-sided structures. However, the sensitivity of ICE was only 82.8 % as it is difficult to differentiate thrombi, myxomatous changes and true infective endocarditis on the basis of echocardiographic findings alone [39]. Additionally ICE is a much more invasive procedure as compared to TEE.

Differentiating a lead thrombus from "true" vegetation on the basis of echocardiography can be very difficult. Thrombi often develop on intra-cardiac portion of device leads. For instance, lead thrombi were found in up to 33 % of ventricular leads and 48 % of atrial leads on autopsy of patients with CIEDs irrespective of cause of death [40]. In another investigation by Supple et al. [41], 86 patients who presented for ablation procedures were examined with ICE. Twenty six (30%) of the patients were found to have lead thrombi on ICE. The thrombi were mobile and more commonly in the right atrium. Clinically these patients did not have any signs of embolism or infection. Anti-coagulation with warfarin was not associated with absence of lead thrombi. Similarly, in a retrospective study from Tufts Medical Center [42], 177 TEEs were performed in patients with a pre-existing cardiac devices, 25 of them were positive for a mass or stranding on the device leads. However, only eight of these patients were adjudicated to have CIED-IE and 72 %

of the patients with a lead associated mass did not have any other evidence suggestive of endocarditis. Therefore, while TEE is a very sensitive test for CIED-IE, it is not very specific and correlation with the patient's overall clinical presentation is critical for appropriate diagnosis.

WBC Scintigraphy, when employing SPECT CT imaging, could be helpful in differentiating cases of bacteremia alone from infections where the CIED is involved as well. In one study [43], 63 patients with suspected CIED infection underwent WBC Scintigraphy with SPECT imaging. Thirty-two of these patients were found to have CIED infection confirmed by positive cultures of extracted device or by clinical follow up. Thirty of these 32 patients (94%) had positive results by WBC Scintigraphy and there were two only false negatives and no false positive results. The scan also helped in outlining the extent of infection by showing if the infected area involved only the generator pocket or affected the leads as well. It was found to have a sensitivity of 94% and a negative predictive value of 94% [43].

There are some data suggesting that 18F-fluorodeoxyglucose Positron emission tomography–computed tomography (^{18}F-FDG PET/CT) may be useful in diagnosing CIED-IE [44–46]. In a larger study designed to look at the role of ^{18}F-FDG PET/CT in CIED infection diagnosis, patients were divided into three groups [47]. Group A consisted of 42 patients with suspected CIED infection, Group B had 12 control patients without signs of infection who had recently undergone device implantation, and Group C comprised of 12 patients who had undergone placement of a CIED more than 6 months ago and did not have any signs of infection. All patients underwent ^{18}F-FDG PET/CT scans. No activity was seen in patients in Group C and minimum activity was seen in Group B patients. Among the patients in Group A, 35 were found to have true CIED infection and 31 of them had positive ^{18}F-FDG PET/CT scans. Six patients were found to have superficial infection and were treated with antibiotics only. Excellent correlation was seen between sites of ^{18}F-FDG uptake and the localization of infection at the time of the extraction in the 24 patients who underwent complete device removal. Only one false positive was seen, in a patient who had a Dacron pouch in place around the generator [47]. Hence the reliability of this approach in patients with an antibiotic mesh or envelope is not known. It is also unclear how prolonged use of antibiotics would affect the results of this particular imaging modality.

Identification of the causative microorganisms is critical for choosing optimal antimicrobial therapy. Therefore, once the decision has been made to remove the device, cultures of the pocket tissue, deep pocket swab, and device surface swab should be obtained at the time of extraction. Also, lead tips should be sent for culture as well. In the case of pocket site infections, culture of tissue from the pocket has a higher yield than swabs from the pocket site [48]. Also, lead tip cultures are not always reliable in the presence of a pocket infection as lead tips can potentially get contaminated during extraction through an infected pocket environment [49]. Sonication of the extracted device to disrupt biofilm on the device surfaces can improve the microbiological diagnosis of infection. In a study done by Oliva et al. [50], 20 patients underwent extraction of CIED due to infection. The sonicate fluid cultures were more sensitive than traditional culture (67 % versus 50 %) and bacterial counts were found to be higher in sonicate fluid cultures as compared to the conventional culture [50]. In a more recent study, Nagpal et al. [51] studies the effectiveness of sonication technique in a prospective study of 42 subjects with clinically non-infected devices and 35 patients with infected CIEDs enrolled over 12 months. In the infected group, significant bacterial growth was observed in 54 % of sonicate fluids, significantly greater than the sensitivities of pocket swab (20 %), device swab (9 %), or tissue (9 %) culture. Of note, majority of patients had received antibiotics prior to device removal in this study. In cases of CIED-IE, sonicate fluid culture yield was 42 %, compared to 11 % for pocket swabs and 5 % for pocket tissue cultures. Therefore, sonication may be the only way to confirm lead infection in patients who have positive blood cultures but no signs of pocket infection and no lead vegetations noted on echocardiography.

Management

No randomized clinical trials have been conducted to compare medical management only versus device removal along with antimicrobial therapy. However, based on high relapse rates seen in patients treated with device retention [33, 52, 53], removal of the infected CIED is considered the mainstay of treatment [25, 53]. The role of antimicrobial therapy is adjuvant [33]. In one study [54] of CIED infections associated with *S. aureus* bacteremia (SAB), mortality rate was up to 47 % if device was not removed versus 16 % in patients with complete extraction. Overall treatment failure (death, infection recurrence) was more common in cases with device retention (52 %) versus complete device removal (25 %). In two separate investigations addressing specifically CIED-IE cases, patients in whom the device was retained had a mortality rate ranging from 31 to 66 %, in comparison to those who underwent complete device removal and the mortality rate was as low as 13 % [12, 55]. In another study from Mayo Clinic, conservative management of CIED infection was associated with a seven-fold increase in 30-day mortality in multivariate analysis [56].

Infected device removal should be done if the patient is hemodynamically stable to tolerate lead extraction procedure. It should not be delayed due to the presence of a bloodstream infection. In afore cited study by Le et al. [56], delayed CIED removal (4 days versus 15.8 days) was associated with a three-fold increase in 1 year mortality. In general, patients in whom TEE reveals evidence of valvular endocarditis (right or left sided) alone, without any vegetation on the CIED leads, it should be assumed that the cardiac device is infected and should be extracted. If the patient is scheduled to undergo heart valve repair or replacement, the removal of the CIED leads can be done at the same time. However, a plan on how the patient will be "bridged" prior to re-implantation should be in place.

Because the majority of CIED infections are caused by gram-positive organisms (primarily staphylococci), vancomycin should be given empirically [33, 53]. Empiric gram-negative coverage with an anti-pseudomonas agent may also be considered in patients who present with severe sepsis or shock. A antimicrobial therapy can then be modified on the basis of culture and *in-vitro* susceptibility data as they become available. If the cultured organism is oxacillin susceptible and the patient does not have a beta lactam allergy, then vancomycin can be discontinued and cefazolin or nafcillin inititated. For gram negative and other organisms the therapy needs to be modified accordingly. In patients with prosthetic valve involvement, gentamicin for first 2 weeks of therapy and rifampin for the entire duration of therapy should be added to the regimen if infection is caused by staphylococci.

There are limited data looking at the optimal duration of antibiotic therapy in this patient population. It is generally recommended that the patient should be treated for at least 2 weeks after removal of the infected cardiac device. However, if the patient continues to have positive blood cultures more than 24 h after removal of the CIED while on appropriate antimicrobial therapy, he should be given a 4-week course of parenteral antibiotic therapy [33]. The antimicrobial therapy should also be prolonged if the patient has evidence of valvular endocarditis, osteomyelitis or septic emboli. In general, patients with CIED-IE should be treated with a parenteral agent for the entire duration of therapy [33].

See Fig. 14.2 for an algorithm for the management of cardiac device infections.

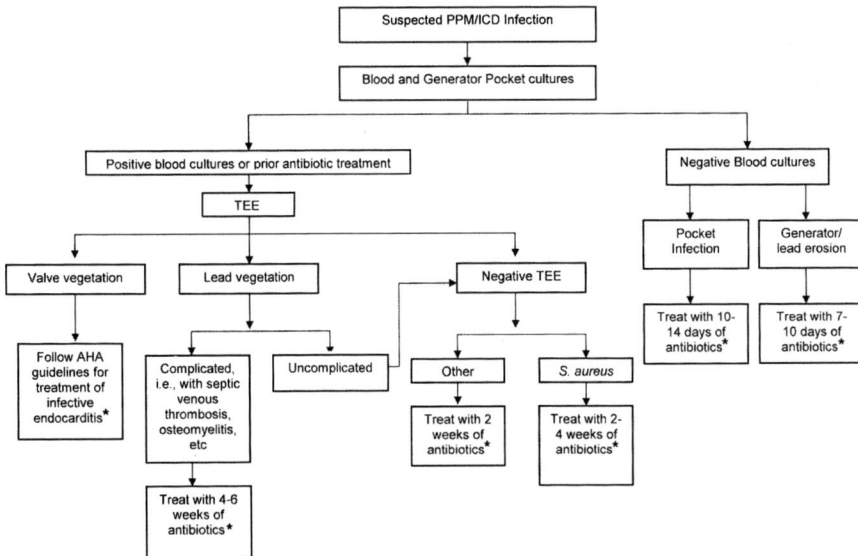

Fig. 14.2 Approach to the management of cardiac device infections (From Sohail et al. [29]. Reprinted with permission from Elsevier Limited)

Lead Extraction

Extraction of infected leads is a procedure that electrophysiologists and cardiac surgeons are encountering with a higher frequency in their practice today. This is largely due to the overall increase in the number of CIED being implanted and the disproportionate increase in the number of CIED infections [25, 58].

CIED leads, which are less than 1 year old, can usually be explanted using a stylus and manual traction to free the lead of its attachment and adhesions. However, leads that have been in place for longer periods of time tend to develop a fibrotic encasement and their removal is more complex. Attempts to remove these leads using stylus and manual traction alone can result in lead breakage, leftover lead fragments and potential damage to the heart. These older leads are now removed using extraction dilators and power sheaths [30]. These power sheaths employ a radio-frequency probe or laser, attached to the tip of the sheath that is threaded transvenously over the lead. This helps in breaking scar tissue and enables subsequent removal of the lead [59, 60]. Regardless of equipment used, lead extraction is an intricate procedure that can be associated with serious complications such as bleeding, stroke, pulmonary embolism and even death [59, 60]. Complicated device removal is associated with an increase in 30-day patient mortality [52, 56]. However, the benefit of device removal outweighs the risks associated with retention of device in most circumstances.

Size of CIED lead vegetation is another concern during percutaneous extraction for CIED-IE. As power sheaths are advanced over the leads, vegetations attached to lead break off and embolize to the pulmonary vasculature. In our experience, most infected leads can be safely removed percutaneously even if the vegetation size is up to 2 cm [12]. Few patients may experience transient hypotension during the procedure or post-operatively but clinically significant pulmonary embolism is rare. However, for lead vegetation size >2 cm, cardiac surgery consultation should be sought when planning lead extraction.

Open Heart Surgery

If the patient needs to undergo open-heart surgery for another reason such as valve replacement or perivalvular abscess, then the CIED leads should be removed during the same procedure. Otherwise open-heart surgery is reserved for cases where percutaneous lead extraction is unsuccessful or not an option due to presence of very large vegetations (>2 cm) [30, 33, 53] due to concern for potential pulmonary embolism [33].

Conservative Management

Patients with infected CIEDs who refuse to undergo extraction or are not candidates for complete device removal due to clinical issues, such as advanced age, limited life-span, or co-morbid conditions are typically managed with long-term suppressive antibiotic therapy [30, 33, 53]. This should be considered as a palliative approach and not a preferred option. The choice of suppressive antimicrobial therapy should be guided by susceptibility testing. This also highlights the importance of isolating causative pathogens for CIED infection. In cases of multi-drug resistant organisms, options for long-term oral antimicrobials can be limited and infectious diseases physician should be consulted to guide therapy. There is a paucity of data regarding the optimal duration or dosage of therapy in this population. Additionally placing patients on long-term suppressive therapy raises the risk of selection of more resistant organisms and *C. difficile* infection. Data regarding relapse of infection in these patients while on long term antibiotic therapy are also not available.

Re-implantation of Cardiac Device

Prior to reimplantation, all patients should be assessed for the need of ongoing CIED therapy. Published data suggest that up to 30 % of the patients no longer need a new cardiac device after removal of an infected device [53]. This is largely due to improvement in the clinical condition of the patient that served as an original indication for CIED therapy, hence obviating the need for a replacement device. Occasionally, it may be due to lack of an appropriate indication at the time of initial device placement. There are no prospective trial data on the ideal time for re-implantation. It is typically recommended that the patients should not undergo the replacement procedure until their blood cultures (drawn after removal of the device), have been negative for a minimum of 72 h [33, 53]. However, for a patient who has evidence of valvular endocarditis on echocardiography, it is recommended that a new device should not be implanted for at least 2 weeks [33, 53]. New CIED generator and leads should be placed on the side contralateral to the prior CIED pocket if possible. If the new device has to be implanted on the same side as the current infection, then a tunneled lead should be placed in the abdomen subcutaneously. Another alternative is placement of epicardial leads, especially if delaying CIED placement for 2 weeks (in cases of CIED-IE) is not feasible, in cases of septic venous thrombosis involving the superior vena cava or other vascular access complications.

See Fig. 14.3 for recommendations for reimplantation of CIED in patients with cardiac device infection.

Outcomes

CIED infections are associated with significant morbidity and mortality in device recipients. Device infection resulted in two-fold higher in-hospital mortality in one investigation [4]. However, device infection may also impact long-term survival. In a cohort of Medicare beneficiaries, the increased risk for mortality in patients with

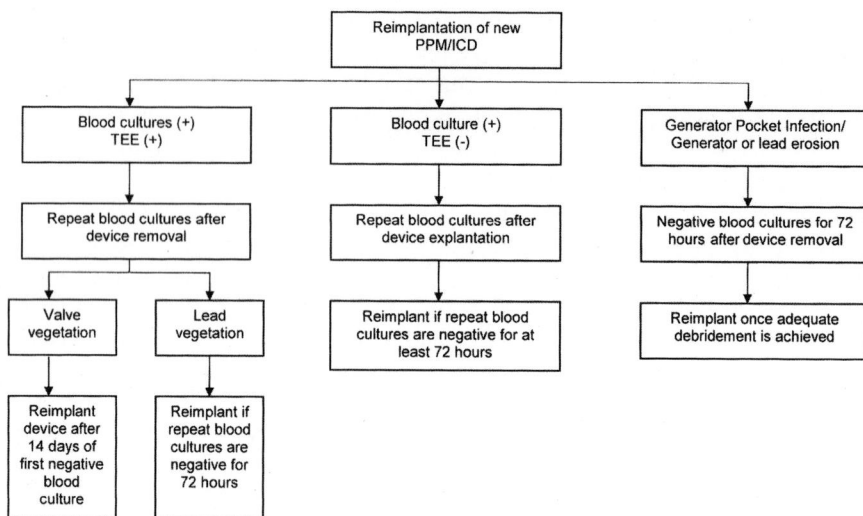

Fig. 14.3 Recommendations for reimplantation of CIED in patients with cardiac device infection (From Sohail et al. [29]. Reprinted with permission from Elsevier Limited)

CIED infection persisted for up to 3 years after the initial hospitalization for device infection [61]. Women with CIED infection had a significantly reduced long-term survival as compared to men (67.3 % versus 72.9 %) in a sub-group analysis of the Medicare beneficiary cohort [62]. Mortality associated with CIED infection varies based on clinical presentation, ranging from 3.7 % in-hospital mortality in patients without endocarditis and up to 14 % in patients with CIED-IE [29].

In a retrospective study of 415 patients with CIED infections, chronic corticosteroid therapy, heart failure and presence of CIED-IE on presentation were associated with increased short-term (<30 days) mortality [63]. Patients receiving chronic corticosteroid therapy had a four-fold increase and those with CIED-IE had a 5.6-fold increase in short-term mortality. Predictors of long-term mortality (>30 days) included renal dysfunction, system revision, malignancy, older age, and all factors affecting short-term mortality. Every 10-year increase in age was also associated with a 20 % increase in risk of death [63]. Other studies have reported associated between mortality and presence of renal dysfunction, older age, presence of thrombocytopenia and cultures being positive for MRSA [4, 7, 30, 64, 65].

Prevention

The use of preventive strategies to reduce the rate of CIED infections is essential due to its significant morbidity and mortality. Moreover, these infections are associated with significant financial burden for patients and payers. In one study, the standardized adjusted incremental and total admission costs for infection were $14

360–$16 498 and $28 676–$53 349 for pacemakers and implantable cardioverter-defibrillators respectively [66]. Also, in 2012 the Center for Medicare and Medicaid services (CMS) added surgical site infection after CIED implantation as a hospital acquired infection; hence, hospitals are no longer eligible to seek payment for managing these infections [67].

Achieving a good hemostasis at the time of implantation and using aseptic technique is the key to prevention of CIED infections [30]. The administration of pre-operative antibiotics has been shown to significantly reduce the risk of surgical site infections in CIED recipients [15, 68, 69]. There is no evidence to suggest that use of postoperative antibiotics has any utility in prevention of infection. The use of prophylactic antibiotics to prevent secondary seeding of cardiac devices from invasive dental, gastrointestinal or genitourinary procedures is also not recommended [25].

Use of an antimicrobial pouch or envelope, impregnated with minocycline and rifampin, that elutes antibiotics locally at the generator site was associated with reduced risk of pocket infections in a retrospective study where the infection rate within the first 6 months was significantly lower in patients who received the envelope (1.1 %) as compared to that in patients without pouch placement (3.6 %) [67]. However, prospective, randomized trial data are needed before any specific recommendations can be made about the pouch's use in routine practice.

References

1. Epstein AE, Dimarco JP, Ellenbogen KA, Estes 3rd NA, Freedman RA, Gettes LS, et al. ACC/AHA/HRS 2008 guidelines for device-based therapy of cardiac rhythm abnormalities: executive summary. Heart Rhythm. 2008;5(6):934–55.
2. Mond HG, Irwin M, Morillo C, Ector H. The world survey of cardiac pacing and cardioverter defibrillators: calendar year 2001. Pacing Clin Electrophysiol. 2004;27(7):955–64.
3. Zhan C, Baine WB, Sedrakyan A, Steiner C. Cardiac device implantation in the United States from 1997 through 2004: a population-based analysis. J Gen Intern Med. 2008;23 Suppl 1:13–9.
4. Voigt A, Shalaby A, Saba S. Rising rates of cardiac rhythm management device infections in the United States: 1996 through 2003. J Am Coll Cardiol. 2006;48(3):590–1.
5. Cabell CH, Heidenreich PA, Chu VH, Moore CM, Stryjewski ME, Corey GR, et al. Increasing rates of cardiac device infections among medicare beneficiaries: 1990–1999. Am Heart J. 2004;147(4):582–6.
6. Greenspon AJ, Patel JD, Lau E, Ochoa JA, Frisch DR, Ho RT, et al. 16-year trends in the infection burden for pacemakers and implantable cardioverter-defibrillators in the United States 1993 to 2008. J Am Coll Cardiol. 2011;58(10):1001–6.
7. de Bie MK, van Rees JB, Thijssen J, Borleffs CJ, Trines SA, Cannegieter SC, et al. Cardiac device infections are associated with a significant mortality risk. Heart Rhythm. 2012; 9(4):494–8.
8. Klug D, Balde M, Pavin D, Hidden-Lucet F, Clementy J, Sadoul N, et al. Risk factors related to infections of implanted pacemakers and cardioverter-defibrillators: results of a large prospective study. Circulation. 2007;116(12):1349–55.

9. Uslan DZ, Sohail MR, St Sauver JL, Friedman PA, Hayes DL, Stoner SM, et al. Permanent pacemaker and implantable cardioverter defibrillator infection: a population-based study. Arch Intern Med. 2007;167(7):669–75.

10. Trappe HJ, Pfitzner P, Klein H, Wenzlaff P. Infections after cardioverter-defibrillator implantation: observations in 335 patients over 10 years. Br Heart J. 1995;73(1):20–4.

11. Arber N, Pras E, Copperman Y, Schapiro JM, Meiner V, Lossos IS, et al. Pacemaker endocarditis. Report of 44 cases and review of the literature. Medicine. 1994;73(6):299–305.

12. Sohail MR, Uslan DZ, Khan AH, Friedman PA, Hayes DL, Wilson WR, et al. Infective endocarditis complicating permanent pacemaker and implantable cardioverter-defibrillator infection. Mayo Clin Proc. 2008;83(1):46–53.

13. Johansen JB, Jorgensen OD, Moller M, Arnsbo P, Mortensen PT, Nielsen JC. Infection after pacemaker implantation: infection rates and risk factors associated with infection in a population-based cohort study of 46299 consecutive patients. Eur Heart J. 2011;32(8):991–8.

14. Le KY, Sohail MR, Friedman PA, Uslan DZ, Cha SS, Hayes DL, et al. Clinical predictors of cardiovascular implantable electronic device-related infective endocarditis. Pacing Clin Electrophysiol. 2011;34(4):450–9.

15. Sohail MR, Uslan DZ, Khan AH, Friedman PA, Hayes DL, Wilson WR, et al. Risk factor analysis of permanent pacemaker infection. Clin Infect Dis. 2007;45(2):166–73.

16. Bloom H, Heeke B, Leon A, Mera F, Delurgio D, Beshai J, et al. Renal insufficiency and the risk of infection from pacemaker or defibrillator surgery. Pacing Clin Electrophysiol. 2006; 29(2):142–5.

17. Tompkins C, McLean R, Cheng A, Brinker JA, Marine JE, Nazarian S, et al. End-stage renal disease predicts complications in pacemaker and ICD implants. J Cardiovasc Electrophysiol. 2011;22(10):1099–104.

18. Al-Khatib SM, Lucas FL, Jollis JG, Malenka DJ, Wennberg DE. The relation between patients' outcomes and the volume of cardioverter-defibrillator implantation procedures performed by physicians treating Medicare beneficiaries. J Am Coll Cardiol. 2005;46(8):1536–40.

19. Mela T, McGovern BA, Garan H, Vlahakes GJ, Torchiana DF, Ruskin J, et al. Long-term infection rates associated with the pectoral versus abdominal approach to cardioverter-defibrillator implants. Am J Cardiol. 2001;88(7):750–3.

20. Da Costa A, Lelievre H, Kirkorian G, Celard M, Chevalier P, Vandenesch F, et al. Role of the preaxillary flora in pacemaker infections: a prospective study. Circulation. 1998;97(18): 1791–5.

21. Sohail MR, Palraj BR, Khalid S, Uslan DZ, Al-Saffar F, Friedman PA, et al. Predicting risk of endovascular device infection in patients with Staphylococcus aureus bacteremia (PREDICT-SAB). Circ Arrhythm Electrophysiol. 2015;8(1):137–44.

22. Madhavan M, Sohail MR, Friedman PA, Hayes DL, Steckelberg JM, Wilson WR, et al. Outcomes in patients with cardiovascular implantable electronic devices and bacteremia caused by gram-positive cocci other than Staphylococcus aureus. Circ Arrhythm Electrophysiol. 2010;3(6):639–45.

23. Uslan DZ, Sohail MR, Friedman PA, Hayes DL, Wilson WR, Steckelberg JM, et al. Frequency of permanent pacemaker or implantable cardioverter-defibrillator infection in patients with gram-negative bacteremia. Clin Infect Dis. 2006;43(6):731–6.

24. Darouiche RO. Device-associated infections: a macroproblem that starts with microadherence. Clin Infect Dis. 2001;33(9):1567–72.

25. Baddour LM, Epstein AE, Erickson CC, Knight BP, Levison ME, Lockhart PB, et al. A summary of the update on cardiovascular implantable electronic device infections and their management: a scientific statement from the American Heart Association. J Am Dent Assoc. 2011;142(2):159–65.

26. Vaudaux PE, Francois P, Proctor RA, McDevitt D, Foster TJ, Albrecht RM, et al. Use of adhesion-defective mutants of Staphylococcus aureus to define the role of specific plasma proteins in promoting bacterial adhesion to canine arteriovenous shunts. Infect Immun. 1995; 63(2):585–90.

27. Hoiby N, Bjarnsholt T, Moser C, Bassi GL, Coenye T, Donelli G, et al. ESCMID guideline for the diagnosis and treatment of biofilm infections 2014. Clin Microbiol Infect. 2015;21 Suppl 1:S1–25.
28. Vuong C, Otto M. Staphylococcus epidermidis infections. Microbes Infect. 2002;4(4):481–9.
29. Sohail MR, Uslan DZ, Khan AH, Friedman PA, Hayes DL, Wilson WR, et al. Management and outcome of permanent pacemaker and implantable cardioverter-defibrillator infections. J Am Coll Cardiol. 2007;49(18):1851–9.
30. Mulpuru SK, Pretorius VG, Birgersdotter-Green UM. Device infections: management and indications for lead extraction. Circulation. 2013;128(9):1031–8.
31. Nagpal A, Baddour LM, Sohail MR. Microbiology and pathogenesis of cardiovascular implantable electronic device infections. Circ Arrhythm Electrophysiol. 2012;5(2):433–41.
32. Viola GM, Awan LL, Darouiche RO. Nonstaphylococcal infections of cardiac implantable electronic devices. Circulation. 2010;121(19):2085–91.
33. Baddour LM, Epstein AE, Erickson CC, Knight BP, Levison ME, Lockhart PB, et al. Update on cardiovascular implantable electronic device infections and their management: a scientific statement from the American Heart Association. Circulation. 2010;121(3):458–77.
34. Le KY, Sohail MR, Friedman PA, Uslan DZ, Cha SS, Hayes DL, et al. Clinical features and outcomes of cardiovascular implantable electronic device infections due to staphylococcal species. Am J Cardiol. 2012;110(8):1143–9.
35. Athan E, Chu VH, Tattevin P, Selton-Suty C, Jones P, Naber C, et al. Clinical characteristics and outcome of infective endocarditis involving implantable cardiac devices. J Am Med Assoc. 2012;307(16):1727–35.
36. Massoure PL, Reuter S, Lafitte S, Laborderie J, Bordachard P, Clementy J, et al. Pacemaker endocarditis: clinical features and management of 60 consecutive cases. Pacing Clin Electrophysiol. 2007;30(1):12–9.
37. Hickson LJ, Gooden JY, Le KY, Baddour LM, Friedman PA, Hayes DL, et al. Clinical presentation and outcomes of cardiovascular implantable electronic device infections in hemodialysis patients. Am J Kidney Dis. 2014;64(1):104–10.
38. Victor F, De Place C, Camus C, Le Breton H, Leclercq C, Pavin D, et al. Pacemaker lead infection: echocardiographic features, management, and outcome. Heart. 1999;81(1):82–7.
39. Narducci ML, Pelargonio G, Russo E, Marinaccio L, Di Monaco A, Perna F, et al. Usefulness of intracardiac echocardiography for the diagnosis of cardiovascular implantable electronic device-related endocarditis. J Am Coll Cardiol. 2013;61(13):1398–405.
40. Novak M, Dvorak P, Kamaryt P, Slana B, Lipoldova J. Autopsy and clinical context in deceased patients with implanted pacemakers and defibrillators: intracardiac findings near their leads and electrodes. Europace. 2009;11(11):1510–6.
41. Supple GE, Ren JF, Zado ES, Marchlinski FE. Mobile thrombus on device leads in patients undergoing ablation: identification, incidence, location, and association with increased pulmonary artery systolic pressure. Circulation. 2011;124(7):772–8.
42. Downey BC, Juselius WE, Pandian NG, Estes 3rd NA, Link MS. Incidence and significance of pacemaker and implantable cardioverter-defibrillator lead masses discovered during transesophageal echocardiography. Pacing Clin Electrophysiol. 2011;34(6):679–83.
43. Erba PA, Sollini M, Conti U, Bandera F, Tascini C, De Tommasi SM, et al. Radiolabeled WBC scintigraphy in the diagnostic workup of patients with suspected device-related infections. J Am Coll Cardiol Img. 2013;6(10):1075–86.
44. de Lima PG, Siciliano RF, Camargo RA, Bueno FL, Junior JS, Costa R, et al. Pacemaker-related infection detected by (18)F-fluorodeoxyglucose positron emission tomography-computed tomography. Int J Infect Dis. 2014;19:87–90.
45. Vos FJ, Bleeker-Rovers CP, van Dijk AP, Oyen WJ. Detection of pacemaker and lead infection with FDG-PET. Eur J Nucl Med Mol Imaging. 2006;33(10):1245.
46. Khamaisi M, Medina A, Mazouz B, Bocher M. Imaging coronary sinus infection in pacemaker electrode with [18F]-fluorodeoxyglucose positron emission tomography. J Cardiovasc Electrophysiol. 2008;19(12):1327–8.

47. Sarrazin JF, Philippon F, Tessier M, Guimond J, Molin F, Champagne J, et al. Usefulness of fluorine-18 positron emission tomography/computed tomography for identification of cardio-vascular implantable electronic device infections. J Am Coll Cardiol. 2012;59(18):1616–25.
48. Dy Chua J, Abdul-Karim A, Mawhorter S, Procop GW, Tchou P, Niebauer M, et al. The role of swab and tissue culture in the diagnosis of implantable cardiac device infection. Pacing Clin Electrophysiol. 2005;28(12):1276–81.
49. Sohail MR. Concerning diagnosis and management of pacemaker endocarditis. Pacing Clin Electrophysiol. 2007;30:829.
50. Oliva A, Nguyen BL, Mascellino MT, D'Abramo A, Iannetta M, Ciccaglioni A, et al. Sonication of explanted cardiac implants improves microbial detection in cardiac device infec-tions. J Clin Microbiol. 2013;51(2):496–502.
51. Nagpal A, Patel R, Greenwood-Quaintance KE, Baddour LM, Lynch DT, Lahr BD, et al. Usefulness of sonication of cardiovascular implantable electronic devices to enhance micro-bial detection. Am J Cardiol. 2015;115(7):912–7.
52. del Rio A, Anguera I, Miro JM, Mont L, Fowler Jr VG, Azqueta M, et al. Surgical treatment of pacemaker and defibrillator lead endocarditis: the impact of electrode lead extraction on outcome. Chest. 2003;124(4):1451–9.
53. Dababneh AS, Sohail MR. Cardiovascular implantable electronic device infection: a stepwise approach to diagnosis and management. Cleve Clin J Med. 2011;78(8):529–37.
54. Chamis AL, Peterson GE, Cabell CH, Corey GR, Sorrentino RA, Greenfield RA, et al. *Staphylococcus aureus* bacteremia in patients with permanent pacemakers or implantable cardioverter-defibrillators. Circulation. 2001;104(9):1029–33.
55. Cacoub P, Leprince P, Nataf P, Hausfater P, Dorent R, Wechsler B, et al. Pacemaker infective endocarditis. Am J Cardiol. 1998;82(4):480–4.
56. Le KY, Sohail MR, Friedman PA, Uslan DZ, Cha SS, Hayes DL, et al. Impact of timing of device removal on mortality in patients with cardiovascular implantable electronic device infections. Heart Rhythm. 2011;8(11):1678–85.
57. Baddour LM, Wilson WR, Bayer AS, Fowler Jr VG, Bolger AF, Levison ME, et al. Infective endocarditis: diagnosis, antimicrobial therapy, and management of complications: a statement for healthcare professionals from the Committee on Rheumatic Fever, Endocarditis, and Kawasaki Disease, Council on Cardiovascular Disease in the Young, and the Councils on Clinical Cardiology, Stroke, and Cardiovascular Surgery and Anesthesia, American Heart Association: endorsed by the Infectious Diseases Society of America. Circulation. 2005; 111(23):e394–434.
58. Jarwe M, Klug D, Beregi JP, Le Franc P, Lacroix D, Kouakam C, et al. Single center experi-ence with femoral extraction of permanent endocardial pacing leads. Pacing Clin Electrophysiol. 1999;22(8):1202–9.
59. Buch E, Boyle NG, Belott PH. Pacemaker and defibrillator lead extraction. Circulation. 2011;123(11):e378–80.
60. Zhou X, Jiang H, Ma J, Bakhai A, Li J, Zhang Y, et al. Comparison of standard and modified transvenous techniques for complex pacemaker lead extractions in the context of cardiac implantable electronic device-related infections: a 10-year experience. Europace. 2013; 15(11):1629–35.
61. Rizwan Sohail M, Henrikson CA, Jo Braid-Forbes M, Forbes KF, Lerner DJ. Increased long-term mortality in patients with cardiovascular implantable electronic device infections. Pacing Clin Electrophysiol. 2015;38(2):231–9.
62. Sohail MR, Henrikson CA, Braid-Forbes MJ, Forbes KF, Lerner DJ. Comparison of mortality in women versus men with infections involving cardiovascular implantable electronic device. Am J Cardiol. 2013;112(9):1403–9.
63. Habib A, Le KY, Baddour LM, Friedman PA, Hayes DL, Lohse CM, et al. Predictors of mor-tality in patients with cardiovascular implantable electronic device infections. Am J Cardiol. 2013;111(6):874–9.
64. Margey R, McCann H, Blake G, Keelan E, Galvin J, Lynch M, et al. Contemporary manage-ment of and outcomes from cardiac device related infections. Europace. 2010;12(1):64–70.

65. Deharo JC, Quatre A, Mancini J, Khairy P, Le Dolley Y, Casalta JP, et al. Long-term outcomes following infection of cardiac implantable electronic devices: a prospective matched cohort study. Heart. 2012;98(9):724–31.
66. Sohail MR, Henrikson CA, Braid-Forbes MJ, Forbes KF, Lerner DJ. Mortality and cost associated with cardiovascular implantable electronic device infections. Arch Intern Med. 2011;171(20):1821–8.
67. Mittal S, Shaw RE, Michel K, Palekar R, Arshad A, Musat D, et al. Cardiac implantable electronic device infections: incidence, risk factors, and the effect of the AigisRx antibacterial envelope. Heart Rhythm. 2014;11(4):595–601.
68. Da Costa A, Kirkorian G, Cucherat M, Delahaye F, Chevalier P, Cerisier A, et al. Antibiotic prophylaxis for permanent pacemaker implantation: a meta-analysis. Circulation. 1998;97(18):1796–801.
69. Bertaglia E, Zerbo F, Zardo S, Barzan D, Zoppo F, Pascotto P. Antibiotic prophylaxis with a single dose of cefazolin during pacemaker implantation: incidence of long-term infective complications. Pacing Clin Electrophysiol. 2006;29(1):29–33.

Chapter 15
Right-Heart Endocarditis

Isidre Vilacosta, Carmen Olmos Blanco, Cristina Sarriá Cepeda,
Javier López Díaz, Carlos Ferrera Durán,
and José Alberto San Román Calvar

Introduction

Right-heart endocarditis is characterized by the presence of infective lesions in the endocardium of right-heart structures or in any sort of catheter, lead, or prosthetic material housed within the right-heart. Right-heart endocarditis accounts for 5–12 % of cases of infective endocarditis (IE) [1, 2]. According to the type of patient who hosts the infective process, we can distinguish four different types of right-heart endocarditis: IE in intravenous drug users (IVDU); IE in patients with pacemakers, implantable cardiac defibrillators, or central venous catheters; IE in patients with right-heart congenital abnormalities; and IE in patients who are not IVDU, who have no implanted cardiac devices or other catheters, and who have no left-sided endocarditis, the so called "three noes" IE group. In this chapter, we will focus on IE in IVDU and in those patients with no predisposing condition for a right-heart infection, the "three noes" group. IE in patients with implantable cardiac devices and in those with congenital heart disease is covered in other chapters.

I. Vilacosta, MD, PhD (✉) • C. Olmos Blanco, MD, PhD • C. Ferrera Durán, MD
Department of Cardiology, Hospital Clínico San Carlos, Madrid, Spain
e-mail: i.vilacosta@gmail.com; Carmen.olmosblanco@gmail.com; Carlosferreraduran@gmail.com

C. Sarriá Cepeda, MD, PhD
Department of Internal Medicine and Infectious Diseases, Hospital Universitario de la Princesa, Madrid, Spain
e-mail: csarriac@gmail.com

J. López Díaz, MD, PhD • J.A. San Román Calvar, MD, PhD
Instituto de Ciencias Del Corazón (ICICOR), Hospital Clínico Universitario de Valladolid, Valladolid, Spain
e-mail: javihouston@yahoo.es; asanroman@secardiologia.es

© Springer International Publishing Switzerland 2016   207
G. Habib (ed.), *Infective Endocarditis*, DOI 10.1007/978-3-319-32432-6_15

Epidemiology, Microbiology, and Pathophysiology

Intravenous drug use is a well recognized predisposing condition for IE. In fact, this condition represents a minor diagnostic Duke criterion for IE [1]. The exact incidence of IE in IVDU is unknown and differs between countries. The incidence of right-heart IE among IVDU may vary from 0.7 to 13/1000 patient-years [3]. Several years ago, Cooper et al. noticed an increase in the number of hospitalizations of IVDU with IE [4]. However, in the last decade, the incidence of IE in IVDU have decreased, being nowadays responsible for one third of all right-heart IE and less than 5 % of all IE episodes [5, 6]. Right-heart IE in IVDU is more frequent in young immunodeficiency virus seropositive and immunosuppressed patients, mainly males [7, 8].

Most infections are community-acquired, and *S. aureus* is the predominant microorganism, with methicillin-resistant strains becoming more prevalent [9]. Nasal colonization, use of contaminated drugs, drug-use paraphernalia, and drug-use environment are risk factors for *S. aureus* infection in this patient population [10]. *Pseudomonas aeruginosa, C. albicans* and other fungi are less frequent. Normal oropharyngeal flora microorganisms (*viridans* group streptococci, *Eikenella corrodens, Haemophilus aphrophilus*, etc.) are also common pathogens. Possibly due to the habit of cleaning their needles with saliva and using it to dissolve the drug, polymicrobial infection is frequent in this scenario [11]. In fact, the main risk factor of polymicrobial IE is intravenous drug use [12]. Remarkably, recurrent IE is more common in IVDU, and the median time interval between episodes is shorter in addicts than in non-addicts [13]. This fact can be at least partly explained by the continuation of drug use in many of these patients. Curiously, alcohol consumption seems to confer protection against IE in IVDU, perhaps by inducing an inhibitory effect on platelet function [14].

The source of bacteremia in IVDU is the autoinoculation of microorganisms by the intravenous injection. In most cases these microorganisms are part of the patient's own flora, although contaminated needle, contaminated drug, drug adulterants or drug diluents (saliva, lemon juice, water, etc.) may be implicated. IVDU may also acquire viral infections (HIV, and B or C hepatitis) and infections due to any other type of circulating microorganism as the result of sharing syringes contaminated by the infected blood of other IVDU.

In addition to contaminated drug solutions and reduced injection hygiene, abnormalities on the immune system may also play a role in the pathophysiology of IE in IVDU [14–16]. There is an overwhelming preponderance for tricuspid valve involvement in this clinical context, but the reason is still unknown [11, 17, 18]. One of the hypotheses is that the physical discharge of particulate matter contained in injected drugs or adulterants might lead to endothelial injury [11]. An attempt to reproduce the disease using the experimental model in rabbits was not successful [19]. Vasospasm caused by injected diluents or illicit drugs, and drug-induced thrombus formation and subsequent bacterial aggregation are just some of many other potential explanations [20]. The affected valve, usually the tricuspid, is almost always previously normal [21]. Whilst the tricuspid valve is the usual site of infection in IVDU, pulmonary and Eustachian valve infection may also be observed, and should not be forgotten that left-sided IE is not uncommon in this group of patients.

The "three noes" group represents about 15 % of all patients with isolated right-heart IE [5, 6]. They are usually middle-age men, older than IVDU, and whereas in IVDU the infection is mainly community acquired, in the "three noes" group, 50 % of episodes are nosocomial [5]. Comorbidities (chronic renal failure, diabetes mellitus, chronic obstructive pulmonary disease, chronic anemia, and cancer) are more frequently present in this group [5, 22, 23]. Some of these patients had the presence of an intravascular catheter, which is most probably the source of bacteremia. In many others there is no apparent source of infection [5, 22–27].

Diagnosis and Complications

History, clinical examination, blood cultures, and echocardiography remain the cornerstones of diagnosis. The usual clinical presentation of right-heart IE is persistent fever, chills, and multiple septic pulmonary emboli, which may manifest with dyspnea, chest pain, cough or hemoptysis [1]. Chest pain is often pleuritic, and cough, when present, may be nonproductive or associated with blood-streaked sputum [20]. Pulmonary septic emboli may be complicated by pulmonary infarction, abscess formation, pneumothorax, and pleural effusion. Since right-heart murmurs often go undetected and IE peripheral stigmata are absent, diagnosis can be delayed, so high-suspicion index is of paramount importance. This is even more important in the "three noes" group of patients. In a series of isolated native tricuspid valve IE, in non-addicted patients, and in the absence of intracardiac catheters or cardiac anomalies, Nandakumar and Raju suggested that right-sided IE must be considered in any patient with the "tricuspid syndrome" consisting of recurrent pulmonary events, anemia, and microscopic hematuria [23]. In our series, this syndrome was present in 28 % of patients from the "three noes" group [5]. Likewise, fever, multiple pulmonary emboli, and sustained bacteremia by *S. aureus* are signs of clinical alert for right-heart IE [28].

Chest X-ray may reveal findings consistent with pulmonary embolism due to septic emboli from the right heart [15]. Chest computed tomography and 18F-FDG-PET/CT scanning will demonstrate multiple infiltrates with cavities in both lung fields (Fig. 15.1a–d), suggesting the presence of multiple pulmonary embolisms and lung abscesses [29]. When systemic emboli occur, paradoxical embolism or associated left-sided IE should be considered [1].

In right-heart IE, heart failure is much less common than in patients with left-sided IE [6, 30]. Right-heart failure can be caused by severe right-sided valvular regurgitation (Fig. 15.2) or obstruction [1]. The existence of pulmonary hypertension will contribute to right-heart failure.

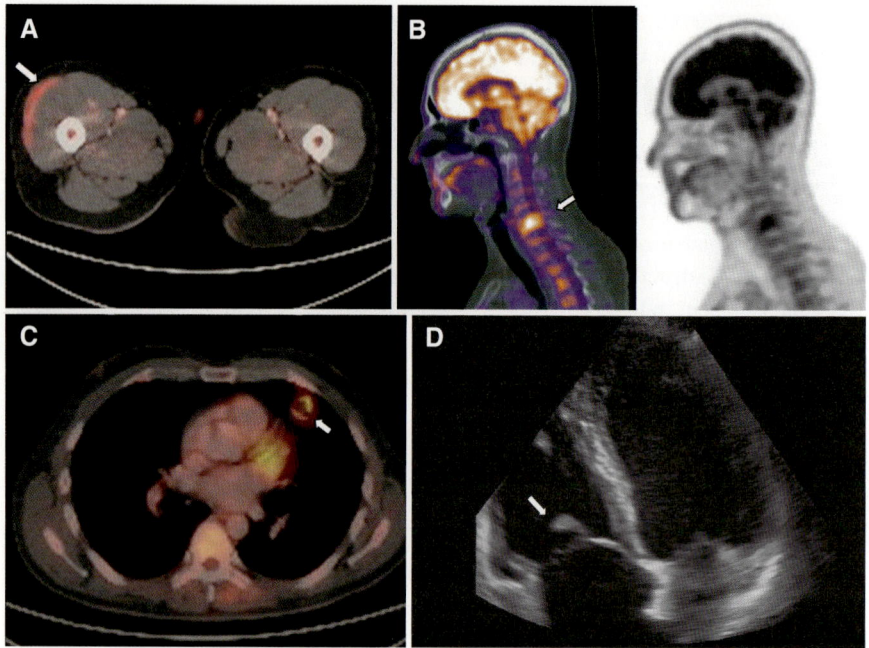

Fig. 15.1 Sagittal 18-F-FDG-PET/CT image (**b**) demonstrating FDG accumulation at the level of C5/C6 (*arrow*) (spondylodiscitis) in a patient with *S. aureus* tricuspid valve endocarditis from the "three noes" group, with no risk factors. In addition, a septic pulmonary embolus (**c**, *arrow*), and a focus of myositis (**a**, *arrow*) are well documented. Transthoracic echocardiogram, four-chamber view (**d**), showing a vegetation (*arrow*) attached to the tricuspid valve

Blood Cultures

As in left-sided IE, positive blood cultures, in combination with clinical and echocardiographic findings, establishes the diagnosis. Therefore, even in patients that are acutely ill, three or more blood cultures should be obtained before antibiotic therapy is initiated. Those cases that are clinically stable and not very ill can be safely observed without antibiotics while the results of blood cultures are awaited. The volume and number of blood cultures is critical because bacteremia in IE is often of low level. Three or more blood cultures (8–12 ml each) should be drawn with careful antiseptic conditions [31]. The modified Duke criteria will effectively classify most of these patients in either definite or possible IE [32]. However, diagnosis of IE in the emergency department remains challenging and is current standard practice to admit IVDU with fever of unclear etiology for blood cultures and echocardiography. A prediction rule for IE in febrile injection drug users has been developed [33]. According to these authors, if patients have no murmur, no tachycardia, and a clear-cut skin infection, they have a low likelihood of IE and may be considered "ruled out" for this disease. On the other hand, any febrile IVDU who have any of these three criteria (murmur, tachycardia, and no identifiable skin infection) should undergo further evaluation for IE [33].

Fig. 15.2 Anatomic
image of the heart of an
IVDU. Four-chamber
view. Two vegetations,
one in the atrial side of the
mitral valve (*arrow*), and
the other in the atrial side
of the tricuspid valve
(*arrow*) are well seen

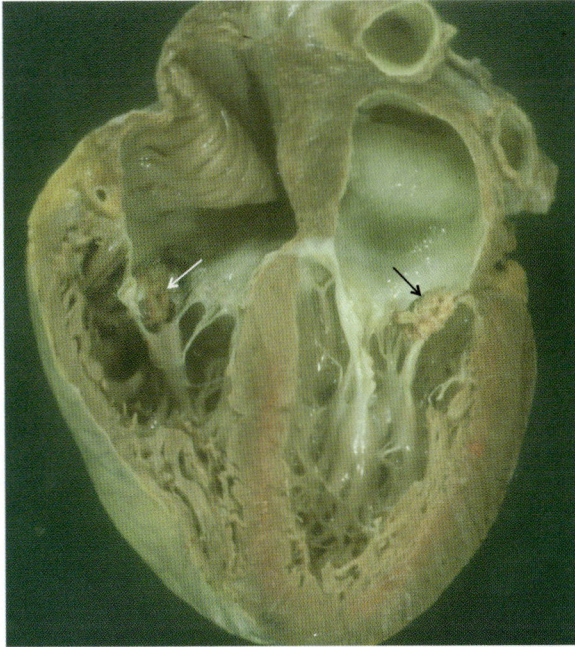

In our series, causative microorganisms more often isolated in IVDU with right-heart IE were *S. aureus*, followed by coagulase-negative staphylococci, most of them methicillin-sensitive [5]. In other series, methicillin-resistant strains are becoming more prevalent [9]. In contrast to previous series of right-sided IE in IVDU, where *viridans* streptococci were responsible of 25 % of the episodes, we did not found any case as the only microorganism responsible for the infection. Streptococci were isolated in combination with other microorganisms (polymicrobial IE). In any case, the isolated microorganisms in IVDU with IE will depend on the country studied, the type of illicit drug, and the type of solvent used, among other factors [12].

With regards to the microbiology of the "three noes" group, staphylococci were the most common pathogens, but the frequency was much lower than in IVDU, and the number of streptococci much higher. In addition, methicillin-resistant staphylococci were frequent (33 %), suggesting a health care related source of infection [5].

Echocardiography

With blood cultures, echocardiography is the other mainstay in the diagnosis of right-heart IE. Transthoracic echocardiography (TTE) has a high sensitivity for the detection of right-heart vegetations (approximately 90 %) [7, 34]. TTE is at least equivalent to transesophageal echocardiography (TEE) for detecting right-sided vegetations in patients with a high pre-test probability [18]. In the patients herein studied, right-sided vegetations are usually attached to normal structures (tricuspid,

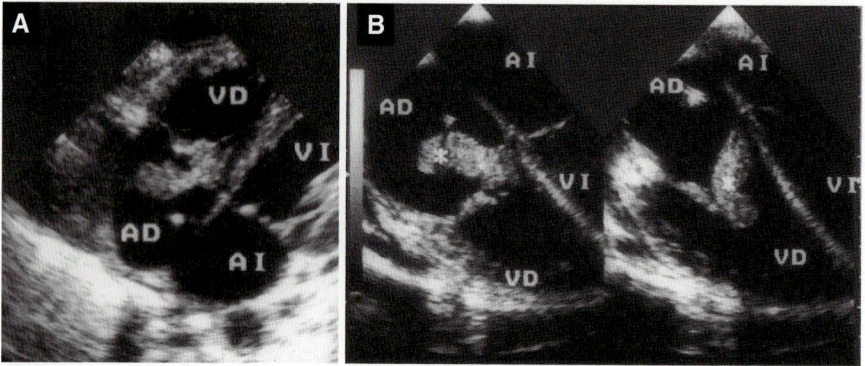

Fig. 15.3 Transthoracic (**a**) and transesophageal (**b**) images of an IVDU with tricuspid valve endocarditis. A giant vegetation attached to the septal leaflet of the tricuspid valve is well seen in both echo modalities. In transesophageal echocardiography, the vegetation is seen prolapsing into the right ventricle in diastole and back into the right atrium in systole. The *asterisk* shows the vegetation. *AD* right atrium, *AI* left atrium, *VI* left ventricle, *VD* right ventricle

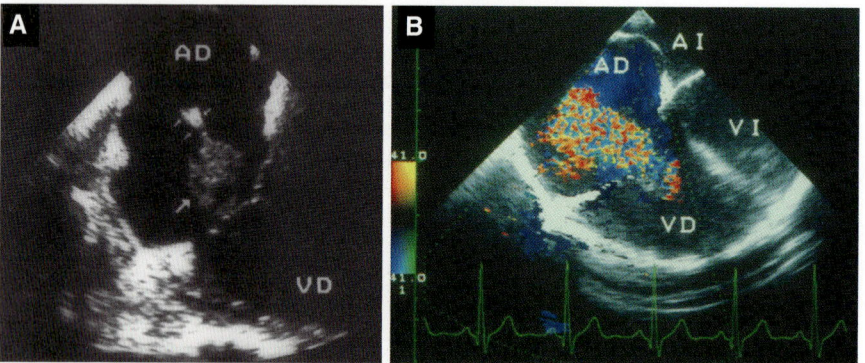

Fig. 15.4 Transesophageal echocardiographic image showing a huge tricuspid valve vegetation with a papillary muscle head (*small arrows*) attached to it (**a**). Transesophageal echocardiographic image with color flow Doppler (**b**) demonstrating a broad jet of reverse and turbulent flow across the tricuspid valve in systole consistent with severe tricuspid regurgitation. *AD* right atrium, *AI* left atrium, *VI* left ventricle, *VD* right ventricle

Eustachian, pulmonary or Thebesian valves; Figs. 15.3a, b and 15.4a, b) [5, 35–38]. Even the right atrial or ventricular endocardium can be a site for a vegetation to settle [6]. Similar to vegetations on the left-sided valves, they tend to be localized on the atrial side of the tricuspid valve and the ventricular side of the pulmonary valve, in the path of the regurgitant jet [39]. Vegetations are usually larger than those found in left-sided IE, which is probably related to the lower right chamber pressures enabling the rapid growth of vegetations [6, 7, 39].

Periannular complications are very rarely encountered in right-heart endocarditis [18]. Most series do not report the rate of periannular complications in IVDU with IE. However, these complications have been found in patients with the "three noes"

IE group [5]. Mobile normal right-sided structures (as the Chiari network) may mimic vegetations, and operators must be aware of their locations and appearance so as to not confound them with vegetations.

As in left-sided IE, older or healed right-sided vegetations tend to be more echo-genic, but there are no means to confidently distinguish between new and old veg-etations [39]. Therefore, we have to be aware that the finding of vegetations on an IVDU is not sufficient to make the diagnosis of active IE, and that these findings must always be interpreted in the clinical context. In a recent well conducted study with a large population of active, asymptomatic IVDU from Denmark, the authors showed that valvular abnormalities (leaflet thickening or moderate to severe valvu-lar regurgitation) assessed by TTE were very prevalent (20 %) in IVDU without a medical history of IE, and vegetations were seen in 5 % of subjects [3]. Interestingly, the high prevalence of vegetations in this group of asymptomatic subjects without a history of IE, but exposed repeatedly to bacteremia, might suggest that as pulmo-nary symptoms are so common in right-heart IE and its prognosis as favorable, it is likely that sometimes IE in IVDU may go unnoticed or misdiagnosed as a pulmo-nary infection and either treated effectively with a short-course of antibiotics or even show spontaneous healing [3].

As already mentioned, the additional value of TEE in this setting has been ques-tioned [18]. Nonetheless, vegetations and some complications can be more pre-cisely characterized by TEE (Figs. 15.3a, b and 15.4a, b). The reasons why TEE is not superior to TTE in this context are the following: (1) IVDU are young and thin patients with good transthoracic acoustic windows; (2) right-heart vegetations are larger than those from the left-side heart and thus can be easily seen with TTE [6], and (3) right-heart valves are anterior structures that are closer to the transthoracic probe than to the transesophageal probe [7, 18].

According to some authors, pulmonary vegetations are better detected by TEE, and some cases of Eustachian valve IE have also been better visualized by TEE than by TTE [40, 41]. On the basis of the previous background, in IVDU suspected of having IE, we recommend performing TEE in the situations listed in Table 15.1. According to the European guidelines, TEE is not mandatory in right-heart IE when TTE findings are clear-cut [1, 39].

The role of TTE and TEE in patients from the "three noes" group has not been assessed [5]. As long as no information on this topic is available, our current diag-nostic workup in this group of patients is being guided by a Bayesian-based decision-making approach: patients with moderate to high probability of having IE and negative results on TTE should undergo TEE. When vegetations are well seen on TTE and the clinical course is uncomplicated, it may not be worth proceeding with TEE [7].

Sungur et al. compared findings from intraoperative live/real time three-dimensional transesophageal echocardiography (3D-TEE) with conventional TEE in ten patients who underwent surgery for native tricuspid valve IE [35]. Unlike conventional TEE, 3D-TEE allowed *en face* visualization of the three tricuspid valve leaflets from both, atrial and ventricular aspects. This permitted a better detec-tion of the number of vegetations, their attachment site, and their dimensions [35].

Table 15.1 Indications of transesophageal echocardiography in IVDU suspected of having infective endocarditis

Poor acoustic transthoracic window
Suspicion of left-sided valve infection
Suspicion of pulmonary valve infection
Right-heart prosthetic valves
Abscesses or other complications
Negative results on transthoracic echocardiogram and:
Moderate to high clinical suspicion
Central intravenous catheters

According to the results of this small preliminary series, 3D-TEE might have a role when planning for a surgical intervention.

Antimicrobial Therapy

On admission, the initial selection of empiric antimicrobial therapy in IVDU should rely upon the suspected microorganism, type of drug and solvent used by the addict, and the infection location. Importantly, antibiotics should only be initiated after blood cultures have been obtained [1]. *S. aureus* must always be covered with penicillinase-resistant penicillins, vancomycin or daptomycin, depending on the local prevalence of methicillin-resistant *S. aureus* (MRSA).

In pentazocine addict patients, an anti-*Pseudomonas* agent should be added because infection with *P. aeruginosa* is frequently found due to contamination during drug manipulation [42]. If the IVDU is addicted to brown heroin dissolved in lemon juice, *Candida* spp. should be considered and antifungal treatment added [43]. Contamination from non-skin flora and polymicrobial infection should be suspected in IVDU with non-sterile injection drug use practices [12, 44, 45]. It should be pointed out that the bacteria implicated in many IVDU with polymicrobial infections are anaerobes primarily found in the oral cavity [12]. Thus, in these cases, adding an antistreptococcal agent is correct.

Once the infecting microorganism and sensitivity results are known, antibiotic therapy has to be appropriately adjusted.

In IVDU with methicillin-susceptible *S. aureus* infection, the standard therapy for IE due to this microorganism is adequate. Penicillinase resistant penicillin (cloxacillin) regimens are superior to glycopeptide (vancomycin) containing regimens [1]. There are consistent data showing that a 2-week antibiotic treatment may be sufficient, and that the addition of an aminoglycoside may not always be necessary. Two-week treatment with oxacillin or cloxacillin without gentamicin is effective for most patients with right-heart IE when there are no complications and the risk of recurrences is low [46, 47]. See Table 15.2 [1].

The standard 4-week regimen therapy should be used in the situations listed in Table 15.3 [1].

Table 15.2 IVDU with right-heart IE candidates to a 2-week antibiotic treatment should fulfill the following items

Methicillin-susceptible S. aureus
Native right-heart valve infection
Good response to treatment
Vegetations <20 mm
Absence of metastatic foci of infection or empyema
Absence of cardiac and extracardiac complications
Absence of left-sided valve infection
Absence of severe immunosuppression (<200 CD4 cells/mm^3) with or without AIDS.

Data from: Habib et al. [1]

Table 15.3 Clinical situations in which the standard 4-week antibiotic regimen should be used

Slow clinical (>72 h) response to initial antibiotic therapy
Persistent positive blood cultures (≥48 h)
Right-heart failure
Methicillin-resistant S. aureus (MRSA) polymicrobial infection
Acute respiratory failure
Systemic septic metastatic foci
Multiple pulmonary embolisms
Extracardiac complications (e.g. acute renal failure, arthritis, empyema, discytis…)
Therapy with antibiotic other than penicillinase-resistant penicillins
Associated left-sided endocarditis
Severe immunosuppression (CD4 count <200 cells/mm^3)

Data from Habib et al. [1]

Vancomycin has long been recommended as the treatment of choice for MRSA isolates [48], but this drug is far from being a "perfect" antibiotic. It does have limited tissue penetration, is slowly bactericidal, and has an increased drug clearance in IVDU. Therefore, it should not be used for short course treatment in patients with *S. aureus* IE. Different studies have demonstrated that mortality associated with MRSA bacteremia is significantly higher when vancomycin is used for treatment of infection with strains with a vancomycin MIC > 1 mcg/ml [49]. Thus, vancomycin should be considered a second-choice drug in patients with infecting MRSA strains having MIC > 1 mcg/ml. In these cases, daptomycin is probably the drug of choice.

One randomized controlled study has demonstrated non-inferiority of daptomycin when compared with standard therapy in the treatment of *S. aureus* infections, including right-sided IE [50]. Nowadays, when using daptomycin, most authors recommend using high doses (10 mg/kg/24 h) and combining it with cloxacillin or fosfomycin to avoid the development of drug resistance [51].

When intravenous route therapy is not possible, right-heart IE in IVDU may be treated with oral ciprofloxacin (750 mg b.i.d.) plus rifampicin (300 mg b.i.d.)

Table 15.4 Surgical indications in right-heart endocarditis

Right heart failure secondary to severe tricuspid regurgitation with poor response to diuretics.
Recurrent septic pulmonary emboli with persisting right-sided, large (>20 mm), vegetations.
IE caused by microorganisms difficult to eradicate (fungi, P. aeruginosa, etc.) with persisting signs of infection despite adequate antimicrobial therapy

From Habib et al. [1]. With permission of Oxford University Press

provided that the strain is fully susceptible to both drugs, it is a non-complicated case, and patient adherence is monitored carefully [52].

For organisms other than *S. aureus*, antibiotic therapy in IVDU with IE does not differ from that in non-addicts.

Little evidence is available regarding antibiotics in the three "noes" group. Initially, staphylococci, methicillin-susceptible and methicillin-resistant, and streptococci should be covered. Once the microorganism has been identified a standard 4-week course of susceptible antibiotics should be provided.

Surgery

Right-heart IE should be resolved conservatively in most cases. Indications for surgery in IVDU are practically the same as for the "three noes" group but in the former we are even more conservative since IVDU have a much higher incidence of recurrences due to continued drug use. Surgical indications are listed in Table 15.4 [1, 17, 53]. The main surgical principles are: (1) debridement of vegetations and infected tissue; (2) valve repair whenever possible, avoiding prosthetic material; (3) elimination of valve regurgitation [54].

When valve repair is not technically feasible, tricuspid valve replacement should be performed [29]. It is worth mentioning that residual mild to moderate tricuspid regurgitation will be well tolerated by the right ventricle in most patients, and that in the tricuspid position, prosthetic valve complications such as thrombus and pannus formation are more frequent than in mitroaortic position, while structural valve degeneration is less extensive [55]. In the case of IVDU, more bioprosthetic valves are implanted because of anticipated noncompliance with the anticoagulation regimen.

Tricuspid valve excision (valvectomy) can be considered in IVDU when valve repair is not possible due to extensive valvular damage, and provided that pulmonary pressure is normal or mildly elevated. Some of these patients will develop post-operative right-heart failure, especially if pulmonary pressure is markedly elevated (e.g., after multiple pulmonary emboli). In these cases, after infection eradication, a second-stage operation with tricuspid valve replacement can be performed several years later after patient rehabilitation and drug use discontinuation [56].

Gaca et al. retrospectively analyzed the current techniques and outcomes for isolated tricuspid valve IE in 910 patients using the Society of Thoracic Surgeons adult cardiac database [57]. In 286 patients the infection was cured, whereas in 624 was still active (patients were receiving antibiotics) at the time of operation. The median age was 40 years; moderate to severe tricuspid insufficiency was present in 78 % of patients, but information on how many were IVDU is missing. There were 490 tricuspid valve replacements, 354 repairs, and 66 valvectomy procedures during the study period [57]. Most patients undergoing valve replacement received a bioprosthetic valve (91.8 %). In the group with valve repair, 34 % of patients received only an annuloplasty ring, and 60 % had no device implanted. The operative mortality in this series was 7.3 % with no significant differences in mortality among valvectomy (12 %), repair (7.6 %), and replacement (6.3 %) [57]. As documented in this series, tricuspid valvectomy is nowadays an infrequent operation, with only 66 cases during the 5-year study period. Compared to the active group, healed patients experienced a trend toward lower operative mortality and lower complication rates.

Tricuspid valve replacement by a cryopreserved mitral homograft is another choice following valvectomy [58]. Its main drawbacks are low availability, and that is technically challenging. Finally, implantation of a stentless aortic bioprosthesis in an upside-down orientation in the tricuspid position is another alternative [59].

As in tricuspid valve IE, in the infrequent case of pulmonary valve IE, pulmonary valve replacement should be avoided, but if necessary, use of a pulmonary homograft is preferred [1].

As expected, reoperation rates for recurrent IE seem to be higher in IVDU (17 %) than in non-IVDU (5 %) [60]. Recently, Dawood et al. analyzed 56 patients who underwent surgery for tricuspid valve IE. Overall operative mortality was low (7.1 %) [61]. Recurrent tricuspid valve IE occurred in 21 % of patients with valve replacement, and in 0 % of patients who underwent valve repair. Thus, in this series, use of valve repair was strongly protective against recurrent tricuspid valve IE [61].

Prognosis

The prognosis of patients with right-heart IE will mainly depend on the sort of patient studied [1]. In a retrospective study with a large cohort of IVDU (220 cases) with native valve IE, 14 patients died (6 %); vegetation size was available in 50 % of cases. In a multivariable analysis restricted to right-sided IE, the variables associated with in-hospital mortality that achieved statistical significance were vegetation size > 2 cm and fungal etiology [62]. De Rosa et al. retrospectively analyzed 263 IVDU in a multicenter study from Italy, including 100 cases of HIV positive patients. One hundred and fifteen cases (43 %) had also left-sided involvement. On multivariate analysis, only left-sided IE and age greater than 35 years were independently associated with mortality [63]. HIV infection did not have a significant effect on mortality. Other studies are in agreement with the results of this multicenter study pointing out that mortality seems to depend more on the side of the heart involved than on the HIV status, even in those cases who have undergone surgery [64–67]. However, those patients with severe immunosuppression (CD4 count <200 cells/mm^3) have a worse prognosis [8].

Musci et al. reviewed the 20-year experience of surgical treatment of right-sided IE in their institution. There was a highly significant difference between the survival rates of patients operated on due to right-sided IE alone compared to right and left-sided IE. The 30 day, 1, 5, 10, and 20-year survival rate after right-sided IE operation was 96.2%, 88.4%, 73.5%, 70.4%, and 70.4%, respectively, compared to 72%, 67.8%, 50.8%, 35.6%, and 35.6% after operation for right and left-sided IE. In this series, risk factors for early mortality were priority of surgery, age over 40 years, and left heart involvement [66].

We found significant differences in in-hospital mortality among the different groups of patients with right-heart IE, 17% in IVDU, 3% in device carriers (pacemakers and defibrillators), and 30% in the "three noes "group. So in-hospital mortality in this last group is high and similar to that of left-sided IE [5]. Interestingly, in a retrospective review of 133 cases of definite *S. aureus* IE, Fernández Guerrero et al. found that while in-hospital mortality of right-sided IE in IVDU was 3.7%, mortality in patients with right-sided IE associated with intravenous infected catheters was 82%, much higher than that of left-sided IE [65]. This high mortality rate in non-IVDU ("three noes" group) might be related to the following factors: diagnosis delay, frequent and severe comorbidities, worse clinical condition at admission (septic shock), high prevalence of methicillin-resistant staphylococci, and high rate of persistent infection [5].

Conclusions

In summary, right-heart IE remains common among IVDU. A new group of patients with right-heart IE, the "three noes," has been recently documented. Diagnostic clinical features of right-heart IE include respiratory symptoms, *S. aureus* bacteremia, and fever of unclear origin. TTE is especially valuable in this scenario. Many IVDU with right-heart IE have a relatively benign clinical course, and most of them may be conservatively managed. Nonetheless, 5–10% of cases will still need surgery, and, in them, a conservative approach is recommended. Recurrences are high in IVDU. Patients from the "three noes" group have more comorbidities, health care related infections, and higher mortality.

Just as in left-sided IE, a multidisciplinary approach including cardiologists, cardiac surgeons, cardiac imaging specialists, microbiologists, and infectious disease specialists is recommendable in right-heart IE.

References

1. Habib G, Hoen B, Tornos P, Thuny F, Prendergast B, Vilacosta I, et al. Guidelines on the prevention, diagnosis, and treatment of infective endocarditis (new version 2009): the task force on the prevention, diagnosis, and treatment of infective endocarditis of the European Society of Cardiology (ESC). Endorsed by the European Society of Clinical Microbiology and

Infectious Diseases (ESCMID) and by the International Society of Chemotherapy (ISC) for infection and cancer. Eur Heart J. 2009;30(19):2369–413.

2. Leone S, Ravasio V, Durante-Mangoni E, Crapis M, Carosi G, Scotton PG, et al. Epidemiology, characteristics, and outcome of infective endocarditis in Italy: the Italian Study on Endocarditis. Infection. 2012;40(5):527–35.

3. Axelsson A, Søholm H, Dalsgaard M, Helweg-Larsen J, Ihlemann N, Bundgaard H, et al. Echocardiographic findings suggestive of infective endocarditis in asymptomatic Danish injection drug users attending urban injection facilities. Am J Cardiol. 2014;114(1):100–4.

4. Cooper HL, Brady JE, Ciccarone D, Tempalski B, Gostnell K, Friedman SR. Nationwide increase in the number of hospitalizations for illicit injection drug use-related infective endocarditis. Clin Infect Dis. 2007;45(9):1200–3.

5. Ortiz C, López J, García H, Sevilla T, Revilla A, Vilacosta I, et al. Clinical classification and prognosis of isolated right-sided infective endocarditis. Medicine. 2014;93(27):e137.

6. Yuan S-M. Right-sided infective endocarditis: recent epidemiologic changes. Int J Clin Exp Med. 2014;7(1):199–218.

7. San Román JA, Vilacosta I, López J, Revilla A, Arnold R, Sevilla T, et al. Role of transthoracic and transesophageal echocardiography in right-sided endocarditis: one echocardiographic modality does not fit all. J Am Soc Echocardiogr. 2012;25(8):807–14.

8. Ribera E, Miró JM, Cortés E, Cruceta A, Merce J, Marco F, et al. Influence of human immunodeficiency virus 1 infection and degree of immunosuppression in the clinical characteristics and outcome of infective endocarditis in intravenous drug users. Arch Intern Med. 1998;158(18):2043–50.

9. Saydain G, Singh J, Dalal B, Yoo W, Levine DP. Outcome of patients with injection drug use-associated endocarditis admitted to an intensive care unit. J Crit Care. 2010;25(2):248–53.

10. Bassetti S, Battegay M. *Staphylococcus aureus* infections in injection drug users: risk factors and prevention strategies. Infection. 2004;32(3):163–9.

11. Miró JM, del Río A, Mestres CA. Infective endocarditis in intravenous drug abusers and HIV-1 infected patients. Infect Dis Clin North Am. 1997;16(2):273–95.

12. Sousa C, Botelho C, Rodrigues D, Azeredo J, Oliveira R. Infective endocarditis in intravenous drug abusers: an update. Eur J Clin Microbiol Infect Dis. 2012;31(11):2905–10.

13. Baddour LM. Twelve-year review of recurrent native-valve infective endocarditis: a disease of the modern antibiotic era. Rev Infect Dis. 1988;10(6):1163–70.

14. Wilson LE, Thomas DL, Astemborski J, Freedman TL, Vlahov D. Prospective study of infective endocarditis among injection drug users. J Infect Dis. 2002;185(12):1761–6.

15. Moss R, Munt B. Injection drug use and right sided endocarditis. Heart. 2003;89(5):577–81.

16. Frontera JA, Gradon JD. Right-side endocarditis in injection drug users: review of proposed mechanisms of pathogenesis. Clin Infect Dis. 2000;30(2):374–9.

17. Hecht SR, Berger M. Right-sided endocarditis in intravenous drug users. Prognostic features in 102 episodes. Ann Intern Med. 1992;117(7):560–6.

18. San Román JA, Vilacosta I, Zamorano JL, Almería C, Sánchez-Harguindey L. Transesophageal echocardiography in right-sided endocarditis. J Am Coll Cardiol. 1993;21(5):1226–30.

19. Sande MA, Lee BL, Millills J, Chambers HF. Endocarditis in intravenous drug users. In: Kaye D, editor. Infective endocarditis. 2nd ed. New York: Raven; 1992.

20. Levine DP, Brown PD. Infections in injection drug users. In: Mandell GL, Bennett JE, Dolin R, editors. Principles and practice of infectious diseases. 7th ed. Philadelphia: Churchill Livingstone/Elsevier; 2010.

21. Dressler FA, Roberts WC. Infective endocarditis in opiate addicts: analysis of 80 cases studied at necropsy. Am J Cardiol. 1989;63(17):1240–57.

22. Naidoo DP. Right-sided endocarditis in the non-drug addict. Postgrad Med J. 1993;69 (814):615–20.

23. Nandakumar R, Raju G. Isolated tricuspid valve endocarditis in non addicted patients: a diagnostic challenge. Am J Med Sci. 1997;314(3):207–12.

24. Kido T, Nakata Y, Aoki K, Hata N, Hazama S. Infective endocarditis of the tricuspid valve in a non-drug user. Jpn J Med. 1991;30(2):154–6.

25. Edmond JJ, Eykyn SJ, Smith LD. Community acquired staphylococcal pulmonary valve endocarditis in non-drug users: case report and review of the literature. Heart. 2001;86(6):E17.
26. Hamza N, Ortiz J, Bonomo RA. Isolated pulmonic valve infective endocarditis: a persistent challenge. Infection. 2004;32(3):170–5.
27. González-Juanatey C, Testa-Fernández A, López-Alvarez M. Isolated pulmonary native valve infectious endocarditis due to Enterococcus faecalis. Int J Cardiol. 2006;113(1):E19–20.
28. De Alarcón A, Villanueva JL. Endocarditis in parenteral drug addicts. Right-sided endocarditis. Influence of HIV infection. Rev Esp Cardiol. 1998;51 Suppl 2:71–8.
29. Akinosoglou K, Apostolakis E, Koutsogiannis N, Leivaditis V, Gogos CA. Right-sided infective endocarditis: surgical management. Eur J Cardiothorac Surg. 2012;42(3):470–9.
30. Wang TKM, Oh T, Voss J, Pemberton J. Characteristics and outcomes for right heart endocarditis: six-year cohort study. Heart Lung Circ. 2014;23(7):625–7.
31. Que Y-A, Moreillon P. *Staphylococcus aureus* (including *staphylococcal* toxic shock). In: Mandell GL, Bennett JE, Dolin R, editors. Principles and practice of infectious diseases. 7th ed. Philadelphia: Churchill Livingstone/Elsevier; 2010.
32. Li JS, Sexton DJ, Mick N, Nettles R, Fowler Jr VG, Ryan T, et al. Proposed modifications to the Duke criteria for the diagnosis of infective endocarditis. Clin Infect Dis. 2000;30(4):633–8.
33. Chung-Esaki H, Rodriguez RM, Alter H, Cisse B. Validation of a prediction rule for endocarditis in febrile injection drug users. Am J Emerg Med. 2014;32(5):412–6.
34. Weisse AB, Heller DR, Schimenti RJ, Montgomery RL, Kapila R. The febrile parenteral drug user: a prospective study in 121 patients. Am J Med. 1993;94(3):274–80.
35. Sungur A, Hsiung MC, Meggo Quiroz LD, Oz TK, Haj Asaad A, Joshi D, et al. The advantages of live/real time three-dimensional transesophageal echocardiography in the assessment of tricuspid valve infective endocarditis. Echocardiography. 2014;31(10):1293–309.
36. Vilacosta I, San Román JA, Roca V. Eustachian valve endocarditis. Br Heart J. 1990;64(5):340–1.
37. San Román JA, Vilacosta I, Sarriá C, Garcimartín I, Rollán MJ, Fernández-Avilés F. Eustachian valve endocarditis: is it worth searching for? Am Heart J. 2001;142(6):1037–40.
38. Kwan C, Chen O, Radionova S, Sadiq A, Moskovits M. Echocardiography: a case of coronary sinus endocarditis. Echocardiography. 2014;31(9):E287–8.
39. Habib G, Badano L, Tribouilloy C, Vilacosta I, Zamorano JL. Recommendations for the practice of echocardiography in infective endocarditis. Eur J Echocardiogr. 2010;11(2):202–19.
40. Winslow T, Foster E, Adams JR, Schiller NB. Pulmonary valve endocarditis: improved diagnosis with biplane transesophageal echocardiography. J Am Soc Echocardiogr. 1992;5(2):206–10.
41. Sawhney N, Palakodeti V, Raisinghani A, Rickman LS, DeMaria AN, Blanchard DG. Eustachian valve endocarditis: a case series and analysis of the literature. J Am Soc Echocardiogr. 2001;14(11):1139–42.
42. Botsford KB, Weistein RA, Nathan CR, Kabins SA. Selective survival in pentazocine and tripelennamine of *Pseudomonas aeruginosa* serotype O11 from drug addicts. J Infect Dis. 1985;151(2):209–16.
43. Bisbe J, Miró JM, Latorre X, Moreno A, Mallolas J, Gatell JM, et al. Disseminated candidiasis in addicts who use brown heroin: report of 83 cases and review. Clin Infect Dis. 1992;15(6):910–23.
44. Oh S, Havlen PR, Hussain N. A case of polymicrobial endocarditis caused by anaerobic organisms in an injection drug user. J Gen Intern Med. 2005;20(10):C1–2.
45. Raucher B, Dobkin J, Mandel L, Edberg S, Levi M, Miller M. Occult polymicrobial endocarditis with *Haemophilus parainfluenzae* in intravenous drug abusers. Am J Med. 1989;86(2):169–72.
46. Fortun J, Navas E, Martínez-Beltran J, Pérez-Molina J, Martin-Davila P, Guerrero A, et al. Short-course therapy for right-sided endocarditis due to *Staphylococcus aureus* in drug abusers: cloxacillin versus glycopeptides in combination with gentamycin. Clin Infect Dis. 2001;33(1):120–5.
47. Ribera E, Gómez-Jimenez J, Cortes E, del Valle O, Planes A, González-Alujas T, et al. Effectiveness of cloxacillin with and without gentamicin in short-term therapy for right-sided

Staphylococcus aureus endocarditis. A randomized, controlled trial. Ann Intern Med. 1996;125(12):969–74.

48. Liu C, Bayer A, Cosgrove SE, Daum RS, Fridkin SK, Gorwitz RJ, et al. Clinical practice guidelines by the infectious diseases society of America for the treatment of methicillin-resistant *Staphylococcus aureus* infections in adults and children. Clin Infect Dis. 2011;52(3):e18–55.

49. Soriano A, Marco F, Martínez JA, Pisos E, Almela M, Dimova VP, et al. Influence of vancomycin minimum inhibitory concentration on the treatment of methicillin-resistant *Staphylococcus aureus* bacteremia. Clin Infect Dis. 2008;46(2):193–200.

50. Fowler Jr VG, Boucher HW, Corey GR, Abrutyn E, Karchmer AW, Rupp ME, et al. Daptomycin versus standard therapy for bacteremia and endocarditis caused by *Staphylococcus aureus*. N Engl J Med. 2006;355(7):653–65.

51. Rose WE, Leonard SN, Sakoulas G, Kaatz GW, Zervos MJ, Sheth A, et al. Daptomycin activity against *Staphylococcus aureus* following vancomycin exposure in an in vitro pharmacodynamic model with simulated endocardial vegetations. Antimicrob Agents Chemother. 2008;52(3):831–6.

52. Al-Omari A, Cameron DW, Lee C, Corrales-Medina VF. Oral antibiotic therapy for the treatment of infective endocarditis: a systematic review. BMC Infect Dis. 2014;14:140.

53. Aris A, Pomar JL, Saura E. Cardiopulmonary bypass in HIV-positive patients. Ann Thorac Surg. 1993;55(5):1104–7.

54. Byrne JG, Rezai K, Sánchez JA, Bernstein RA, Okum E, Leacche M, et al. Surgical management of endocarditis: the society of thoracic surgeons clinical practice guideline. Ann Thorac Surg. 2011;91(6):2012–9.

55. Nakano K, Ishibashi-Ueda H, Kobayashi J, Sasako Y, Yagihara T. Tricuspid valve replacement with bioprostheses: long-term results and causes of valve dysfunction. Ann Thorac Surg. 2001;71(1):105–9.

56. Arbulu A, Holmes RJ, Asfaw I. Surgical treatment of intractable right-sided infective endocarditis in drug addicts: 25 years' experience. J Heart Valve Dis. 1993;2(2):129–37.

57. Gaca JG, Sheng S, Daneshmand M, Scott Rankin J, Williams ML, O'Brien SM, et al. Current outcomes for tricuspid valve infective endocarditis surgery in North America. Ann Thorac Surg. 2013;96(4):1374–81.

58. Mestres CA, Miró JM, Paré JC, Pomar JL. Six-year experience with cryopreserved mitral homografts in the treatment of tricuspid valve endocarditis in HIV-infected drug addicts. J Heart Valve Dis. 1999;8(5):575–7.

59. Cardarelli MG, Gammie JS, Brown JM, Poston RS, Pierson III RN, Griffith BP. A novel approach to tricuspid valve replacement: the upside down stentless aortic bioprosthesis. Ann Thorac Surg. 2005;80(2):507–10.

60. Kaiser S, Melby SJ, Zierer A, Schuessler RB, Moon MR, Moazami N, et al. Long-term outcomes in valve replacement surgery for infective endocarditis. Ann Thorac Surg. 2007;83(1):30–5.

61. Dawood MY, Cheema FH, Ghoreishi M, Foster NW, Villanueva RM, Salenger R, et al. Contemporary outcomes of operations for tricuspid valve infective endocarditis. Ann Thorac Surg. 2015;99(2):539–46.

62. Martín-Dávila P, Navas E, Fortún J, Moya JL, Cobo J, Pintado V, et al. Analysis of mortality and risk factors associated with native valve endocarditis in drug users: the importance of vegetation size. Am Heart J. 2005;150(5):1099–106.

63. De Rosa FG, Cicalini S, Canta F, Audagnotto S, Cecchi E, Di Perri G. Infective endocarditis in intravenous drug users from Italy: the increasing importance in HIV-infected patients. Infection. 2007;35(3):154–60.

64. Lemma M, Vanelli P, Beretta L, Botta M, Antinori A, Santoli C. Cardiac surgery in HIV-positive intravenous drug addicts: influence of cardiovascular bypass on the progression to AIDS. Thorac Cardiovasc Surg. 1992;40(5):279–82.

65. Fernández Guerrero ML, González López JJ, Goyenechea A, Fraile J, de Górgolas M. Endocarditis caused by *Staphylococcus aureus*: a reappraisal of the epidemiologic, clinical,

and pathologic manifestations with analysis of factors determining outcome. Medicine (Baltimore). 2009;88(1):1–22.

66. Musci M, Siniaswki H, Pasic M, Grauhan O, Weng Y, Meyer R, et al. Surgical treatment of right-sided active infective endocarditis with or without involvement of the left heart: 20-year single center experience. Eur J Cardiothorac Surg. 2007;32(1):118–25.

67. Ortiz-Bautista C, López J, García-Granja PE, Sevilla T, Vilacosta I, Sarriá C, et al. Current profile of infective endocarditis in intravenous drug users: the prognostic relevance of the valves involved. Int J Cardiol. 2015;187:472–4.

Chapter 16
Non-bacterial Thrombotic Endocarditis

Patrizio Lancellotti

Introduction

Non-bacterial thrombotic endocarditis (NBTE) was first described in 1888 by Zeigler [1], who introduced the word "thromboendocarditis" to describe deposition of fibrin on cardiac valves. It was Gross and Friedberg [2] in 1936 who coined the term "nonbacterial thrombotic endocarditis." Under the same entity, NBTE comprises several denominations, namely marantic endocarditis, Libman-Sacks endocarditis, or verrucous endocarditis [3]. NBTE is characterised by the presence of sterile vegetations, which consist of fibrin and platelet aggregates, on cardiac valves. These vegetations are associated neither with bacteraemia nor with destructive changes of the underlying valve [3]. The aetiology and the pathogenesis of NBTE are not fully elucidated; several mechanisms play a role. The common factor is endothelial damage and subsequent exposure of the subendothelial connective tissue to the circulating platelets [4]. Factors implicated in the initiation are: (a) immune complexes, (b) hypoxia, (c) hypercoagulability, and (d) carcinomatosis [4].

Epidemiology

NBTE is a rare condition representing <2 % of all endocarditis. NBTE was most often found post-mortem with rates in autopsy series ranging from 0.9 to 1.6 % [5, 6]. However, pathologic studies may underestimate the prevalence of NBTE because

Electronic supplementary material The online version of this chapter (doi:10.1007/978-3-319-32432-6_16) contains supplementary material, which is available to authorized users.

P. Lancellotti, MD, PhD
Department of Cardiology, University of Liège, Liège, Belgium
e-mail: plancellotti@chu.ulg.ac.be

Table 16.1 Diseases associated with NBTE

Malignancies	Solid tumours (pancreas, lung)
	Haematological malignancies (lymphoma)
Chronic diseases	Tuberculosis
	Acquired immune deficiency syndrome (AIDS)
	Uraemia
Connective tissue disorders	Systemic lupus erythematosis
	Antiphospholipids antibodies syndrome
Hypercoagulation states	Trauma from indwelling catheters
	Advanced age
Hypercoagulation states, Immunes complex	Septicaemia
	Severe burns

of inadequate evaluation of specimens. Its prevalence is likely underestimated. With the advent of imaging, and especially of echocardiography, NBTE has also been detected during life. It has been reported in every age group, most commonly affecting patients between the fourth and eighth decades of life with no sex predilection [7]. NBTE is a condition associated with numerous diseases such as cancer, connective tissue disorders (i.e., systemic lupus erythematosus patients possessing antiphospholipid antibodies and named Libman-Sacks endocarditis), autoimmune disorders, hypercoagulable states, septicaemia, severe burns, and chronic diseases such as tuberculosis, uraemia or acquired immune deficiency syndrome [8] (Table 16.1). In patients with systemic lupus erythematosus, observational studies using transthoracic echocardiography have reported prevalence rates of 6–11 %, with higher rates (43 %) observed when transesophageal echocardiography was performed [9].

Symptoms and Signs

Vegetations themselves do not cause symptoms. Lesions are thus usually clinically silent, without significant valvular dysfunction. When such dysfunction does occur, however, valvular regurgitation and, rarely, stenosis may result in heart failure and arrhythmias, such as atrial fibrillation. Fever and a heart murmur are sometimes present. Symptoms often result from the underlying disease or from embolization and depend on the organ affected (e.g., brain, kidneys, spleen). Secondary infective endocarditis, although uncommon, can also complicate valvular abnormalities and can cause neurologic and systemic complications. The risk of systemic emboli is increased substantially in the presence of mitral stenosis, atrial fibrillation, or both.

Diagnosis

It is essential to differentiate NBTE from infective endocarditis and other causes of valvular morphological changes. See Table 16.2 for the differential diagnoses for NBTE. However, differentiation from culture-negative infective endocarditis may be

Table 16.2 Differential diagnosis for non-bacterial thrombotic endocarditis

Infective endocarditis
Degenerative valvular disease
Fibroelastoma
Rheumatic valvular disease
Löffler's endocarditis
Lambl excrescences (normal variant) (filiform strands that originate at valve closure sites; they are thought to be normal variants, but some reports have proposed embolic potential)

difficult but is important. The same initial diagnostic work-up as for infective endo-carditis is recommended. NBTE should be suspected when chronically ill patients develop symptoms suggesting arterial embolism. The presence of a new murmur or a change in a pre-existing murmur, although infrequent, in the setting of a predispos-ing disease should alert the clinician to consider NBTE. Serial blood cultures and echocardiography should be done. Negative blood cultures and valvular vegetations suggest the diagnosis [10]. However, the condition is not always easily recognized on echocardiographic images. Post-mortem studies described mulberry like clusters of verrucae on the ventricular surface of the posterior mitral leaflet, often with adher-ence of the mitral leaflet and chordae to the mural endocardium. The lesions typically consist of accumulations of immune complexes and mononuclear cells. Examination of embolic fragments after embolectomy can also help make the diagnosis.

In practice, the diagnosis of NBTE is difficult and relies on strong clinical suspi-cion in the context of (a) a disease process known to be associated with NBTE, (b) the presence of a heart murmur, (c) negative blood culture, (d) the presence of veg-etations not responding to antibiotic treatment, and (e) evidence of multiple sys-temic emboli [11].

Laboratory Findings

Comprehensive haematological and coagulation studies (full blood count, pro-thrombin time, partial thromboplastin time, fibrinogen, thrombin time, D-dimers and cross-linked fibrin degradation products) should be performed to search for a potential causes. CRP is rarely increased and often there is no leucocytosis. Multiple blood cultures should be undertaken to rule out infective endocarditis, although negative blood cultures can be observed in infective endocarditis (e.g., prior antibi-otic therapy, HACEK group, fungi, etc.). Polymerase chain reaction (PCR) using nucleic acid target or signal amplification along with sequence analysis of the blood and tissue targeting common microorganism (Tropheryma whippelii, Coxiella bur-netti, and species of Bartonella, Chlamydia, Brucella, Legionella, Mycobacteria and Mycoplasma) should be performed. They can facilitate detection of culture negative endocarditis [12]. Immunological assays for antiphospholipid syndrome (lupus anticoagulant, anticardiolipin antibodies, and anti-β2-glycoprotein 1 antibodies with at least one must be positive for the diagnosis of antiphospholipid syndrome on ≥ 2 occasions 12 weeks apart) should be undertaken in patients presenting with

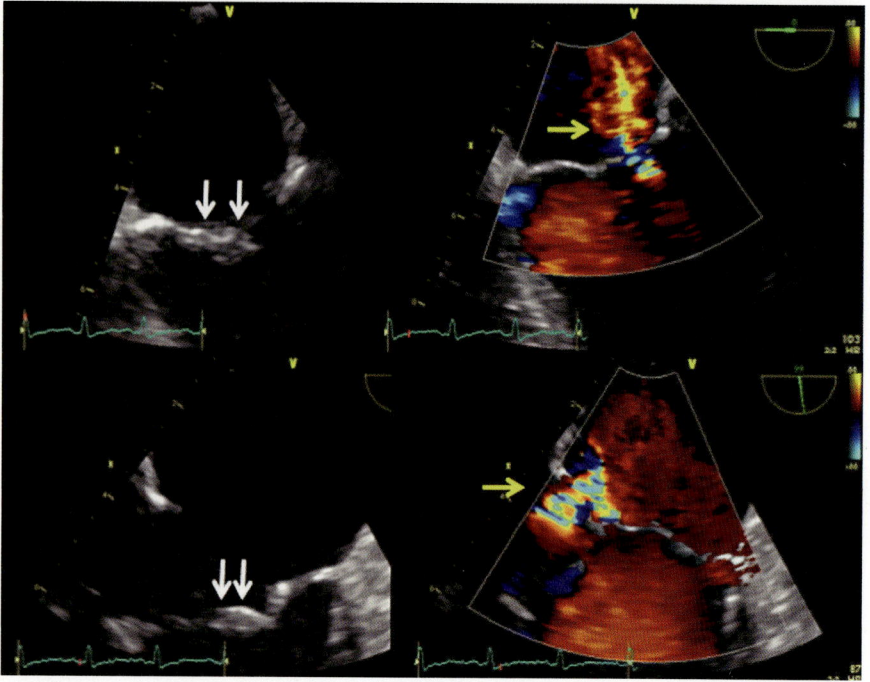

Fig. 16.1 Example of NBTE in a patient with lung cancer. Transesophageal echocardiogram, 4-chamber 0° view. There is a small mobile mass (*white arrow*) seen at the tip of the anterior mitral valve leaflet leading to moderate mitral regurgitation (*yellow arrow*)

recurrent systemic emboli or known systemic lupus erythematous [13]. Other features such as rheumatoid factor, antinuclear antibody and a comprehensive workup for systemic lupus erythematosus or malignancies can be indicated.

Echocardiography

Valvular vegetations in NBTE are usually small (0.1–2 cm in diameter), broad based, and irregularly shaped [14, 15] (Fig. 16.1). They have little inflammatory reaction at the site of attachment, which make them more friable and detachable (Table 16.3). Following embolization, small remnants on affected valves (≤3 mm) may result in false negative echocardiography results. Transthoracic echocardiography is the first line imaging but transoesophageal echocardiography should be ordered in case of high suspicion of NTBE [16]. 3D transoesophageal echocardiography can provide clinically relevant additive information that complements 2D imaging for the detection and characterization of NBTE [17]. Left-sided (mitral more than aortic) and bilateral vegetations are more consistent with NTBE than with infective endocarditis [18] (Fig. 16.2, Video 16.1). Valvular regurgitation is noted most commonly in patients with leaflet thickening, which is thought to

Table 16.3 Anatomical – echocardiographic – histologic findings

General features	Vegetation's characteristics	Histologic findings
Left heart valves only Vegetation-like lesions Diffuse valve thickening No abscess formation	Usually small vegetations Non destructive Changing from one day to another Sessile or pediculated	**Active verrucae** – Consist of clumps of fibrin on and within the valvular leaflet tissue, which is focally necrotic, with plasma cells and lymphocytes **Combined active and healed lesions** – Contain vascularized, fibrous tissue adjacent to fibrinous and necrotic areas **Healed lesions** – Consist of dense, vascularized, fibrous tissue

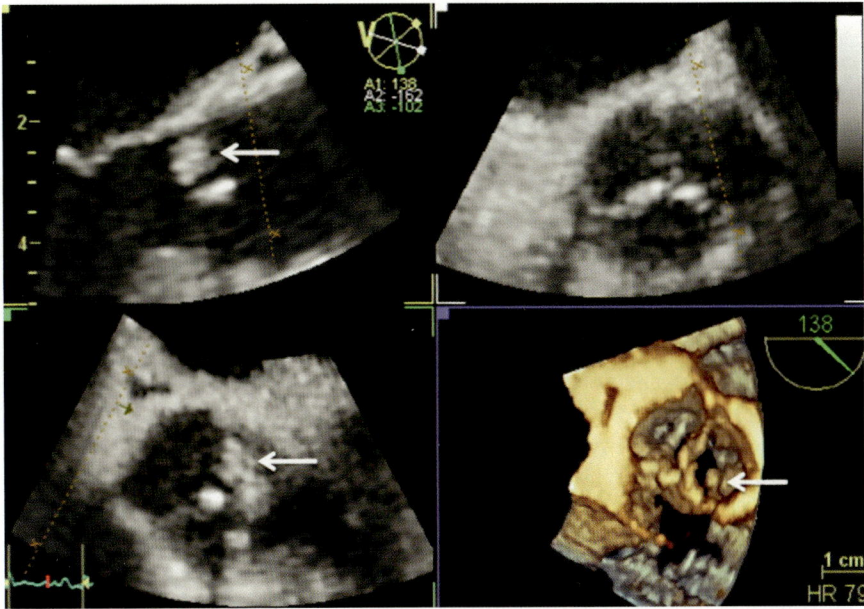

Fig. 16.2 Example of NBTE in a patient with systemic lupus erythematosis with cerebral embolism. 3D transesophageal echocardiogram showing a small mass (*white arrow*) attached to the aortic cusp without significant regurgitation (Video 16.1)

represent the chronic healed phase of disease. Pure mitral regurgitation is the most common valvular abnormality, followed by aortic regurgitation, combined mitral stenosis and regurgitation, and combined aortic stenosis and regurgitation [19].

Prognosis

The prognosis is generally poor, more because of the seriousness of predisposing disorders and associated comorbidities (e.g., renal failure, myocardial dysfunction) than the cardiac lesion. However, longitudinal data of valvular abnormalities are limited. Very few series reported no progression of mild or moderate regurgitation to severe regurgitation over a 2–3-year period and reported only isolated cases of mildly progressive stenosis [20]. The likely prevalence of secondary infective endocarditis is low, but it has not been widely reported. Potential contributing factors to infective endocarditis are connective tissue disorders connective tissue disorders such systemic lupus erythematosus, medications prescribed for these diseases, and underlying valvular abnormalities.

Treatment

NTBE is first managed by treating the underlying pathology. For instance, with the introduction of steroid therapy for systemic lupus erythematosus, improved longevity of patients appears to have changed the spectrum of valvular disease. Conversely, in patients with advanced and non-curable cancers, surgery is unlikely to influence the final outcome and also not prevent recurrent embolization. If there is no contraindication, these patients should be anticoagulated with heparin/warfarin, although there is little evidence to support this strategy [21]. In NTBE, the use of direct thrombin or factor Xa inhibitors has not been evaluated. In antiphospholipid syndrome, life-long anticoagulation is indicated. A trial comparing rivaroxaban (an inhibitor of factor Xa) and warfarin in patients with thrombotic antiphospholipid syndrome is currently in progress [22]. However, the risk of anticoagulation is haemorrhagic conversion of embolic events. Computed tomography or magnetic resonance imaging of the brain should be performed in patients with NBTE and cerebral attack before anticoagulation to rule out intracranial haemorrhage. There are no guidelines for surgical intervention in patients with NBTE. Surgical intervention, valve debridement and/or reconstruction, is often not recommended unless the patient present recurrent thromboembolism despite well-conducted anticoagulation [23]. Other indications for valve surgery are the same as for infective endocarditis (i.e. congestive cardiac failure due to valvular dysfunction). In the context of cancer, a multidisciplinary approach is recommended [24].

References

1. Lopez JA, Ross RS, Fishbein MC. Nonbacterial thrombotic endocarditis. A review. Am Heart J. 1987;113:773–84.
2. Gross L, Friedberg CK. Nonbacterial thrombotic endocarditis. Classification and general description. Arch Intern Med. 1936;58:620–40.
3. Libman E, Sacks B. A hitherto undescribed form of valvular and mural endocarditis. Arch Intern Med. 1924;33:701–37.
4. Silbiger JJ. The valvulopathy of non-bacterial thrombotic endocarditis. J Heart Valve Dis. 2009;18:159–66.
5. Eiken PW, Edwards WD, Tazelaar HD, et al. Surgical pathology of nonbacterial thrombotic endocarditis in 30 patients, 1985–2000. Mayo Clin Proc. 2001;76:1204.

6. El-Shami K, Griffiths E, Streiff M. Nonbacterial thrombotic endocarditis in cancer patients: pathogenesis, diagnosis, and treatment. Oncologist. 2007;12:518.
7. Borowski A, Ghodsizad A, Cohnen M, Gams E. Recurrent embolism in the course of marantic endocarditis. Ann Thorac Surg. 2005;79:2145–7.
8. Habib G, Cohen P, Milandre L, Gayraud D, Giuliani P, Harlé JR, Scheiner C, Casalta JP, Ferracci A, Luccioni R. Non bacterial thrombotic endocarditis (marantic endocarditis). Apropos of a case and value of transoesophageal echocardiography. Arch Mal Coeur Vaiss. 1996;89:261–4.
9. Roldan CA, Shively BK, Crawford MH. An echocardiographic study of valvular heart disease associated with systemic lupus erythematosus. N Engl J Med. 1996;335:1424.
10. Fournier PE, Thuny F, Richet H, Lepidi H, Casalta JP, Arzouni JP, Maurin M, Célard M, Mainardi JL, Caus T, Collart F, Habib G, Raoult D. Comprehensive diagnostic strategy for blood culture-negative endocarditis: a prospective study of 819 new cases. Clin Infect Dis. 2010;51:131–40.
11. Mazokopakis EE, Syros PK, Starakis IK. Nonbacterial thrombotic endocarditis (marantic endocarditis) in cancer patients. Cardiovasc Hematol Disord Drug Targets. 2010;10:84–6.
12. Moore JE, Millar BC, Yongmin X, Woodford N, Vincent S, Goldsmith CE, McClurg RB, Crowe M, Hone R, Murphy PG. A rapid molecular assay for the detection of antibiotic resistance determinants in cause of infective endocarditis. J Appl Microbiol. 2001;90:719–26.
13. Lisnevskaia L, Murphy G, Isenberg D. Systemic lupus erythematosus. Lancet. 2014;384:1878–88.
14. Asopa S, Patel A, Khan OA, Sharma R, Ohri SK. Non-bacterial thrombotic endocarditis. Eur J Cardiothorac Surg. 2007;32:696–701.
15. Reisner SA, Brenner B, Haim N, Edoute Y, Markiewicz W. Echocardiography in nonbacterial thrombotic endocarditis: from autopsy to clinical entity. J Am Soc Echocardiogr. 2000;13:876–81.
16. Roldan CA, Qualls CR, Sopko KS, Sibbitt Jr WL. Transthoracic versus transesophageal echocardiography for detection of Libman-Sacks endocarditis: a randomized controlled study. J Rheumatol. 2008;35:224–9.
17. Roldan CA, Tolstrup K, Macias L, Qualls CR, Maynard D, Charlton G, Sibbitt WL Jr. J Am Soc Echocardiogr. 2015;28(7):770–9.
18. Dutta T, Karas MG, Segal AZ, Kizer JR. Yield of transesophageal echocardiography for non-bacterial thrombotic endocarditis and other cardiac sources of embolism in cancer patients with cerebral ischemia. Am J Cardiol. 2006;97:894–8.
19. Edoute Y, Haim N, Rinkevich D, Brenner B, Reisner SA. Cardiac valvular vegetations in cancer patients: a prospective echocardiographic study of 200 patients. Am J Med. 1997;102:252–8.
20. Moyssakis I, Tektonidou MG, Vasilliou VA, Samarkos M, Votteas V, Moutsopoulos HM. Libman-Sacks endocarditis in systemic lupus erythematosus: prevalence, associations, and evolution. Am J Med. 2007;120:636–42.
21. Salem DN, Stein PD, Al-Ahmad A, Bussey HI, Horstkotte D, Miller N, Pauker SG. Antithrombotic therapy in valvular heart disease – native and prosthetic: the seventh ACCP conference on antithrombotic and thrombolytic therapy. Chest. 2004;126:457S–82.
22. Giles I, Khamashta M, D'Cruz D, Cohen H. A new dawn of anticoagulation for patients with antiphospholipid syndrome? Lupus. 2012;21:1263–5.
23. Dandekar UP, Watkin R, Chandra N, Santo KC, Bhudia S, Pitt M, et al. Aortic valve replacement for Libman-Sacks endocarditis. Ann Thorac Surg. 2009;88:669–71.
24. Habig G, Lancellotti P, Antunes MJ, et al. ESC 2015 guidelines on the management of infective endocarditis. Eur Heart J. 2015;36(44):3075–128.

Chapter 17
Infective Endocarditis in Congenital Heart Disease

Joey Mike Kuijpers, Berto J. Bouma, and Barbara J.M. Mulder

Introduction

The population of children and adults with congenital heart disease (CHD) is expanding, largely due to improved surgical and medical management and consequent prolonged survival of these patients [1, 2]. With longer survival and more complex surgical management, often involving prosthetics, CHD has become an important substrate for infective endocarditis (IE), especially in younger patients. This has contributed greatly to the evolving epidemiology of IE in the population overall. Despite recommendations for prophylaxis in the highest risk patients, IE remains a feared and serious complication in CHD patients [3–5]. Systematic studies of IE in the setting of CHD are scarce, and current knowledge stems mainly from retrospective studies and case series. On the background of this limitation, the clinical entity of CHD-related IE will be reviewed in this chapter.

Epidemiology

The incidence of IE in children and adults with CHD is greater than that in the general population, but varies significantly between different types of CHD (see section in this chapter on "Predisposing Defects and Risk Factors"). In paediatric CHD, the overall incidence rate of IE is an estimated 4.1 episodes per 10,000 person-years (versus 3.9–6.4 episodes per 1000,000 person-years in general) [6, 7]. The incidence rate in adult CHD (ACHD) is estimated at 11 episodes per 10,000 person-years (versus 17–62 episodes per 1000,000 person-years in general) [8, 9]. As in IE

J.M. Kuijpers, MD, MSc • B.J. Bouma, MD, PhD • B.J.M. Mulder, MD, PhD (✉)
Department of Cardiology, Academic Medical Center, Amsterdam, The Netherlands
e-mail: joeyks@gmail.com; b.j.bouma@amc.uva.nl; b.j.mulder@amc.uva.nl

© Springer International Publishing Switzerland 2016
G. Habib (ed.), *Infective Endocarditis*, DOI 10.1007/978-3-319-32432-6_17

in general, male ACHD patients are affected approximately twice as often as females, while the incidence is equal between the sexes in children [6, 8, 9].

As the population of CHD patients at risk for IE is growing [1], the contribution of CHD-associated IE to overall incidence is proportionately large and likely to increase [10]. Underlying CHD is found in 30–80 % of children and in 25 % of adults admitted for IE [7, 10–12]. In paediatric patients, the age distribution of IE occurrence peaks in infancy and late adolescence. In ACHD, median age at IE occurrence is in the early thirties, while this is around age 50 for adult IE patients in general [8, 9, 12].

Predisposing Defects and Risk Factors

As in other structural heart disease, the predisposition for IE in CHD is dependent on the presence of a substrate for valvular or mural endothelial damage and that of susceptible foreign surfaces. This is mainly determined by an interplay between the type of defect, its repair status, and the presence of prosthetic material used for repair or palliation. Recent cardiac surgery is a risk factor of particular importance to CHD patients, while other general risk factors, namely previous IE, early infancy and male sex among adults also apply to CHD patients.

Type of Defect, Repair Status, and Prosthetic Material

Defect types that cause turbulent blood flow are a major determinant of IE risk. Specifically, unrepaired defects associated with high risk for IE are complex cyanotic CHD, ventricular septal defect (VSD) and left ventricular outflow tract (LVOT) obstructions [6, 9, 13].

The effect of repair status on IE risk in patients with CHD is dependent on whether or not the repair was complete and, strongly, on the use of prosthetic material. Specifically, implantation of prosthetic conduits, shunts or valves is of major influence on IE risk, as these prosthetics themselves cause turbulent flow and provide susceptible surfaces. Complete repair without the implantation of prosthetic conduits, shunts or valves, either surgical or interventional, eliminates abnormal blood flow and consequently decreases or eliminates risk for IE. However, the risk is high in the first months after repair, due to remaining endothelial damage and the presence of foreign surfaces such as patches or closure devices that are in direct contact with blood. When the endothelium has recovered, and these foreign surfaces have become endothelialized, generally within six months, the risk for IE is assumed to be low [14, 15]. Relatively new but increasingly performed transcatheter device closures of atrial septal defects (ASDs) and ventricular septal defects (VSDs) are likely to confer the same short-term risk as surgical repairs. Despite some reported late occurrences of IE after such interventions, long-term risk is probably low [14,

16]. If residual defects remain, so will the potential for endocardial infection, as associated turbulent flow patterns will cause continued endothelial damage or hamper endothelialization of foreign surfaces. Repair or palliation with implantation of prosthetic conduits, shunts or valves does not reduce, and may even increase IE risk. As management of complex cyanotic CHD often involves such procedures, associated survival benefits are offset by a high lifetime risk for IE [9, 13]. The effect on IE risk may vary with type of material and mode of implantation. Specifically for prosthetic pulmonary valves, percutaneous implantation and bovine jugular vein material are particularly associated with high risk [17].

From the above it can be deduced that the emphasis for risk assessment in the current era of widely accessible surgical and interventional reparative and palliative procedures is on the presence of prosthetics or residual defects, while defect type and location are of importance in unrepaired CHD. From this viewpoint, the contemporary risk-profile of patients with specific defects is discussed below.

Complex Cyanotic Defects

Complex cyanotic CHD, either unrepaired, repaired or palliated, is associated with a contemporary IE risk of up to 21 and 58 cases per 10,000 person-years for paediatric and adult patients, respectively [6, 9]. As reparative strategies differ between defects, the risk differs strongly between types of repaired cyanotic defects. An illustrative example is the risk difference between tetralogy of Fallot (ToF) and the somewhat similar lesion pulmonary atresia (PA) with a VSD. Unrepaired, both carry a high risk for IE. After correction of ToF, involving a prosthetic patch but generally no shunts or conduits, IE occurs practically only in those with residual defects and those who did require palliative shunts [13, 18]. Contrastingly, after repair of PA with a VSD, involving a right ventricle to pulmonary artery conduit, risk is an estimated 115 cases per 10,000 patient-years [9, 13]. Patients with functionally univentricular hearts often undergo palliative procedures that frequently involve the use of prosthetics. Thus, patients with palliated univentricular physiologies are at high lifetime risk for IE [19, 20].

Ventricular Septal Defect

Estimates of IE risk in patients with an open VSD vary from 19 to 38 cases per 10,000 person-years. Importantly, risk is independent of defect size, and small asymptomatic VSDs should not be underestimated in their infective potential. Complete repair almost fully eliminates risk, with IE occurrence mostly restricted to patients in the first six months after patch closure and those with residual defects [13, 18, 21]. In adults, but not in children, VSD is associated with increased IE risk. This might be explained by greater frequency of complex lesions in adults. Indeed, the risk for IE is reportedly twice as high if there is coexisting aortic regurgitation [6, 9, 21].

Left Ventricular Outflow Tract Obstruction

Both repaired and unrepaired, congenital LVOT obstruction, specifically aortic valve stenosis, is a high-risk lesion. The risk for IE may be higher in those treated surgically (41–72 cases per 10,000 person-years) than in those treated medically (16 cases per 10,000 person-years), a difference probably partially explained by the implantation of a prosthetic valve. However, surgical intervention is associated with greater defect severity. Indeed, greater severity is a stronger predictor of IE risk than is surgical management [13, 21]. Coarctation of the aorta is a low-risk lesion, although IE does occur after surgical repair or on a coexisting abnormal aortic valve [9, 13]. Bicuspid aortic valve (BAV), a morphological abnormality present in 0.5–2 % of the population [22], is a frequently found condition underlying IE [12]. IE was reported to occur in 10–30 % of patients in early case series [23]. However, these early studies included mainly symptomatic patients, and their high risk reflects valvular dysfunction rather than the valve deformation itself. Indeed, in later studies including asymptomatic and uncomplicated patients, incidence was only 0.3 % per year [24]. Of note, in a large clinical ACHD cohort, IE incidence was approximately 21 cases per 10,000 person-years in BAV patients. This underlines that once it has become clinically overt due to valve degeneration or insufficiency, BAV should be regarded a high-risk lesion [9].

Other Defects

Both repaired and unrepaired isolated right-sided lesions are associated with a relatively low IE risk in both children and adults. In patients with pulmonary stenosis, risk is increased after implantation of a prosthetic pulmonary valve, with greater risk after percutaneous than after surgical implantation [17]. Regardless of repair status, isolated secundum ASD is a low-risk lesion, although risk is greater than in the population in general. This may be attributable to coexistent (valvular) lesions. PDA frequently underlies IE in young children, but rarely in older patients, as closure practically eliminates risk [6, 9, 13].

Risk Factors

Naturally, the risk for IE is associated with medical conditions, procedures and lifestyle habits that induce bacteraemia. A potential event of transient bacteraemia can be identified in only a minority of cases. Dental procedures or infection, cardiac surgery, cardiac catheterisation and non-cardiac invasive procedures are frequent causes in CHD-related cases of IE. Cutaneous infections may be an underestimated source of bacteraemia [19, 25, 26]. As is found in general, previous IE is an important predisposing factor for recurrent episodes of IE in CHD patients, and male gender is associated with greater risk among adults [4, 9]. In paediatric CHD patients, the risk for IE is highest in early childhood. This is probably due to multiple age-related risk factors, such as frequent use of central venous catheters in the young. Moreover, many CHD patients have reparative surgery early in life, increasing risk in the immediate postoperative period, while often decreasing long-term risk. During infancy, IE affects particularly those with complex cyanotic defects, often after surgery. In older children, simple defects are more frequent [6, 11, 27].

Microbiology

In CHD-related IE, *Streptococcus spp.* are isolated in 40–50%, *Staphylococcus spp.* in approximately 20–30% and Gram-negative bacteria, miscellaneous other bacteria and fungi together in 10–20% of cases, although the relative frequencies of causative organisms differ strongly between reported case series. Incidence of culture-negative IE is about 15% (see section in this chapter on "Microbiological Diagnosis") [19, 25, 28]. This microbiological pattern may differ marginally from that found in general IE, where *Staphylococcal* species show a slight predominance and Gram-negative bacteria and fungi are isolated in under 10% of cases [28, 29]. *Staphylococcus spp.* are relatively frequent in device-related IE and in IE associated with cyanotic CHD [30, 31]. Gram-negative and fungal infections are associated with post-operative and nosocomial IE [25, 32]. With a large proportion of CHD patients undergoing surgery, such organisms can be expected to be increasingly found in cases of CHD-related IE. Moreover, children with CHD may be more susceptible to colonization by certain Gram-negative bacteria [33].

Clinical Course and Complications

Time from the potential or assumed event of transient bacteraemia, if identified, to onset of symptoms is approximately two weeks. This so-called incubation period is rather variable, however, and ranges from less than one to several weeks. Mean time from onset of symptoms to diagnosis and start of appropriate treatment is approximately five weeks over available reports, although this delay may still be up to several months in very indolent cases [18, 26].

Signs and Symptoms

The clinical presentation of CHD-associated IE, often with prolonged low-grade fever accompanied by a variety of (non)specific complaints and findings, is similar to that of IE in general [28]. Cardiac examination may reveal a new or changed murmur. However, especially in the patient with repaired complex CHD, it may not be straightforward to determine whether a murmur is new or changed since prior examination. Graft infection and resultant dysfunction may be reflected in reduced systemic oxygen saturation and functional capacity in such patients [34].

Complications

The general principles regarding risk for complications are likely to apply to CHD patients, although this has never been formally evaluated. Importantly, the presence of prosthetic valves, a systemic-to-pulmonary shunt and cyanotic CHD are associated with greater risk for complications [25, 34, 35].

Congestive heart failure (CHF) is the most common complication of CHD-associated IE, occurring in up to 30–50 % of cases, although its incidence seems to have decreased over the past decades. It is more common in patients with prosthetic valves, and those who have previously undergone cardiac surgery [19, 25, 28, 36]. Perivalvular extension of the infection occurs in about 5 % of CHD-associated IE cases [20, 26, 31], far lower than the 10–40 % reported for IE in general [37]. This may be due to a lower relative frequency of aortic valve involvement, associated with greater risk for perivalvular abscess formation [38]. Alternatively, lower sensitivity of echocardiography in CHD patients may lead to underdiagnosis of this complication (see section in this chapter on "Diagnosis"). Of note, in native aortic valve IE, BAV is associated with increased risk for periannular extension (64 % versus 17 % in tricuspid aortic valves) [39]. Risk for perivalvular extension is very high in prosthetic valve IE (56–100 %) [40]. Clinically overt septic embolization, to either the pulmonary or systemic circulation, occurs in 10–35 % of cases, similar to general incidence and equal between native and prosthetic valve IE. General risk factors for embolization probably apply to CHD-related cases [19, 28, 31, 35].

Diagnosis

The threshold for suspecting IE in patients with CHD should be low, as any delay in diagnosis can adversely affect prognosis. In the febrile patient with a high-risk CHD lesion or intracardiac prosthetics, including valves, conduits and shunts, IE is to be considered.

The sensitivity of the modified Duke criteria may be reduced in the setting of CHD [41–43], as echocardiography is more frequently false-negative in patients with prosthetic material or complex cardiac anatomy and blood cultures are more frequently negative in prosthetic material IE [4, 44]. Thus, the diagnosis often relies more heavily on symptomatology and laboratory findings. The presence of peripheral IE stigmata and, although lacking specificity, that of splenomegaly, elevated

C-reactive protein and microscopic haematuria could be a valuable addition to the current diagnostic criteria, particularly in those with complex lesions and those with surgical prosthetics [42].

Microbiological Diagnosis

The overall 10–15 % incidence of culture negativity in CHD-associated IE is within the range of 2.5–31 % reported for IE in general. In contemporary studies, employing newer techniques for microbiological diagnosis, it is under 10 % [19, 28, 42, 44]. Although culture-negative IE is frequently due to prior antibiotic treatment, infection by uncommon or fastidious micro-organisms increasingly underlays negative blood cultures. This may be of particular importance to CHD patients, as these organisms are relatively common in postoperative and prosthetic material IE [25, 42, 44]. Especially in culture-negative cases with high clinical suspicion, other strategies for identification of uncommon pathogens (e.g., serologic testing, [immuno]histology) should be considered to strengthen diagnosis and target therapy [42, 44].

Imaging

Sensitivity of echocardiography in CHD-associated IE is approximately 70 % overall, but varies greatly with defect complexity and presence of prosthetics. Although lower than in patients with normal anatomy, sensitivity is relatively high in patients with isolated defects [28, 34]. Contrastingly, it may be under 50 % in postoperative cases and in patients with complex lesions or prosthetics [19, 36]. Vegetations on prosthetics outside the heart are particularly difficult to visualize. Especially in adults with complex cardiac anatomy or prosthetics, transoesophageal echocardiography (TOE) may have diagnostic advantages over transthoracic echocardiography (TTE), although this has not been systematically studied (Fig. 17.1a, b). A negative TOE study does not rule out a diagnosis of IE [4, 25, 45].

While the role of alternative modes of imaging (magnetic resonance imaging, MRI; computed tomography, CT; positron emission tomography, PET and radionuclide scanning) for the diagnosis of IE has not been exactly determined to date, they may prove particularly useful in CHD patients, when the diagnostic capacity of echocardiography is compromised due to interference by prosthetics. Indeed, cases of IE in patients with prosthetic valves or shunts in whom the diagnosis could be made by PET/CT after negative or inconclusive TOE have been reported. Moreover, this modality can demonstrate or exclude local extension of the infection, septic embolisms and metastatic infection, and be used for assessment of treatment efficacy during follow-up (Fig. 17.2a, b) [46].

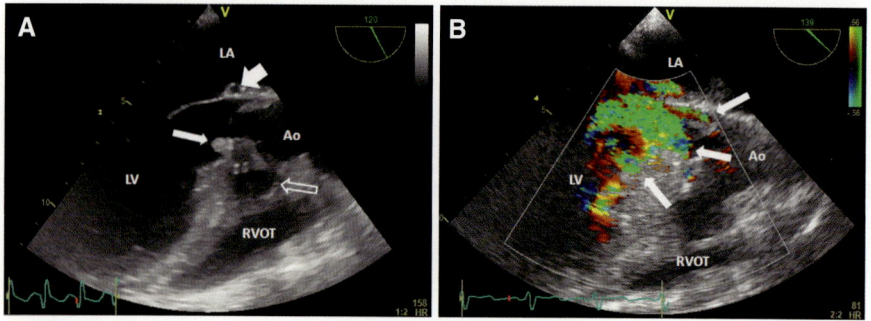

Fig. 17.1 (**a, b**) TEE images of a 19-year-old man with a history of unicuspid aortic valve repair one year earlier, who presented with chest pain. Blood cultures are positive for *Staphylococcus warneri*. (**a**) A mobile structure, suggestive of a vegetation, is visible on the right coronary cusp (RCC; *thin white arrow*). Also seen are an anomalous coronary artery pathway (*thick white arrow*) and pseudoaneurysm involving the RCC (*open arrow*). There are no signs of periannular extension. (**b**) The Doppler image shows aortic regurgitation, with three distinct regurgitant jets: one through the insufficient aortic valve (*middle arrow*) and the aortic commissure (*upper arrow*) and one at the base of the RCC, originating from the pseudoaneurysm (*lower arrow*), indicating valve destruction. Abbreviations: *LA* left atrium, *LV* left ventricle, *Ao* aorta, *RVOT* right-ventricular outflow tract

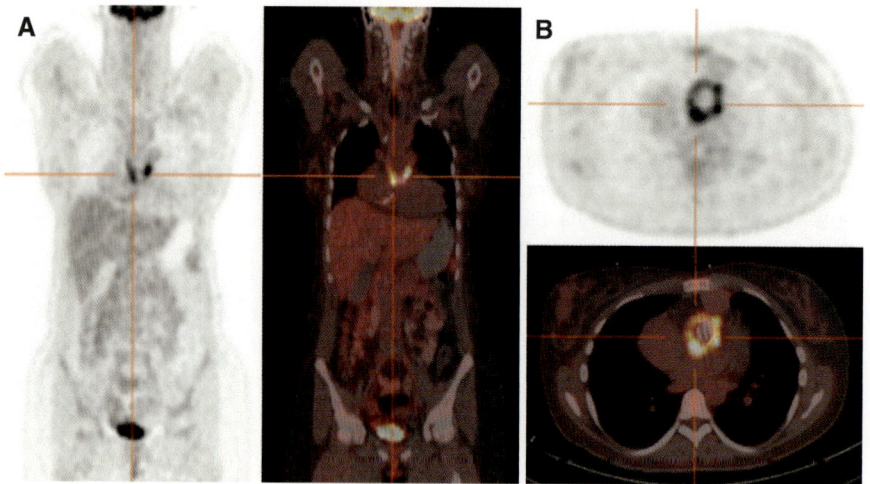

Fig. 17.2 (**a, b**) PET/CT images of a 40-year-old woman, born with pulmonic atresia and a VSD and history of pulmonary homograft implantation, tricuspid reconstruction and a Bentall-procedure after developing aortic dilation and associated aortic insufficiency later in life. She presented with fever, malaise and fatigue. Blood cultures were positive for *Staphylococcus aureus*. Both TTE and TEE did not demonstrate any findings indicative of IE. (**a**) Coronal images. (**b**) Transaxial images, both showing PET (**a**: *left*, **b**: *top*) and PET/CT fused images (**a**: *right*, **b**: *bottom*). The picture shows a focal area of increased FDG uptake at the site of the prosthetic aortic valve and in the wall of the aortic root, very suggestive of an infection

Site of Infection

In CHD-associated IE, the affected structure is more frequently right-sided than in IE in general. Although reports vary considerably regarding distribution of IE location, over one third of CHD-related cases are generally right-sided and about 50% are left-sided. The remainder are either located outside the heart (approximately 20%; e.g., at the site of a PDA, aortic coarctation, implanted conduits) involve both left- and right-sided structures, or are not classified with respect to location. As in general IE, left-sided disease generally involves the valves. Of the right heart structures, the tricuspid valve is the most commonly affected, followed by the pulmonary valve. In contrast to left-sided disease, mural RV structures are also frequently affected, generally the rim or closure patch of a VSD or the RV free wall opposite such a defect. The detail of available reports is insufficient to determine whether affected valves are native or prosthetic, or if differences herein exist between affected sites [4, 19, 25, 28].

Treatment

Treatment of IE in the setting of CHD follows the general principals of targeted antimicrobial therapy and indications for surgery, set out in detail in international guidelines [4, 47].

The rate of surgery during the active phase of CHD-associated IE varies from 10 to 60% across reports [19, 25, 26, 32]. The most frequently reported indications for early surgery are heart failure, (high estimated risk for) embolization, persistent fever, locally uncontrolled infection and removal of infected prosthetics [4, 47]. Development of IE on a conduit or shunt is usually not manageable with antibiotic treatment alone. Generally required surgical explantation of contaminated material is associated with high mortality (see section "Outcome" below) [20, 25, 34]. Elective surgery after completed antibiotic treatment is indicated in a proportion of patients, to repair or replace damaged valves, replace degenerated grafts or to treat congenital defects not diagnosed prior to IE occurrence. These late operations are generally safe [20, 25, 26].

Outcome

Overall mortality of CHD-associated IE is under 10%, which is lower than that reported for IE in patients with acquired heart disease [19, 20, 28]. This may be due to the higher proportion of right-sided IE, known to have a better prognosis [4]. Mortality rates in CHD-associated IE have decreased over the past decades, likely due to earlier and more effective surgical therapy for IE in the setting of CHD, along with general improvements in diagnosis and antimicrobial therapy [19, 32, 34]. Mortality differs between types of CHD, however, and is up to 50 % in those with complex defects. This is probably, at least in part, related to the presence of prosthetics and associated need for surgical intervention [4, 25]. Indeed, surgical mortality remains as high as 40 %, and is greatest in patients with prosthetic-valve IE [19, 20, 25]. Apart from involvement of prosthetic material and need for surgical intervention (indicative of more severe and uncontrolled IE), other factors associated with greater mortality are those also found in general IE: early infancy, nosocomial acquisition, infection by uncommon pathogens, large vegetation size (>20 mm) and the development of complications, particularly heart failure [25, 31, 32, 36]. The main causes of death are also similar to those in IE in general (heart failure, refractory infection, infectious or surgical complications) [19, 20, 26, 36].

Prevention

The focus of the most recent guidelines for the prevention of IE is on the highest risk patients, undergoing the highest risk procedures. The highest risk patients are those at greatest risk for either adverse IE outcome (North-American guidelines) or developing procedure-related IE (European guidelines) [3–5]. Both definitions selected the same CHD patients eligible for prophylaxis: those with valves replaced or repaired using prosthetics and those with cyanotic CHD, either unrepaired or repaired with residual defects or palliative shunts or conduits. After CHD repair with prosthetic material, prophylaxis is recommended for six months. In case of residual defects at the site of foreign material, prophylaxis is recommended beyond this period.

As the impact of bacteraemia resulting from daily activities and poor hygiene is an important determinant of IE risk, maintenance of optimal oral health and regular dental review are of great importance for prevention of IE. Awareness of IE risk and its association with daily oral and skin hygiene is often lacking in CHD patients, while greater awareness is associated with better maintenance of oral health and more frequent dental review. Thus, these issues should be profoundly addressed in education of patients and their caregivers [48, 49].

While the risk of IE is largely determined by the presence of high-velocity and turbulent blood flow patterns, the guidelines do not appreciate assessment of such haemodynamics in determining IE risk. Particularly concerning VSD and LVOT obstructions, this could leave patients at risk [13, 19, 21], which may be of concern to clinicians. Indeed, over a quarter of clinicians caring for CHD patients were found to feel that recent guidelines leave some patients at risk. However, up to 80 % were found to have discontinued prophylaxis for small unrepaired VSDs and native aortic valvar stenoses following publication of the 2007 AHA guidelines. Remarkably, rates of prophylaxis for scenarios that do warrant prophylaxis according to the guidelines decreased: prophylaxis in VSD patients during the first six months after patch closure or with a residual shunt was practiced in only 54 % and

69% (versus 75% and 100% before, respectively) [50]. Although it cannot be deduced whether it is due to unfamiliarity with guidelines, unclear recommendations, individual interpretation of literature or other reasons, this noncompliance does underline that adherence to guidelines could be improved.

Summary

CHD is an important substrate for IE, especially in younger patients, and the expanding population of paediatric and adult CHD patients contributes greatly to overall IE incidence. Simple lesions, such as ASD and isolated right-sided lesions carry a low IE risk. Lesions associated with high-velocity and turbulent blood flow, particularly complex CHD, LVOT obstructions and VSD are associated with high risk. Moreover, the implantation of prosthetic valves, conduits and shunts for repair or palliation is associated with high long-term risk, while risk is practically eliminated after complete repair without such prosthetics. Although right-sided infection is relatively more frequent, the clinical presentation and basis for diagnosis and treatment of CHD-associated IE do not differ from IE in general. However, especially in patients with complex CHD or prosthetics, sensitivity of echocardiography may be reduced and alternative modes of imaging may proof useful tools. Mortality is low (<10%) in CHD-associated IE, relative to mortality in IE in general, but it remains high in those with complex defects or prosthetics and in cases requiring surgery. While antibiotic prophylaxis is indicated in patients at highest risk, the importance of good oral and skin hygiene for the prevention of IE has to be emphasized. Education of patients and caregivers is vital in this respect, as awareness of risk is often lacking.

References

1. Moons P, Bovijn L, Budts W, Belmans A, Gewillig M. Temporal trends in survival to adulthood among patients born with congenital heart disease from 1970 to 1992 in Belgium. Circulation. 2010;122:2264–72.
2. van der Bom T, Zomer AC, Zwinderman AH, Meijboom FJ, Bouma BJ, Mulder BJM. The changing epidemiology of congenital heart disease. Nat Rev Cardiol. 2011;8:50–60.
3. Wilson W, Taubert KA, Gewitz M, Lockhart PB, Baddour LM, Levison M, Bolger A, Cabell CH, Takahashi M, Baltimore RS, Newburger JW, Strom BL, Tani LY, Gerber M, Bonow RO, Pallasch T, Shulman ST, Rowley AH, Burns JC, Ferrieri P, Gardner T, Goff D, Durack DT. Prevention of infective endocarditis guidelines from the American Heart Association: a guideline from the American Heart Association Rheumatic Fever, Endocarditis, and Kawasaki Disease Committee, Council on Cardiovascular Disease in the Young, and the Council on Clinical Cardiology, Council on Cardiovascular Surgery and Anesthesia, and the Quality of Care and Outcomes Research Interdisciplinary Working Group. Circulation. 2007;116:1736–54.
4. Habib G, Hoen B, Tornos P, Thuny F, Prendergast B, Vilacosta I, Moreillon P, de Jesus Antunes M, Thilen U, Lekakis J, Lengyel M, Müller L, Naber CK, Nihoyannopoulos P, Moritz A,

Zamorano JL, ESC Committee for Practice Guidelines. Guidelines on the prevention, diagnosis, and treatment of infective endocarditis (new version 2009): the task force on the prevention, diagnosis, and treatment of infective endocarditis of the European Society of Cardiology (ESC). Endorsed by the European Society of Clinical Microbiology and Infectious Diseases (ESCMID) and the International Society of Chemotherapy (ISC) for Infection and Cancer. Eur Heart J. 2009;30:2369–413.

5. Warnes CA, Williams RG, Bashore TM, Child JS, Connolly HM, Dearani JA, del Nido P, Fasules JW, Graham Jr TP, Hijazi ZM, Hunt SA, King ME, Landzberg MJ, Miner PD, Radford MJ, Walsh EP, Webb GD. ACC/AHA, 2008 guidelines for the management of adults with congenital heart disease: a report of the American College of Cardiology/American Heart Association Task Force on Practice Guidelines (Writing Committee to develop guidelines on the management of adults with congenital heart disease) developed in collaboration with the American Society of Echocardiography, Heart Rhythm Society, International Society for Adult Congenital Heart Disease, Society for Cardiovascular Angiography and Interventions, and Society of Thoracic Surgeons. J Am Coll Cardiol. 2008;52:e143–263.

6. Rushani D, Kaufman JS, Ionescu-Ittu R, Mackie AS, Pilote L, Therrien J, Marelli AJ. Infective endocarditis in children with congenital heart disease cumulative incidence and predictors. Circulation. 2013;128:1412–9.

7. Coward K, Tucker N, Darville T. Infective endocarditis in Arkansan children from 1990 through 2002. Pediatr Infect Dis J. 2003;22:1048–52.

8. Mylonakis E, Calderwood SB. Infective endocarditis in adults. N Engl J Med. 2001;345: 1318–30.

9. Verheugt CL, Uiterwaal CSPM, van der Velde ET, Meijboom FJ, Pieper PG, Veen G, Stappers JLM, Grobbee DE, Mulder BJM. Turning 18 with congenital heart disease: prediction of infective endocarditis based on a large population. Eur Heart J. 2011;32:1926–34.

10. Johnson JA, Boyce TG, Cetta F, Steckelberg JM, Johnson JN. Infective endocarditis in the pediatric patient: a 60-year single-institution review. Mayo Clin Proc. 2012;87:629–35.

11. Day MD, Gauvreau K, Shulman S, Newburger JW. Characteristics of children hospitalized with infective endocarditis. Circulation. 2009;119:865–70.

12. Ma XZ, Li XY, Que CL, Lv Y. Underlying heart disease and microbiological spectrum of adult infective endocarditis in one Chinese university hospital: a 10-year retrospective study. Intern Med J. 2013;43:1303–9.

13. Morris CD, Reller MD, Menashe VD. Thirty-year incidence of infective endocarditis after surgery for congenital heart defect. JAMA. 1998;279:599–603.

14. Inglessis I, Elmariah S, Rengifo-Moreno PA, Margey R, O'Callaghan C, Cruz-Gonzalez I, Baron S, Mehrotra P, Tan TC, Hung J, Demirjian ZN, Buonanno FS, Ning M, Silverman SB, Cubeddu RJ, Pomerantsev E, Schainfeld RM, Dec GW, Palacios IF. Long-term experience and outcomes with transcatheter closure of patent foramen ovale. JACC Cardiovasc Interv. 2013;6:1176–83.

15. Kreutzer J, Ryan CA, Gauvreau K, Van Praagh R, Anderson JM, Jenkins KJ. Healing response to the clamshell device for closure of intracardiac defects in humans. Catheter Cardiovasc Interv. 2001;54:101–11.

16. Slesnick TC, Nugent AW, Fraser CD, Cannon BC. Incomplete endothelialization and late development of acute bacterial endocarditis after implantation of an Amplatzer septal occluder device. Circulation. 2008;117:e326–7.

17. Malekzadeh-Milani S, Ladouceur M, Iserin L, Bonnet D, Boudjemline Y. Incidence and outcomes of right-sided endocarditis in patients with congenital heart disease after surgical or transcatheter pulmonary valve implantation. J Thorac Cardiovasc Surg. 2014;148:2253–9.

18. Li W, Somerville J. Infective endocarditis in the grown-up congenital heart (GUCH) population. Eur Heart J. 1998;19:166–73.

19. Filippo SD, Delahaye F, Semiond B, Celard M, Henaine R, Ninet J, Sassolas F, Bozio A. Current patterns of infective endocarditis in congenital heart disease. Heart. 2006;92:1490–5.

20. Niwa K, Nakazawa M, Tateno S, Yoshinaga M, Terai M. Infective endocarditis in congenital heart disease: Japanese national collaboration study. Heart. 2005;91:795–800.
21. Gersony WM, Hayes CJ, Driscoll DJ, Keane JF, Kidd L, O'Fallon WM, Pieroni DR, Wolfe RR, Weidman WH. Bacterial endocarditis in patients with aortic stenosis, pulmonary stenosis, or ventricular septal defect. Circulation. 1993;87:I121–6.
22. Siu SC, Silversides CK. Bicuspid aortic valve disease. J Am Coll Cardiol. 2010;55: 2789–800.
23. Ward C. Clinical significance of the bicuspid aortic valve. Heart. 2000;83:81–5.
24. Tzemos N, Therrien J, Yip J, et al. Outcomes in adults with bicuspid aortic valves. JAMA. 2008;300:1317–25.
25. Fortún J, Centella T, Martín-Dávila P, Lamas MJ, Pérez-Caballero C, Fernández-Pineda L, Otheo E, Cobo J, Navas E, Pintado V, Loza E, Moreno S. Infective endocarditis in congenital heart disease: a frequent community-acquired complication. Infection. 2013;41:167–74.
26. Knirsch W, Haas NA, Uhlemann F, Dietz K, Lange PE. Clinical course and complications of infective endocarditis in patients growing up with congenital heart disease. Int J Cardiol. 2005; 101:285–91.
27. Ashkenazi S, Levy O, Blieden L. Trends of childhood infective endocarditis in Israel with emphasis on children under 2 years of age. Pediatr Cardiol. 1997;18:419–24.
28. Knirsch W, Nadal D. Infective endocarditis in congenital heart disease. Eur J Pediatr. 2011; 170:1111–27.
29. Fowler VG, Miro JM, Hoen B, Cabell CH, Abrutyn E, Rubinstein E, Corey GR, Spelman D, Bradley SF, Barsic B, Pappas PA, Anstrom KJ, Wray D, Fortes CQ, Anguera I, Athan E, Jones P, van der Meer JTM, Elliott TSJ, Levine DP, Bayer AS, ICE Investigators. Staphylococcus aureus endocarditis: a consequence of medical progress. JAMA. 2005;293:3012–21.
30. Baddour LM, Bettmann MA, Bolger AF, Epstein AE, Ferrieri P, Gerber MA, Gewitz MH, Jacobs AK, Levison ME, Newburger JW, Pallasch TJ, Wilson WR, Baltimore RS, Falace DA, Shulman ST, Tani LY, Taubert KA. Nonvalvular cardiovascular device–related infections. Circulation. 2003;108:2015–31.
31. Ishiwada N, Niwa K, Tateno S, Yoshinaga M, Terai M, Nakazawa M, Cardiology for TJS of P, Cardiac Surgery Joint Working Groups for Guidelines for Prophylaxis D, Disease M of IE in PWCH. Causative organism influences clinical profile and outcome of infective endocarditis in pediatric patients and adults with congenital heart disease. Circ J. 2005;69: 1266–70.
32. Yoshinaga M, Niwa K, Niwa A, Ishiwada N, Takahashi H, Echigo S, Nakazawa M. Risk factors for in-hospital mortality during infective endocarditis in patients with congenital heart disease. Am J Cardiol. 2008;101:114–8.
33. Steelman R, Einzig S, Balian A, Thomas J, Rosen D, Gustafson R, Gochenour L. Increased susceptibility to gingival colonization by specific HACEK microbes in children with congenital heart disease. J Clin Pediatr Dent. 2001;25:91–4.
34. Ferrieri P, Gewitz MH, Gerber MA, Newburger JW, Dajani AS, Shulman ST, Wilson W, Bolger AF, Bayer A, Levison ME, Pallasch TJ, Gage TW, Taubert KA. Unique features of infective endocarditis in childhood. Circulation. 2002;105:2115–26.
35. Thuny F, Disalvo G, Belliard O, Avierinos J-F, Pergola V, Rosenberg V, Casalta J-P, Gouvernet J, Derumeaux G, Iarussi D, Ambrosi P, Calabro R, Riberi A, Collart F, Metras D, Lepidi H, Raoult D, Harle J-R, Weiller P-J, Cohen A, Habib G. Risk of embolism and death in infective endocarditis: prognostic value of echocardiography a prospective multicenter study. Circulation. 2005;112:69–75.
36. Awadallah SM, Kavey R-EW, Byrum CJ, Smith FC, Kveselis DA, Blackman MS. The changing pattern of infective endocarditis in childhood. Am J Cardiol. 1991;68:90–4.
37. Graupner C, Vilacosta I, SanRomán J, Ronderos R, Sarriá C, Fernández C, Mújica R, Sanz O, Sanmartín JV, Pinto AG. Periannular extension of infective endocarditis. J Am Coll Cardiol. 2002;39:1204–11.

38. Daniel WG, Mügge A, Martin RP, Lindert O, Hausmann D, Nonnast-Daniel B, Laas J, Lichtlen PR. Improvement in the diagnosis of abscesses associated with endocarditis by transesophageal echocardiography. N Engl J Med. 1991;324:795–800.
39. Kahveci G, Bayrak F, Pala S, Mutlu B. Impact of bicuspid aortic valve on complications and death in infective endocarditis of native aortic valves. Tex Heart Inst J. 2009;36:111–6.
40. Bayer AS, Bolger AF, Taubert KA, Wilson W, Steckelberg J, Karchmer AW, Levison M, Chambers HF, Dajani AS, Gewitz MH, Newburger JW, Gerber MA, Shulman ST, Pallasch TJ, Gage TW, Ferrieri P. Diagnosis and management of infective endocarditis and its complications. Circulation. 1998;98:2936–48.
41. Durack DT, Lukes AS, Bright DK. New criteria for diagnosis of infective endocarditis: utilization of specific echocardiographic findings. Duke endocarditis service. Am J Med. 1994; 96:200–9.
42. Lamas CC, Eykyn SJ. Blood culture negative endocarditis: analysis of 63 cases presenting over 25 years. Heart. 2003;89:258–62.
43. Li JS, Sexton DJ, Mick N, Nettles R, Fowler VG, Ryan T, Bashore T, Corey GR. Proposed modifications to the Duke criteria for the diagnosis of infective endocarditis. Clin Infect Dis. 2000;30:633–8.
44. Brouqui P, Raoult D. New insight into the diagnosis of fastidious bacterial endocarditis. FEMS Immunol Med Microbiol. 2006;47:1–13.
45. Flachskampf FA, Wouters PF, Edvardsen T, Evangelista A, Habib G, Hoffman P, Hoffmann R, Lancellotti P, Pepi M. Recommendations for transoesophageal echocardiography: EACVI update 2014. Eur Heart J Cardiovasc Imaging. 2014;15:353–65.
46. Bartoletti M, Tumietto F, Fasulo G, Giannella M, Cristini F, Bonfiglioli R, Raumer L, Nanni C, Sanfilippo S, Di Eusanio M, Scotton PG, Graziosi M, Rapezzi C, Fanti S, Viale P. Combined computed tomography and fluorodeoxyglucose positron emission tomography in the diagnosis of prosthetic valve endocarditis: a case series. BMC Res Notes. 2014;7:32.
47. Baddour LM, Wilson WR, Bayer AS, Fowler VG, Bolger AF, Levison ME, Ferrieri P, Gerber MA, Tani LY, Gewitz MH, Tong DC, Steckelberg JM, Baltimore RS, Shulman ST, Burns JC, Falace DA, Newburger JW, Pallasch TJ, Takahashi M, Taubert KA. Infective endocarditis diagnosis, antimicrobial therapy, and management of complications: a statement for healthcare professionals from the Committee on Rheumatic Fever, Endocarditis, and Kawasaki Disease, Council on Cardiovascular Disease in the Young, and the Councils on Clinical Cardiology, Stroke, and Cardiovascular Surgery and Anesthesia, American Heart Association: Endorsed by the Infectious Diseases Society of America. Circulation. 2005;111:e394–434.
48. Barreira JL, Baptista MJ, Moreira J, Azevedo A, Areias JC. Understanding of endocarditis risk improves compliance with prophylaxis. Rev Port Cardiol Orgão Of Soc Port Cardiol Port J Cardiol Off J Port Soc Cardiol. 2002;21:939–51.
49. Moons P, De Volder E, Budts W, De Geest S, Elen J, Waeytens K, Gewillig M. What do adult patients with congenital heart disease know about their disease, treatment, and prevention of complications? A call for structured patient education. Heart. 2001;86:74–80.
50. Pharis CS, Conway J, Warren AE, Bullock A, Mackie AS. The impact of 2007 infective endocarditis prophylaxis guidelines on the practice of congenital heart disease specialists. Am Heart J. 2011;161:123–9.

Chapter 18
Blood Culture-Negative Endocarditis

Pierre-Edouard Fournier, George Watt, Paul N. Newton, Cristiane C. Lamas,
Pierre Tattevin, and Didier Raoult

Introduction

Infective endocarditis (IE) is a severe disease whose incidence has increased over
time despite different prevention strategies and a changing epidemiology, with an
increase in *Staphylococcus aureus* IE and in IE occurring in intravenous drug users,
in older patients, and in those with nosocomial bacteremias or intracardiac devices
[1, 2]. Heart surgery is required in 25–50 % of cases [3], and mortality remains high,

P.-E. Fournier, MD, PhD (✉)
Microbiology Laboratory, Institut Hospitalo-Universitaire Méditerranée-Infection, Hospital
La Timone, Marseille, France
e-mail: Pierre-edouard.fournier@univ-amu.fr

G. Watt, MD, PhD
Department of Internal Medicine, John A. Burns School of Medicine, University of Hawaii at
Manoa, Honolulu, HI, USA
e-mail: gwattth@yahoo.com

P.N. Newton, BM, BCh, DPhil, MRCP, DTM&H
Microbiology Laboratory, Mahosot Hospital, Vientiane, Laos
e-mail: Paul.newton@tropmedres.ac

C.C. Lamas, MD, PhD, MRCP
Department of Valvular Heart Disease, Instituto Nacional de Cardiologia,
Rio de Janeiro, Brazil
e-mail: cristianelamas@gmail.com

P. Tattevin, MD, PhD
Intensive Care Unit and Department of Infectious Diseases, Pontchaillou University Hospital,
Rennes, France
e-mail: Pierre.tattevin@chu-rennes.fr

D. Raoult
Unité de Recherche sur les Maladies Infectieuses et Tropicales Emergentes, UMR CNRS
7278, IRD 198, Institut National de la Santé et de la Recherche Médicale (INSERM) 1095,
Faculté de Médecine, Aix-Marseille Université, Marseille, France
e-mail: Didier.raoult@gmail.com

© Springer International Publishing Switzerland 2016
G. Habib (ed.), *Infective Endocarditis*, DOI 10.1007/978-3-319-32432-6_18

with more than 30 % of patients dying within a year of diagnosis [3, 4]. In 5–69.7 % of cases, depending on the case series, blood cultures (i.e., ≥ three aerobic and anaerobic blood cultures collected over 48 h), the first line microbiological tool for the diagnosis of IE, remain negative, despite more than 1 week of incubation [5]. The importance attributed to culture in the diagnosis of IE is demonstrated by its weight in the Duke criteria [6]. In most cases, the negativity of blood cultures is explained by the empirical administration of antibiotics prior to blood cultures. Fastidious microorganisms are the second cause of BCNE and account for ~5 % of all IE. These include microorganisms that require prolonged incubation and/or specific media, including *Brucella* sp., defective streptococci (*Abiotrophia* sp., *Gemella* sp., *Granulicatella* sp.), *Finegoldia magna*, HACEK bacteria (*Haemophilus* sp., *Actinobacillus* sp., *Cardiobacterium* sp., *Eikenella* sp., *Kingella* sp.), *Legionella* sp., *Listeria* sp., mycobacteria, *Mycoplasma* sp., *Propionibacterium acnes,* and fungi (*Candida* sp., *Aspergillus* sp.), as well as strictly (*Coxiella burnetii, Tropheryma whipplei*) or facultative (*Bartonella* sp.) intracellular bacteria [7]. In addition to IE, endocarditis can also occur as a complication of non-infective diseases such as auto-immune diseases (rheumatoid arthritis, systemic lupus erythematosus), neoplasia (marantic endocarditis) [7, 8], Loeffler's endocarditis and allergic phenomena [8].

Due to the delayed diagnosis, in-hospital complications are more frequent [9–11]. To reduce the diagnostic delay and improve the prognosis, patients should ideally be managed by a multi-disciplinary team involving specialists in cardiology, cardiac imaging, infectious diseases and microbiology [12, 13].

Epidemiology of Blood Culture-Negative IE Worldwide

The incidence of BCNE, as well as that of its causative agents, varies greatly according to countries [7, 10, 14–21]. Globally, the incidence of BCNE follows a North-to-South increase [22]. In Europe, the incidence of BCNE has been reported to be 9 % in France [23], 13 % in the United Kingdom [19], 14 % in Spain [21], 20 % in Japan [20], 24 % in Sweden [24] and 25 % in Italy [25]. By comparison, BCNE accounted for 23 % in Brazil [26], 31 % in India [27], 48 % in Pakistan [17], 50 % in Turkey [28], 54 % in Tunisia [29], 55 % in South Africa [16], 56 % in Algeria [15], 58 % in Morocco [30], 61 % in the Lao PDR [31], 69 % in Thailand [32] and 69.7 % In Egypt [33].

In addition to differences in frequency of BCNE according to countries, differences are also observed in the distribution of identified causative agents of BCNE, notably that of zoonotic microorganisms (in particular *Coxiella burnetii*, *Bartonella* sp. and *Brucella* sp.) [34]. However, these differences may also reflect differences in antibiotic use or study design (microbiological techniques used or studied populations), as shown in the following studies. The proportion of BCNE cases caused by zoonotic agents was 0 in South Africa [16], 6.7 % in the Lao PDR (two cases of *B. henselae* IE) [35], 12.5 % in Italy (3 cases of brucellosis) [36], 9 % in Turkey

(*Brucella* sp. only but neither Q fever nor *Bartonella* sp. were investigated) [28], 10.3 % in Brazil (2 *Bartonella* and 1 *C. burnetii* IE) [37], 11.9 % in Egypt (Q fever, *Bartonella* sp. and *Brucella* sp.) [33], 13 % in southern France (Q fever and *Bartonella* sp. but no *Brucella* sp.) [7], 17 % in Thailand (Q fever, *Bartonella* sp., *Streptococcus suis*, *Erysipelothrix rusiopathiae*, *Campylobacter fetus*) [32], 20 % in the UK (mainly Q fever and *Bartonella* sp. but broad range PCR from valves was not performed) [19].

Main Etiologies of Blood-Culture Negative IE

Infectious Etiologies

Antibiotic administration prior to blood sampling remains the most common cause of BCNE (especially when caused by staphylococci or streptococci). However, as detailed above, a substantial number of cases are caused by intracellular bacteria, including *Coxiella burnetii*, the agent of Q fever, *Bartonella* sp., *Brucella* sp., *Legionella* sp., *Mycoplasma* sp., *Tropheryma whipplei*, the agent of Whipple's disease, other fastidious bacteria such as *Abiotrophia* sp. and *Propionibacterium acnes*, or fungi (mainly *Candida* sp. and *Aspergillus* sp.) [7]. Table 18.1 lists the main risk factors for BCNE caused by fastidious microorganisms.

Table 18.1   Risk factors for BCNE caused by fastidious microorganisms

Pathogen	Risk factors
Aspergillus sp.	Contamination through aerosols in patients with intracardiac devices or prostheses, and/or immunodeficiency
Bartonella sp.	Contact with kittens (*B. henselae*), contact with human body lice (*B. quintana*)
Brucella sp.	Contact with, or occupational exposure to farm animals, especially cattle, sheep and goats, through direct contact or ingestion of unpasteurized and contaminated milk products or insufficiently cooked meat
Candida sp.	Intravenous drug users, parenteral nutrition, multiple complex digestive surgeries, active cancer, and prolonged broad-spectrum antibiotic treatment
Coxiella burnetii	Contamination through aerosols of placental or parturient fluids from infected mammals (sheep, goats), or ingestion of contaminated raw milk products. May be an occupational disease in workers exposed to farm animals
Legionella sp.	Infection through inhalation of aerosols of infected water. Mainly in patients with prosthetic valves
Mycoplasma sp.	Mostly *M. hominis*, within a year following valvular surgery. Suspected nosocomial transmission
Tropheryma whipplei	Males with as yet undetermined specific immunodeficiency, inter-human transmission

Non-infectious Etiologies

Although endocarditis mostly results from infectious causes, this disease may also complicate non-infectious diseases such as autoimmune diseases and neoplasia [7, 8]. The most common form of autoimmune endocarditis is Libman-Sacks endocarditis. This manifestation of systemic lupus erythematous is observed in young adults with a severe lupus and the valvular lesions are mostly mitral [38]. It is associated with primary or secondary antiphospholipid syndrome [39], as antiphospholipid antibodies, notably the anticardiolipin and lupus anticoagulant, favour the formation of non-bacterial thrombotic vegetations. Endocarditis has also been described in other autoimmune conditions such as rheumatoid arthritis or Behçet's disease. In the latter condition, endocarditis, in most cases aortic, is rare but has a poor prognosis [40]. In addition, during rheumatic fever, antibody cross-reactivity following *Streptococcus pyogenes* infection results in damage to endocardium, myocardium and pericardium.

Neoplasia, especially involving lung, pancreas, and colon, can be complicated by the development of thrombotic sterile vegetations (marantic endocarditis) due to hypercoagulable states and, sometimes, with antiphospholipid antibodies. Marantic endocarditis mostly involves the mitral and aortic valves.

Loeffler's endocarditis is a form of restrictive cardiomyopathy with eosinophilic proliferation in endocardial and myocardial tissue, which may be caused by parasites, drug reaction, eosinophilic leukemia or lymphomas. Finally, foreign material rejection or allergic phenomena may be a cause of non-infectious endocarditis in patients with porcine bioprosthetic valves [8].

Diagnostic Strategy

The diagnosis of IE usually relies on the association of an infectious syndrome and evidence of recent endocardial involvement, which is the basis of the various scores developed to date. Currently, the most widely used diagnostic criteria are the Duke University criteria that were notably amended to include Q fever serology as a new major criterion [6, 41]. However, the sensitivity of these modified criteria is limited, especially in the early stages of the disease, in cases of negative blood culture and in the presence of prosthetic valve or pacemaker/defibrillator leads. Therefore, other scoring systems, in particular using a combination of non-specific clinical signs and biological results, have been proposed to improve the early diagnosis of IE [19, 42].

In addition, special attention should be paid to the medical history of the patient that may point towards a specific diagnosis. In particular, the following epidemio-clinical clues may facilitate the diagnosis. *Bartonella quintana* should be suspected in homeless, alcoholic and/or patients coming from Maghreb; *Tropheryma whipplei* in patients >50 y-o with chronic arthralgias; *Coxiella burnetii* in patients >40 y-o with bicuspid aortic valve; *Brucella* sp. in patients coming from South America and

Turkey; allergy to pork in patients with a relapsing BCNE and a porcine bioprosthesis; lupus erythematosus in young women; rheumatoid arthritis in older women with
arthralgias; marantic endocarditis in patients >40 y-o with embolic phenomena.

However, despite the progresses made in identifying the agents of BCNE permitted by the use of improved scoring systems, the increased use of cardiac surgery in
the acute phase of endocarditis and the diversification of the diagnostic techniques
used, such as polymerase chain reaction (PCR) techniques, immunohistochemistry,
systematic serologies, magnetic resonance imaging and molecular imaging, the
ratio of BCNE without any etiological diagnosis remains elevated [3].

Nevertheless, the precise microbiological diagnosis being mandatory in order to
guide therapy and improve patient management, the timing and type of tests may be
standardized in a diagnostic kit designed to contain all vials and tubes required for
blood culture, serological screening of the most common agents of BCNE, PCR
from blood, and detection of auto-antibodies or anti-pork IgE (Table 18.1) [5, 8].

See Fig. 18.1 for an algorithm for a polyphasic diagnostic strategy for the identification of the causative agents of blood culture-negative endocarditis.

Blood Cultures

Significant improvements have been made in blood culture over the past decades
[43], notably permitted by enhanced automated systems (that enable cultivating
most pathogens including *Candida* sp., deficient streptococci and HACEK group
bacteria) [44]. These include the recommendations that three sets of blood cultures
consisting of ≥10 mL of blood per vial should be collected prior to antibiotic administration [45] and that extended incubation of vials should only be performed when
cultures remain sterile after 48–72 h [46].

Serology

In cases of BCNE caused by fastidious organisms, the diagnosis may be obtained by
serology for *C. burnetii*, *Bartonella* sp., *Brucella melitensis*, *Legionella pneumophila*, and *Aspergillus* sp. [7]. The former two agents being the most common worldwide [7], these assays should be prioritized. An IgG titer to phase I >1:800 was
demonstrated to have a 98 % positive predictive value (PPV) for Q fever endocarditis and this value is currently considered as a major Duke criterion [6, 47]. Similarly,
an IgG titer >1:800 to *Bartonella henselae* or *B. quintana* has a PPV >95 % for
endocarditis caused by these microorganisms [48]. Assays for the other agents
should be used according to the local epidemiology (see above). Regarding IE
caused by *Mycoplasma* species, less than ten cases have been published to date, all
but one caused by *M. hominis*, and none of which have been diagnosed by serology
[49]. The usefulness of testing patients for antibodies to *Chlamydia* species appears

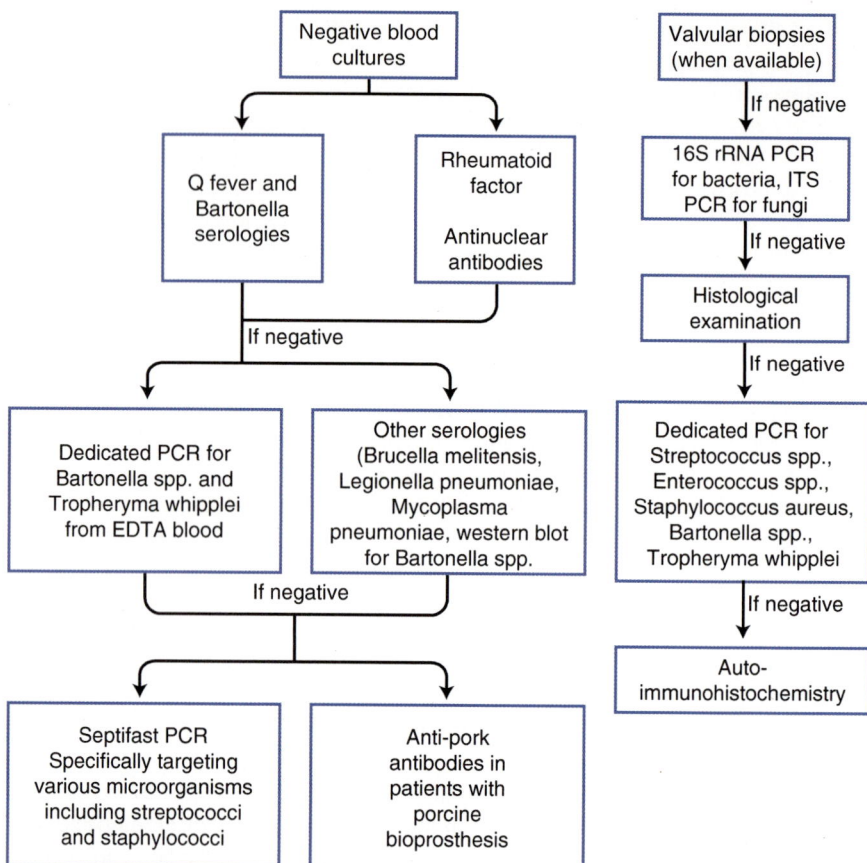

Fig. 18.1 Polyphasic diagnostic strategy for the identification of the causative agents of blood culture-negative endocarditis

even more limited. Indeed, due to serological cross-reactivity between *Chlamydia* and *Bartonella* species, most published cases of serologically-diagnosed *Chlamydia* IE were probably *Bartonella* infections [7]. Therefore, serology assays for these microorganisms do not appear to be useful.

The role of mannan:anti-mannan antibodies and (1,3)-β-d-glucans in the diagnosis of *Candida* sp. endocarditis seems promising but remains to be defined [50].

Table 18.2 lists diagnostic assays available for fastidious microorganisms [49].

Valve Culture

When valvular surgery is necessary, it is essential to obtain valve samples for histology, culture, and molecular detection assays. Valvular biopsies may remain culture-positive longer than blood in the case of early antibiotic therapy.

Table 18.2 Diagnostic procedures for BCNE caused by fastidious microorganisms

Pathogen	Diagnostic procedure
Aspergillus sp.	Serum galactomannan, 1,3 β-D glucan
	Culture, immunohistology and PCR from valvular biopsies
Bartonella sp.	Blood cultures
	Serology: IgG ≥1:800 or positive western blot
	Culture, immunohistology and PCR from valvular biopsies
Brucella sp.	Blood cultures
	Serology
	Culture, immunohistology and PCR from valvular biopsies
Candida sp.	Serum 1,3 β-D glucan
	Culture, immunohistology and PCR from valvular biopsies
Coxiella burnetii (agent of Q fever)	Serology: IgG to phase I>1:800
	Tissue culture, immunohistology and PCR from valvular biopsies or blood
Legionella sp.	Blood cultures
	Serology
	Urinary antigen
	Culture, immunohistology and PCR from valvular biopsies
Mycoplasma sp.	Culture, immunohistology and PCR from valvular biopsies
Tropheryma whipplei (agent of Whipple's disease)	Histology and PCR from valvular biopsies

Polymerase Chain Reactions

Polymerase chain reaction (PCR) and sequencing, especially when targeting broad range genomic targets such as 16S rRNA for bacteria or ITS for fungi, may enable the identification of any bacterium or fungi, respectively [51]. Such systems have demonstrated excellent sensitivity and specificity [52, 53]. In cases when a specific microorganism is suspected, dedicated real-time PCR (RT-PCR) assays may be used [37, 54]. Alternatively, multiplexed RT-PCR assays such as the LightCycler SeptiFast system that enables detection of 25 bacteria or fungi may be used when all other assays are negative [55]. It should be reminded that a positive PCR from a valvular specimen may not systematically be synonym of infection, as bacterial DNA, notably from streptococci or enterococci, may persist for months to years in cardiac valves following an efficiently treated IE episode [56]. PCR may also be performed from EDTA blood, although its sensitivity is lower compared to amplification form valvular biopsies [7, 57].

Histology

A number of special stains may help guide the etiologic diagnosis. As examples, the periodic acid–Schiff (PAS), Giemsa and Warthin–Starry, Ziehl-Neelsen and Gimenez stains enable detecting *T. whipplei*, *Bartonella* sp., *mycobacteria* and *C. burnetii* or *Legionella* sp., respectively. When histologic lesions are consistent with IE but other assays are negative, auto-immunohistochemistry using the patient's serum may detect otherwise unidentified bacteria [58].

Other Laboratory Assays

Antinuclear and antiphospholipid antibodies and rheumatoid factor may be searched in patients with a history of chronic athro-myalgias [7]. In patients with porcine valvular bioprosthesis who develop relapsing IE without any identified causative microorganism, the presence of anti-pork antibodies should be investigated [8].

PET-CT

Positron emission tomography-computed tomography (PET-CT) exhibiting a higher sensitivity than CT alone for the detection and evaluation of infections, it was demonstrated to be a valuable tool for the diagnosis of IE [59]. Saby et al. even proposed that PET-CT might be considered as a major diagnostic criterion [60]. It may especially be useful in pauci-symptomatic patients, as may be the case in *Bartonella* or *T. whipplei* infections [61, 62], or in suspected marantic endocarditis when it may detect the primitive tumor [63].

Treatment

Empirical Treatment

The empirical treatment of BCNE is similar to that of culture positive IE. The most common causative agents of IE (staphylococci, streptococci, and enterococci) being also common agents of BCNE, an antibiotic therapy active on these agents should be administered immediately after blood cultures. The European or American guidelines recommend an association of amoxicillin-clavulanic acid (or amoxicillin-sulbactam)+gentamicin for native valve IE, vancomycin+gentamicin+rifampin in patients with a valve prosthesis implanted in the past year, or oxacillin or (flu)cloxacillin+gentamicin in intravenous drug users [43, 64].

Specific Treatments

As in cases of blood culture-positive IE, the antibiotic therapy should systematically be tailored to the identified agent. This is especially important for fastidious microorganisms, many of which are not susceptible to the empirical therapy (Table 18.3).

Table 18.3 Treatment of BCNE caused by fastidious microorganisms

Pathogen	Proposed therapy	References
Aspergillus sp.[a]	Voriconazole i.v. (12 mg/day for 24 h, then 8 mg/kg/day) or liposomal amphotericin B i.v. (3–5 mg/kg/day) for ≥12 weeks (valvular surgery is mandatory for cure)	[78]
Bartonella sp.[a]	Ceftriaxone (2 g/day) or ampicillin (or amoxicillin, 12 g/day) i.v. or doxycycline (200 mg/day) p.o. for 6 weeks + gentamicin (3 mg/kg/day) i.v. for 2–3 weeks	[68]
Brucella sp.	Doxycycline (200 mg/day) + cotrimoxazole (960 × 2/day) + rifampin (300–600 mg/day) p.o. for ≥3 months	[79]
Candida sp.[a]	Echinocandin or liposomal amphotericin B i.v. (3–5 mg/kg/day) +/− 5-fluorocytosine (200–600 mg/kg/day). Lifelong fluconazole when surgery is contraindicated	[50]
Coxiella burnetii (agent of Q fever)	Doxycycline (200 mg/day, to be adapted to serum level) + hydroxychloroquine (200–600 mg/day, to be adapted to serum level) p.o. or doxycycline (200 mg/day, to be adapted to serum level) + plus ofloxacin (400 mg/day) p.o. for ≥18 months	[65]
Legionella sp.[b]	Erythromycin (3 g/day) i.v. for 2 weeks, then p.o. for 4 weeks + rifampin (300–1200 mg/day) or ciprofloxacin (1.5 g/day) p.o. for 6 weeks or levofloxacin (1.5 g/day) i.v. for 2 weeks, then p.o. for 4 weeks	[49]
Mycoplasma sp.	Doxycycline (200 mg/day) for 6 weeks	[70–73]
Tropheryma whipplei (agent of Whipple's disease)	Doxycycline (200 mg/day, to be adapted to serum level) + hydroxychloroquine (200–600 mg/day, to be adapted to serum level) p.o. for ≥18 months	[54]

i.v. intravenous, *p.o.* per os
[a]Valvular surgery is often required
[b]Newer fluoroquinolones are more potent than ciprofloxacin against *Legionella* sp.

IE due to *C. burnetii* should be treated with a combination of oral doxycycline and hydroxychloroquine for a minimum of 18 months [65]. Hydroxychloroquine increases the phagolysosome pH (from 4.7 to 5.8) and improves tetracycline-induced bacterial killing. The plasma levels of both drugs should be monitored throughout the treatment (objective: 0.8–1.2 mg/L for hydroxychloroquine, and ≥5 mg/L for doxycycline). It should be noted that the same therapy, prescribed for 1 year, was demonstrated to efficiently prevent the development of endocarditis in patients with a valvular defect who develop acute Q fever [66, 67].

IE due to *Bartonella* sp. should be treated with a combination of a β-lactam (amoxicillin, ceftriaxone) and an aminoglycosides (gentamicin) for at least 2 weeks, and then the β-lactam alone for an additional 4 weeks [68]. Up to 90 % of patients may undergo surgical valve replacement.

IE due to *T. whipplei* should be treated with a combination of oral doxycycline and hydroxychloroquine for 18 months [54]. The rationale for using this combined therapy and for monitoring plasma levels of both drugs is similar to that for *C. burnetii* endocarditis. Trimethoprim-sulfamethoxazole, once considered as the reference antibiotic for Whipple's disease, should no longer be used as *T. whipplei* is naturally resistant to trimethoprim, and the bacterium develops resistance to sulfamethoxazole during treatment, resulting in relapses [69]. Surgical valve replacement may be required for successful therapy.

The European guidelines for the management of IE recommend the use of newer fluoroquinolones for 6 months as antibiotic regiment for *Mycoplasma* endocarditis [43]. However, among the published cases of *Mycoplasma* endocarditis, the three patients treated with doxycycline recovered [70–73] *vs* only one of four patients who received other antibiotics [74–77]. Therefore, doxycycline, rather than fluoroquinolones, should be used for these infections.

Conclusion

Blood culture-negative endocarditis is a severe disease that remains a diagnostic challenge. As several fastidious agents of endocarditis require a specific antibiotic therapy, diagnostic assays should be diversified and adapted to local epidemiology and to the patient's medical and exposure history.

Disclosure P. Tattevin was supported financially by Abbott Laboratories, Astellas, AstraZeneca, Aventis, Bristol-Myers Squibb, Galderma, Gilead Sciences, Janssen-Cilag, MSD, Novartis, Pfizer, and the medicines company ViiV- Healthcare for research, for the organization of scientific meetings, trainings, and/or to attend national and international conferences.

C. Lamas was supported by Novartis Laboratories to attend national and international conferences.

References

1. Martin JM, Neches WH, Wald ER. Infective endocarditis: 35 years of experience at a children's hospital. Clin Infect Dis. 1997;24:669–75.
2. Sandre RM, Shafran SD. Infective endocarditis: review of 135 cases over 9 years. Clin Infect Dis. 1996;22:276–86.
3. Murdoch DR, Corey GR, Hoen B, Miro JM, Fowler Jr VG, Bayer AS, et al. Clinical presentation, etiology, and outcome of infective endocarditis in the 21st century: the International Collaboration on Endocarditis-Prospective Cohort Study. Arch Intern Med. 2009;169(5):463–73.
4. Moreillon P, Que YA. Infective endocarditis. Lancet. 2004;363(9403):139–49.
5. Raoult D, Casalta JP, Richet H, Khan M, Bernit E, Rovery C, et al. Contribution of systematic serological testing in diagnosis of infective endocarditis. J Clin Microbiol. 2005;43 (10):5238–42.
6. Li JS, Sexton DJ, Mick N, Nettles R, Fowler VGJ, Ryan T, et al. Proposed modifications to the duke criteria for the diagnosis of infective endocarditis. Clin Infect Dis. 2000;30:633–8.
7. Fournier PE, Thuny F, Richet H, Lepidi H, Casalta JP, Arzouni JP, et al. Comprehensive diagnostic strategy for blood culture-negative endocarditis: a prospective study of 819 new cases. Clin Infect Dis. 2010;51(2):131–40.
8. Fournier PE, Thuny F, Grisoli D, Lepidi H, Vitte J, Casalta JP, et al. A deadly aversion to pork. Lancet. 2011;377(9776):1542.
9. Murashita T, Sugiki H, Kamikubo Y, Yasuda K. Surgical results for active endocarditis with prosthetic valve replacement: impact of culture-negative endocarditis on early and late outcomes. Eur J Cardiothorac Surg. 2004;26(6):1104–11.

10. Zamorano J, Sanz J, Almeria C, Rodrigo JL, Samedi M, Herrera D, et al. Differences between endocarditis with true negative blood cultures and those with previous antibiotic treatment. J Heart Valve Dis. 2003;12(2):256–60.
11. Zamorano J, Sanz J, Moreno R, Almeria C, Rodrigo JL, Samedi M, et al. Comparison of outcome in patients with culture-negative versus culture-positive active infective endocarditis. Am J Cardiol. 2001;87(12):1423–5.
12. Chambers J, Sandoe J, Ray S, Prendergast B, Taggart D, Westaby S, et al. The infective endocarditis team: recommendations from an international working group. Heart. 2014;100(7):524–7.
13. Botelho-Nevers E, Thuny F, Casalta JP, Richet H, Gouriet F, Collart F, et al. Dramatic reduction in infective endocarditis-related mortality with a management-based approach. Arch Intern Med. 2009;169(14):1290–8.
14. Werner M, Andersson R, Olaison L, Hogevik H. A 10-year survey of blood culture negative endocarditis in Sweden: aminoglycoside therapy is important for survival. Scand J Infect Dis. 2008;40(4):279–85.
15. Benslimani A, Fenollar F, Lepidi H, Raoult D. Bacterial zoonoses and infective endocarditis, Algeria. Emerg Infect Dis. 2005;11(2):216–24.
16. Koegelenberg CF, Doubell AF, Orth H, Reuter H. Infective endocarditis in the Western Cape Province of South Africa: a three-year prospective study. QJM. 2003;96(3):217–25.
17. Tariq M, Alam M, Munir G, Khan MA, Smego Jr RA. Infective endocarditis: a five-year experience at a tertiary care hospital in Pakistan. Int J Infect Dis. 2004;8(3):163–70.
18. Marks P, Gogova M, Kromery VJR. Culture negative endocarditis: data from the national survey in Slovakia. Postgrad Med J. 2002;78:61–2.
19. Lamas CC, Eykyn SJ. Blood culture negative endocarditis: analysis of 63 cases presenting over 25 years. Heart. 2003;89(3):258–62.
20. Nakatani S, Mitsutake K, Hozumi T, Yoshikawa J, Akiyama M, Yoshida K, et al. Current characteristics of infective endocarditis in Japan: an analysis of 848 cases in 2000 and 2001. Circ J. 2003;67(11):901–5.
21. Ferrera C, Vilacosta I, Fernandez C, Lopez J, Olmos C, Sarria C, et al. Reassessment of blood culture-negative endocarditis: its profile is similar to that of blood culture-positive endocarditis. Rev Esp Cardiol (Engl Ed). 2012;65(10):891–900.
22. Brouqui P, Raoult D. New insight into the diagnosis of fastidious bacterial endocarditis. FEMS Immunol Med Microbiol. 2006;47(1):1–13.
23. Selton-Suty C, Celard M, Le Moing V, Doco-Lecompte T, Chirouze C, Iung B, et al. Preeminence of Staphylococcus aureus in infective endocarditis: a 1-year population-based survey. Clin Infect Dis. 2012;54(9):1230–9.
24. Hoen B, Selton-Suty C, Lacassin F, Etienne J, Briançon S, Leport C, et al. Infective endocarditis in patients with negative blood cultures: analysis of 88 cases from a one-year nationwide survey in France. Clin Infect Dis. 1995;20:501–6.
25. Cecchi E, Forno D, Imazio M, Migliardi A, Gnavi R, Dal Conte I, et al. New trends in the epidemiological and clinical features of infective endocarditis: results of a multicenter prospective study. Ital Heart J. 2004;5(4):249–56.
26. Siciliano RF, Mansur AJ, Castelli JB, Arias V, Grinberg M, Levison ME, et al. Community-acquired culture-negative endocarditis: clinical characteristics and risk factors for mortality. Int J Infect Dis. 2014;25:191–5.
27. Garg N, Kandpal B, Garg N, Tewari S, Kapoor A, Goel P, et al. Characteristics of infective endocarditis in a developing country-clinical profile and outcome in 192 Indian patients, 1992–2001. Int J Cardiol. 2005;98(2):253–60.
28. Cetinkaya Y, Akova M, Akalin HE, Ascioglu S, Hayran M, Uzuns O, et al. A retrospective review of 228 episodes of infective endocarditis where rheumatic valvular disease is still common. Int J Antimicrob Agents. 2001;18(1):1–7.
29. Letaief A, Boughzala E, Kaabia N, Ernez S, Abid F, Ben CT, et al. Epidemiology of infective endocarditis in Tunisia: a 10-year multicenter retrospective study. Int J Infect Dis. 2007; 11(5):430–3.
30. Bennis A, Zahraoui M, Azzouzi L, Soulami S, Mehadji BA, Tahiri A, et al. [Bacterial endocarditis in Morocco]. Ann Cardiol Angeiol (Paris). 1995;44(7):339–44.

31. Mirabel M, Rattanavong S, Frichitthavong K, Chu V, Kesone P, Thongsith P, et al. Infective endocarditis in the Lao PDR: clinical characteristics and outcomes in a developing country. Int J Cardiol. 2015;180:270–3.

32. Watt G, Lacroix A, Pachirat O, Baggett HC, Raoult D, Fournier PE, et al. Prospective comparison of infective endocarditis in Khon Kaen, Thailand and Rennes, France. Am J Trop Med Hyg. 2015;92(4):871–4.

33. El-Kholy AA, El-Rachidi NG, El-Enany MG, AbdulRahman EM, Mohamed RM, Rizk HH. Impact of serology and molecular methods on improving the microbiologic diagnosis of infective endocarditis in Egypt. Infection. 2015;43(5):523–9.

34. Tleyjeh IM, Abdel-Latif A, Rahbi H, Scott CG, Bailey KR, Steckelberg JM, et al. A systematic review of population-based studies of infective endocarditis. Chest. 2007;132(3):1025–35.

35. Rattanavong S, Fournier PE, Chu V, Frichitthavong K, Kesone P, Mayxay M, et al. Bartonella henselae endocarditis in Laos – 'the unsought will go undetected'. PLoS Negl Trop Dis. 2014;8(12):e3385.

36. Lupis F, Giordano S, Pampinella D, Scarlata F, Romano A. Infective endocarditis: review of 36 cases. Infez Med. 2009;17(3):159–63.

37. Lamas CC, Ramos RG, Lopes GQ, Santos MS, Golebiovski WF, Weksler C, et al. Bartonella and Coxiella infective endocarditis in Brazil: molecular evidence from excised valves from a cardiac surgery referral center in Rio de Janeiro, Brazil, 1998 to 2009. Int J Infect Dis. 2013; 17(1):e65–6.

38. Jain D, Halushka MK. Cardiac pathology of systemic lupus erythematosus. J Clin Pathol. 2009;62(7):584–92.

39. Zuily S, Regnault V, Selton-Suty C, Eschwege V, Bruntz JF, Bode-Dotto E, et al. Increased risk for heart valve disease associated with antiphospholipid antibodies in patients with systemic lupus erythematosus: meta-analysis of echocardiographic studies. Circulation. 2011;124 (2):215–24.

40. Geri G, Wechsler B, Thi Huong DL, Isnard R, Piette JC, Amoura Z, et al. Spectrum of cardiac lesions in Behcet disease: a series of 52 patients and review of the literature. Medicine (Baltimore). 2012;91(1):25–34.

41. Durack DT, Lukes AS, Bright DK. New criteria for diagnosis of infective endocarditis: utilization of specific echocardiographic findings. Duke Endocarditis Service. Am J Med. 1994;96(3):200–9.

42. Richet H, Casalta JP, Thuny F, Merrien J, Harle JR, Weiller PJ, et al. Development and assessment of a new early scoring system using non-specific clinical signs and biological results to identify children and adult patients with a high probability of infective endocarditis on admission. J Antimicrob Chemother. 2008;62(6):1434–40.

43. Habib G, Hoen B, Tornos P, Thuny F, Prendergast B, Vilacosta I, et al. Guidelines on the prevention, diagnosis, and treatment of infective endocarditis (new version 2009): the Task Force on the Prevention, Diagnosis, and Treatment of Infective Endocarditis of the European Society of Cardiology (ESC). Endorsed by the European Society of Clinical Microbiology and Infectious Diseases (ESCMID) and the International Society of Chemotherapy (ISC) for Infection and Cancer. Eur Heart J. 2009;30(19):2369–413.

44. Baron EJ, Miller JM, Weinstein MP, Richter SS, Gilligan PH, Thomson Jr RB, et al. Executive summary: a guide to utilization of the microbiology laboratory for diagnosis of infectious diseases: 2013 recommendations by the Infectious Diseases Society of America (IDSA) and the American Society for Microbiology (ASM)(a). Clin Infect Dis. 2013;57(4):485–8.

45. Weinstein MP, Mirrett S, Wilson ML, Reimer LG, Reller LB. Controlled evaluation of 5 versus 10 milliliters of blood cultured in aerobic BacT/Alert blood culture bottles. J Clin Microbiol. 1994;32(9):2103–6.

46. Wilson ML, Mirrett S, Reller LB, Weinstein MP, Reimer LG. Recovery of clinically important microorganisms from the BacT/Alert blood culture system does not require testing for seven days. Diagn Microbiol Infect Dis. 1993;16(1):31–4.

47. Fournier PE, Casalta JP, Habib G, Messana T, Raoult D. Modification of the diagnostic criteria proposed by the Duke Endocarditis Service to permit improved diagnosis of Q fever endocarditis. Am J Med. 1996;100(6):629–33.
48. Fournier PE, Mainardi JL, Raoult D. Value of microimmunofluorescence for diagnosis and follow-up of Bartonella endocarditis. Clin Diagn Lab Immunol. 2002;9(4):795–801.
49. Brouqui P, Raoult D. Endocarditis due to rare and fastidious bacteria. Clin Microbiol Rev. 2001;14(1):177–207.
50. Lefort A, Chartier L, Sendid B, Wolff M, Mainardi JL, Podglajen I, et al. Diagnosis, management and outcome of Candida endocarditis. Clin Microbiol Infect. 2012;18(4):E99–109.
51. Katsouli A, Massad MG. Current issues in the diagnosis and management of blood culture-negative infective and non-infective endocarditis. Ann Thorac Surg. 2013;95(4):1467–74.
52. Vondracek M, Sartipy U, Aufwerber E, Julander I, Lindblom D, Westling K. 16S rDNA sequencing of valve tissue improves microbiological diagnosis in surgically treated patients with infective endocarditis. J Infect. 2011;62(6):472–8.
53. Marin M, Munoz P, Sanchez M, del Rosal M, Alcala L, Rodriguez-Creixems M, et al. Molecular diagnosis of infective endocarditis by real-time broad-range polymerase chain reaction (PCR) and sequencing directly from heart valve tissue. Medicine (Baltimore). 2007; 86(4):195–202.
54. Fenollar F, Celard M, Lagier JC, Lepidi H, Fournier PE, Raoult D. Tropheryma whipplei endocarditis. Emerg Infect Dis. 2013;19(11):1721–30.
55. Mencacci A, Leli C, Montagna P, Cardaccia A, Meucci M, Bietolini C, et al. Diagnosis of infective endocarditis: comparison of the LightCycler SeptiFast real-time PCR with blood culture. J Med Microbiol. 2012;61(Pt 6):881–3.
56. Casalta JP, Thuny F, Fournier PE, Lepidi H, Habib G, Grisoli D, et al. DNA persistence and relapses questions on the treatment strategies of Enterococcus infections of prosthetic valves. PLoS One. 2012;7(12):e53335.
57. Casalta JP, Gouriet F, Roux V, Thuny F, Habib G, Raoult D. Evaluation of the LightCycler SeptiFast test in the rapid etiologic diagnosis of infectious endocarditis. Eur J Clin Microbiol Infect Dis. 2009;28:569–73.
58. Lepidi H, Coulibaly B, Casalta JP, Raoult D. Autoimmunohistochemistry: a new method for the histologic diagnosis of infective endocarditis. J Infect Dis. 2006;193(12):1711–7.
59. Thuny F, Gaubert JY, Jacquier A, Tessonnier L, Cammilleri S, Raoult D, et al. Imaging investigations in infective endocarditis: current approach and perspectives. Arch Cardiovasc Dis. 2013;106(1):52–62.
60. Saby L, Laas O, Habib G, Cammilleri S, Mancini J, Tessonnier L, et al. Positron emission tomography/computed tomography for diagnosis of prosthetic valve endocarditis: increased valvular 18F-fluorodeoxyglucose uptake as a novel major criterion. J Am Coll Cardiol. 2013; 61(23):2374–82.
61. Gouriet F, Fournier PE, Zaratzian C, Sumian M, Cammilleri S, Riberi A, et al. Diagnosis of Bartonella henselae prosthetic valve endocarditis in man, France. Emerg Infect Dis. 2014; 20(8):1396–7.
62. Jos SL, Angelakis E, Caus T, Raoult D. Positron emission tomography in the diagnosis of Whipple's endocarditis: a case report. BMC Res Notes. 2015;8:56.
63. Gouriet F, Saby L, Delaunay E, Cammilleri S, Le DY, Riberi A, et al. Incidental diagnosis of colonic tumor by PET/CT in infectious endocarditis. J Infect. 2013;67(1):88–90.
64. Baddour LM, Wilson WR, Bayer AS, Fowler Jr VG, Bolger AF, Levison ME, et al. Infective endocarditis: diagnosis, antimicrobial therapy, and management of complications: a statement for healthcare professionals from the Committee on Rheumatic Fever, Endocarditis, and Kawasaki Disease, Council on Cardiovascular Disease in the Young, and the Councils on Clinical Cardiology, Stroke, and Cardiovascular Surgery and Anesthesia, American Heart Association: endorsed by the Infectious Diseases Society of America. Circulation. 2005;111 (23):e394–434.

65. Raoult D, Houpikian P, Tissot DH, Riss JM, Arditi-Djiane J, Brouqui P. Treatment of Q fever endocarditis: comparison of 2 regimens containing doxycycline and ofloxacin or hydroxychloroquine. Arch Intern Med. 1999;159(2):167–73.
66. Fenollar F, Fournier PE, Carrieri MP, Habib G, Messana T, Raoult D. Risks factors and prevention of Q fever endocarditis. Clin Infect Dis. 2001;33(3):312–6.
67. Million M, Walter G, Thuny F, Habib G, Raoult D. Evolution from acute Q fever to endocarditis is associated with underlying valvulopathy and age and can be prevented by prolonged antibiotic treatment. Clin Infect Dis. 2013;57(6):836–44.
68. Raoult D, Fournier PE, Vandenesch F, Mainardi JL, Eykyn SJ, Nash J, et al. Outcome and treatment of Bartonella endocarditis. Arch Intern Med. 2003;163:226–30.
69. Fenollar F, Rolain JM, Alric L, Papo T, Chauveheid MP, van Beek D, et al. Resistance to trimethoprim/sulfamethoxazole and Tropheryma whipplei. Int J Antimicrob Agents. 2009; 34(3):255–9.
70. Cohen JL, Sloss LJ, Kundsin R, Golightly L. Prosthetic valve endocarditis caused by Mycoplasma hominis. Am J Med. 1989;86:819–21.
71. DiSesa VJ, Sloss LJ, Cohn LH. Heart transplantation for intractable prosthetic valve endocarditis. J Heart Transplant. 1990;9(2):142–3.
72. Fenollar F, Gauduchon V, Casalta JP, Lepidi H, Vandenesch F, Raoult D. Mycoplasma endocarditis: two case reports and a review. Clin Infect Dis. 2004;38(3):e21–4.
73. Jamil HA, Sandoe JA, Gascoyne-Binzi D, Chalker VJ, Simms AD, Munsch CM, et al. Late-onset prosthetic valve endocarditis caused by Mycoplasma hominis, diagnosed using broad-range bacterial PCR. J Med Microbiol. 2012;61(Pt 2):300–1.
74. Blasco M, Torres L, Marco ML, Moles B, Villuendas MC, Garcia Moya JB. Prosthetic valve endocarditis caused by Mycoplasma hominis. Eur J Clin Microbiol Infect Dis. 2000; 19(8):638–40.
75. Dominguez SR, Littlehorn C, Nyquist AC. Mycoplasma hominis endocarditis in a child with a complex congenital heart defect. Pediatr Infect Dis J. 2006;25(9):851–2.
76. Hussain ST, Gordon SM, Tan CD, Smedira NG. Mycoplasma hominis prosthetic valve endocarditis: the value of molecular sequencing in cardiac surgery. J Thorac Cardiovasc Surg. 2013;146(1):e7–9.
77. Scapini JP, Flynn LP, Sciacaluga S, Morales L, Cadario ME. Confirmed Mycoplasma pneumoniae endocarditis. Emerg Infect Dis. 2008;14(10):1664–5.
78. Kalokhe AS, Rouphael N, El Chami MF, Workowski KA, Ganesh G, Jacob JT. Aspergillus endocarditis: a review of the literature. Int J Infect Dis. 2010;14(12):e1040–7.
79. Scarano M, Pezzuoli F, Patane S. Brucella infective endocarditis. Int J Cardiol. 2014; 172(3):e509–10.

Chapter 19
Infective Endocarditis in Special Populations: Patients Under Dialysis

Christine Selton-Suty, Olivier Huttin, François Goehringer, and Luc Frimat

Abbreviations

CKD	Chronic kidney disease
CVC	Central venous catheter
ESRD	End-stage renal disease
HD	Haemodialysis
ICD	Implantable Cardioverter Defibrillator
IE	Infective endocarditis
PD	Peritoneal dialysis
S.aureus	*Staphylococcus aureus*

Introduction

Incidence of infective endocarditis (IE) is well known to vary among different sub-populations of hosts, being estimated around 100 times higher among patients with valvular prostheses than in the general population. Between those two extreme levels of incidence, some specific populations are at intermediate risk and need to be

C. Selton-Suty, MD (✉)
Department of Cardiology, University Hospital of Nancy, Institut Lorrain du Coeur et des Vaisseaux, Vandoeuvre les Nancy, France
e-mail: c.suty-selton@chu-nancy.fr

O. Huttin, MD
Department of Cardiology, University Hospital of Nancy, Vandoeuvre les Nancy, France
e-mail: o.huttin@chu-nancy.fr

F. Goehringer, MD
Department of Infectious and Tropical Diseases, University Hospital of Nancy,
Vandoeuvre les Nancy, France
e-mail: f.goehringer@chu.nancy.fr

L. Frimat, MD, PhD
Department of Nephrology, University Hospital of Nancy, Vandoeuvre les Nancy, France
e-mail: l.frimat@chu.nancy.fr

© Springer International Publishing Switzerland 2016
G. Habib (ed.), *Infective Endocarditis*, DOI 10.1007/978-3-319-32432-6_19

recognized because of particular features linked to specific hosts. This chapter will focus on IE in patients under dialysis.

More than 1.5 million patients with established end-stage renal disease (ESRD) are treated with haemodialysis (HD) over the world with approximately 425,000 patients in Europe and 380,000 in the US [1–3]. IE is the result of a complex interaction between host, exposure, and pathogen, and patients with ESRD have all the ingredients to develop this pathology. Old age, malnutrition, comorbidities favouring development of infection (diabetes mellitus, immunosuppression, etc.) and degenerative heart valve disease are frequent in dialysis patients. Furthermore, vascular access for HD is a perfect gateway for frequent exposures to various pathogens, the most frequent of them being *Staphylococcus aureus (S. aureus)*, which has a special affinity to adhere on valve lesions.

Epidemiology

First description of IE in a dialysis patient dates back to the 1970s by Blagg et al. who reported a case of death following cerebral embolism in a patient with subacute bacterial IE [4].

IE in dialysis patients is a typical form of health-care associated disease. The frequency of this mode of acquisition of IE has been highlighted since the end of the twentieth century in the US [5]. From the Duke Medical Center files, Cabell et al. showed a progressive increase of HD dependence, immunosuppression and *S. aureus* infection over a 6-year period (1992–1998). HD was independently associated with *S. aureus* infection (OR 3.1 [1.6–5.9]) and accounted for 7 % of the cases of IE in 1992, a proportion that increased to around 20 % in 1998 [6].

In the 2008 French epidemiological survey, health-care associated IE represented 27 % of the whole population and dialysis patients accounted only for 2.2 % of the total series of IE patients [7]. An extrapolation based on the French population of patients dependent on HD allowed an estimation of the incidence around 1700–2000 cases of IE/10^6 HD patients [8]. This estimated incidence is 70 times higher than that of IE in the general population (around 30 cases/10^6 inhabitants) but only 0.7 times lower than that of patients with valvular prostheses (around 3000 cases/10^6 patients).

Analysis of the US Renal Data system (1992–97) [9] revealed 2075 new cases of IE among 327,993 new HD patients (0.6 %) and estimated the cumulative incidence at 2670 cases of IE/10^6 HD patients. HD patients had an age-adjusted incidence ratio for IE of 18 and peritoneal dialysis (PD) patients of 11 compared to the general population. The incidence ratio for primary hospitalizations for IE was also around 70 times higher in HD patients than in the general population.

The frequency of HD patients in series of IE varies in the literature and is higher in the US than in the European countries. A monocentric US study estimated the incidence of IE to be 129–174 times higher than in non HD patients, and reported a very high percentage of 35 % of HD patients among 160 IE between 2001 and

2006 [10]. Another European study reported lower frequency of 6 % of HD patients among 241 IE [11]. Many factors can explain this higher frequency of IE among US HD patients, such as old age, high rate of comorbidities (obesity, diabetes mellitus, etc.) and frequent use of central venous catheter as vascular access in the US [12, 13].

In a series of 210 HD patients with *S. aureus* bacteremia, the frequency of patients who developed IE was 17 % [14]. In the French registry VIRSTA which gathered 2008 patients with *S. aureus* bacteremia, 211 patients were HD patients (10.5 %) and 26 (12.3 %) developed IE (versus 11 % in non HD patients, ns) [15].

Predisposing Factors for IE in HD Patients

Factors Linked to the Host

Many characteristics of dialysis patients are well-known to increase the risk of infection: old age, malnutrition with low serum albumin, anaemia, impaired immune defences and comorbidities. Among them, diabetes mellitus is one of the leading causes of HD, reported in 30–50 % of the patients, and is a major risk factor for infection [16–18].

Degenerative valvular disease with valvular and annular calcifications is frequent among ESRD patients, affecting both mitral and aortic valves. The Framingham study analysed a subgroup of 3047 participants who all had echocardiography. Among participants with valvular/annular calcification (9 %), 20 % had chronic kidney disease (CKD) defined as GFR <60 ml/mn/1.73 m^2, compared with 7 % in patients without valvular calcification. After adjustment, participants with CKD had a 60 % increased odds of mitral annular calcification. So, in the community, CKD is associated with presence of valvular calcification even before the onset of dialysis [19].

Among dialysis patients, the percentage of either mitral and/or aortic calcifications varies in the literature from 30 to 75 %, partly depending on the duration on maintenance dialysis (Table 19.1) [20–25]. Interestingly, during the first decade of the millennium, a new paradigm on mineral homeostasis emerged. Due vitamin D and parathyroid hormone disturbances influencing calcium-phosphate metabolism expose CKD patients, in particular HD ones, concurrently to bone and cardiovascular diseases [26].

Other cardiovascular diseases are also frequent in HD patients. Chang [27] compared HD patients who developed IE with HD patients seen at the same center during the same period and showed that IE patients more often had a pacemaker implant (15 vs. 1.1 %, p < 0.01), previous heart surgery (15 vs. 0.4 %, p < 0.01) and congestive heart failure (CHF) (50 vs. 10.4 %, p < 0.05). Furthermore, the duration on maintenance HD (12.9±19.1 vs. 57.9±42.3 months, p < 0.001) and serum albumin at the time of admission (2.91±0.40 vs. 3.96±0.52 g/dL, p < 0.001) were lower in IE patients than in others.

Table 19.1 Frequency of valvular calcifications among patients under dialysis

Author	Period	N	Mitral calcifications %	Aortic calcifications %	Any valvular calcifications %
Choi [20]	Onset of dialysis	258			30
Ikee [21]	On dialysis	112	75	52	
Leskinen [22]	Before dialysis	58			31
	On dialysis	36			50
	Transplanted patients	41			29
	Controls	58			12
Sharma [23]	Before transplantation	140	40		
Raggi [24]	On dialysis	200	46	33	
Ribeiro [25]	On dialysis	92	44	52	
	Controls	92	10	4	

Factors Linked to Exposures

Disruption of dermal barrier to gain access for dialysis results in frequent exposures to infection in dialysis patients. Vascular access is the usual portal of entry of infection in HD patients. In peritoneal dialysis (PD), infection may occur from the catheter entrance through the skin or from digestive translocation directly into the peritoneal cavity. Bacteremia is therefore a common event for both HD and PD patients, occurring in more than 10 % of incident patients over a 7 year period in the series of Powe [17]. The pathogenesis of catheter-related bloodstream infection (CRBSI) includes micro-organisms entry into the bloodstream through the vascular access followed by adherence to catheter, colonization and biofilm formation -which makes them very resistant to antibiotic action- and bacteremia.

There are three main types of vascular access for HD: native arteriovenous fistula (AVF), arteriovenous graft (AVG) and central venous catheter (CVC). CVCs for HD are of two types: acute (non-cuffed non-tunnelled) catheters and chronic (cuffed tunnelled) catheters. AVF use is strongly recommended by guidelines because of lower rates of infectious and thrombotic complications [28].

The incidence of HD-related bacteremia is more than tenfold higher in AVGs than AVFs: 2.5 episodes per 1000 dialysis procedures versus 0.2 [29]. However, the rate of infection is the highest through CVCs. In the late 1990s, the incidence of *S. aureus* bacteremia among patients with tunnelled, cuffed HD catheters was reported to range from 0.6 to 3.9 per 1000 catheter-days [16, 30]. In the United States in 2007–2008, the rate of pooled access-related bloodstream infection in HD patients with a central line was 1.05 cases per 1000 catheter days [28, 31]. In the EPIBACDIAL study, catheters, especially long-term implanted ones, were found to be the leading risk factor of bacteremia among 988 HD patients, with a risk ratio of 7.6 [95 % CI 3.7–15.6] versus fistula [16]. In the study of Chang comparing 20 HD pts with IE to 268 control HD patients, there were more patients dialyzed via non-cuffed dual-lumen catheters in IE patients (55 vs. 0 %, $p < 0.001$), and fewer patients dialyzed via arteriovenous fistula (AVF) (25 vs. 88 %, p < 0.001) than in non-IE HD patients [27]. A Brazilian series of 156 patients with CVC reported 94 infectious episodes (60 %) over a period of 1 year: 39 (25 %) had positive blood cultures at the CVC insertion location of whom 35 were also positive on peripheral blood culture and 27 (17 %) developed IE [32].

Factors Linked to the Pathogens

Episodes of bacteremia are quite frequent among HD patients. The source of micro-organisms is mostly endogen, related to the cutaneous, but also to the nasal or peri-neal flora of the patient, and rarely exogenous. The pathogens which are mainly responsible for bloodstream infections are Staphylococci, Enterococci, Gram-negative enteric bacilli, Pseudomonas aeruginosa, and Candida spp [28].

S. aureus is the main cause of bacteremia among patients receiving HD (up to 75 % of cases) [33]. The annual incidence of S. aureus bacteremia among ESRD patients is very high, reported in the Danish registry to be around 35 per 1000 person-years compared to a rate of 0.5 per 1000 person-years in the general popula-tion [34]. The incidence is the highest among HD patients (46 per 1000 person-years) compared to PD patients (22 per 1000 person-years). Strains of S. aureus that infect HD intravascular devices are indeed particularly virulent and usually resistant to thrombin-induced platelet microbicidal protein [35] thus favouring the adherence on valves. One third of HD patients with S. aureus bacteremia will suffer a distant septic complication (IE, osteomyelitis, epiduritis, arthritis, etc.) [14] or a local one such as septic thrombophlebitis of the vascular access.

The proportion of methicillin-resistant S. aureus isolated in ESRD patients has been increasing with time, with various frequencies reported according to the local bacterial epidemiology of health-care associated infections. This proportion was as high as 20–30 % of all S. aureus strains in the late 1990s [36, 37] but now tends to decrease in the US [38], representing even less than 1 % of S. aureus strains in the Danish registry [34]. Most of the cases of methicillin-resistant S. aureus infections are nosocomial and occur in patients who have been hospitalized in the year prior to infection [38].

Furthermore, HD patients are particularly exposed not only to staphylococcal infections but also to all other nosocomial infections with increased prevalence of multi-resistant micro-organisms in that population. However, these other micro-organisms more rarely cause IE.

Diagnosis

The main clinical and microbiological features of IE in HD patients as described in the literature are summarized in Table 19.2. The diagnosis of IE in an HD patient presenting with a bacteremia is often difficult. Fever is not always present, reported in 40–75% of the series. Biological markers such as anaemia or positive inflammatory

Table 19.2 Main features of IE among HD patients from the literature

| Author | Period | Episodes of IE (pts) | Vascular access | | | Localisation | | | | Micro-organisms | | | Diabetes mellitus | Surgery | Mortality | |
			AF %	AVG %	CVC %	Aortic %	Mitral %	Tricuspid pacemaker %	Multi-valvular %	S. aureus %	Other Staph %	Entero-cocci %	%	%	Initial %	1 year %
Robinson [54]	1990–1997	20/20	5	45	55	30	50	25	?	55	30	10	45	20	30	
Mc Carthy [55]	1983–1987	20/17	10	70	20	25	45	10	0	40	10	20	35	30	45	75
Maraj [56]	1990–2000	32/32	3	38	59	–	++	–	–	80			–	–	25	56
Doulton [57]	1980–2002	30/28	41	11	38	37	43	0	17	57	3	13	28	50	30	46
Jones [58]	1998–2011	42/42	35	0	65	43	31	0	9.5	45	12	12	33	21	14	33(3M)
Kamalakannan [44]	1990–2004	69/69	12	22	67	22	49	10	?	58	14	7	38	22	49	
Nori [37]	1999–2004	54/52	4	13	74	44	52	19	10	40	22	33	42	24	37	
Chang [27]	1990–2004	20/20	25	15	60	10	35	15	5		15	5	45	0	60	
Spies [36]	1990–2001	40/40	60	18	30	20	53	6	20	50	12	23	50	37	52	

? means that this data was not specified in the artilce

Table 19.3 Arguments raising a high suspicion of IE in an HD patient with bacteremia and implying the performance of an early echocardiography

Host-related	CVC as vascular access
	Presence of a pacemaker or Implantable Cardioverter Defibrillator
	Presence of a valvular prosthesis
	Previous episode of IE
Pathogen-related	*S. aureus* bacteremia
	Bacteremia with other micro-organisms potentially responsible of IE (other staphylococci, enterococci, streptococci, candida)
	Recurrent or relapsing bacteremia, whatever the micro-organism
IE-related	Heart failure, new murmur, conduction abnormalities on ECG
	Stroke
	Presence of other clinical signs: cutaneous, spondylodiscitis, pulmonary or other embolism
Dialysis-related	Hypotension during dialysis in a usually hypertensive patient

markers may be related to the bacteremia or to the underlying chronic kidney disease and are not specific. Haematuria is not a valid criterion in patients on dialysis. So the pertinence of Duke criteria is questioned in that specific population.

Even the major microbiological criteria that requires positive blood cultures in the absence of a primary focus is challenged in HD patients where vascular access is often the primary focus of infection. Of note, blood cultures must be drawn not only from the vascular access but also from peripheral veins when possible, in order to reduce the inevitable uncertainty in the interpretation of blood culture results that arises when an organism is recovered that could represent either colonization of the catheter or true infection [39].

As in the general population, echocardiography is the main diagnostic tool in dialysis patients. In order to make an early diagnosis before any hemodynamic and/or embolic complications occur, echocardiography must be performed as soon as possible, especially if arguments raising a high suspicion of IE (summarized in Table 19.3) are present. However, transthoracic echocardiography only may not always be sufficient for the diagnosis, as annular and valvular calcifications may mask vegetations and abscesses. So, transesophageal echocardiography must be discussed in all HD patients with positive blood cultures, and systematically performed in all cases of *S. aureus* bacteremia and in patients with intracardiac devices (pace maker, valvular prostheses). In case of a negative TEE with a remaining high clinical suspicion of IE, echocardiography should be repeated in the next 7–10 days [40]. Left heart valves are the most commonly affected, and multivalvular location is not infrequent, reported in 10–23 % of the series.

Treatment of IE in HD Patients

Therapeutic management of these patients follows several key aspects discussed in the sections below.

Systemic Antibiotic Therapy

Systemic antibiotic therapy usually follows the standard guidelines on IE [40] and on Intravascular Catheter-Related Infection [41]. As HD patients are difficult-to-treat and frail patients, it is recommended that, when feasible, nephrologists collaborate with infectious disease staff to determine optimal antibiotic selection and dosing.

The antibiotic regimen used and duration are the same as for other IEs. Only the dose should be adjusted according to each molecule specific recommendations depending on metabolism of renal elimination. On dialysis days, antibiotics should follow the dialysis session. As for all the IE, antibiotics must be administered intravenously, which can cause venous access problems in these patients with limited venous capital. For empiric antibiotic regimen, in case of Gram positive cocci bacteremia, anti MRSA drugs must be considered such as IV vancomycine or daptomycine [28].

Cardiac Surgery

In a general manner, patients with end stage renal disease (ESRD) undergoing cardiac surgery have very high in-hospital mortality rates (13–36%) and limited life expectancy (15–42 months) [42] and IE may potentially further aggravate this surgical prognosis. Quite recent data from the US Renal Data System report a low rate of only 11% of surgery among more than 11,000 dialysis patients hospitalized for IE over the period 2004–2007 [43]. In the literature, the frequency of surgery is usually around 20–25%, far lower than that of the general IE population. In a small study on 69 HD patients with definite IE, valve surgery was the only independent predictive factor of survival [44]. No studies have specifically addressed the issue of whether surgery must follow the same recommendations in HD patients than in non HD patients. So, the decision of valvular surgery in HD patients should be specifically discussed by a multidisciplinary team including cardiologist, nephrologist, cardiac surgeon and infectious diseases specialist.

Regarding the type of valvular prosthesis to be used, recommendations have changed over time. Although initially thought to have accelerated degeneration in HD patients, bioprosthesis seems to be now the substitute of choice. This shift is mainly due to frequent haemorrhagic complications of mechanical prostheses. Observational data showed no significant differences in survival between biological and mechanical prostheses. Estimated survival at 1 and 3 years was 60 and 50% for biological and 37 and 30% for mechanical prostheses in the US Renal Data System (ns) [43]. Thus, mechanical prostheses should only be considered in young and otherwise healthy HD patients while biological ones should be used in other patients [2].

Treatment of Portal of Entry

Vascular access is the portal of entry of infection in most of the cases. In case of HD through CVC, the removal and replacement of vascular access must be discussed. However, given the limited options for vascular access in many patients receiving chronic HD, loss of vascular access is often not acceptable [14]. Other management options include use of antibiotic lock solution (high concentrations of antibiotic combined with anticoagulant instilled into the catheter lumen) or guidewire exchange of the catheter which are both superior to systemic antibiotics alone [3]. In a small study, Fernandez-Cean suggested that a temporary switch to peritoneal dialysis (PD) could improve the prognosis of patients as compared to the persistent use of the initial vascular access [45]; however, this has not been confirmed in larger series.

Prophylaxis of IE in HD Patients

Usual rules of IE prophylaxis apply to HD patients as most of them have valvular underlying disease [40]. Good oral hygiene and regular dental review must be explained to HD patients. Aseptic measures during venous catheters manipulation and during any invasive procedures are of particular importance in HD patients, in order to reduce the rate of bacteremia and health care-associated IE.

As a general rule, CVCs should be avoided when possible. The choice of one type of CVC must be discussed when used, as there is a large number of available catheters, with very different costs but also characteristics aiming at the reduction of infection and thrombosis [46]. Best practices for catheter care must be applied [47]. The interest of systematic prophylactic antimicrobial lock therapy in HD CVCs is still debated [48, 49]. Some authors reported that HD catheter-care procedure including exit-site disinfection with chlorhexidine gluconate could result in a sustained reduction in bacteraemia rates as compared with standard care [50].

A special attention should be paid to patients with pacemakers and defibrillators: CVC should be avoided and the access site should be on the opposite side to where the implanted device lies wherever possible [28].

Prophylactic vaccination to prevent *S. aureus* infections has been evaluated in patients undergoing HD. However, although the vaccine induced a robust immune response and had an acceptable safety profile, it did not show any protective effect against *S. aureus* bacteremia and further research is needed in that field [51–53].

Prognosis

Estimated mortality in a general population of dialysis patients at 5 years after the onset of dialysis is 50–60 % in patients under 60 years of age and 70–75 % in patients older than 60, around one-third of the expected remaining lifetime of the general population [1].

Infection is the second leading cause of death among ESRD patients and use of CVCs as access is a predictor of all-cause and infection-specific mortality [16]. Among HD patients with IE, initial mortality ranges from 14 to 60% and 1-year mortality is impressive, varying from 45 to 75% (Table 19.2). IE patients undergoing HD have a far higher early and late mortality than other IE patients (early: 43 versus 16%, p=0.03 and late 22 versus 9%, p < 0.05) in the series of Ruiz [11]. Furthermore, mortality of patients operated on for IE is also higher among HD patients than in other IE patients, reported to be as high as 73% in the series of Spies [36]. The US Renal Data System reports survival rates of only 50–60% at 6 months after surgery for IE among 1267 patients operated on for IE and independent predictors of mortality include older age, diabetes mellitus as the cause of ESRD, surgery during index hospitalization, *Staphylococcus* as the causative organism, and dysrhythmias as a comorbid condition [42]. So, IE in HD patients has really an impressively dreadful prognosis.

Conclusion

Bacteremia, especially due to *S. aureus*, occurs frequently in patients under dialysis and is complicated with IE in a relatively small number of cases. However, as IE in HD patients is devastating and associated with a dramatically poor prognosis, an early diagnosis is of crucial importance to avoid hemodynamic and embolic complications that are associated with lethality and difficult therapeutic (mainly surgical) decisions. Echocardiography is the cornerstone of the diagnosis and must be performed very early, especially if arguments raising a high suspicion of IE are present.

Due to the very peculiar features of patients under dialysis with high rate of comorbidities and general frailty, therapeutic decisions should always be discussed by a multidisciplinary team including cardiologist, nephrologist, infectious disease specialists and cardiac surgeons. However, careful clinical monitoring, strict measures of asepsis during dialysis, limitation of CVC use, improvement of nutritional and mineral status, correction of anaemia and successful management of diabetes mellitus are of utmost importance to reduce the incidence of BSI and prevent the development of IE in dialysis patients.

References

1. Noordzij M, Kramer A, Abad Diez JM, Alonso de laTorre R, Arcos Fuster E, Bikbov BT, et al. Renal replacement therapy in Europe: a summary of the 2011 ERA-EDTA Registry Annual Report. Clin Kidney J. 2014;7(2):227–38.
2. Nucifora G, Badano LP, Viale P, Gianfagna P, Allocca G, Montanaro D, et al. Infective endocarditis in chronic haemodialysis patients: an increasing clinical challenge. Eur Heart J. 2007;28(19):2307–12.

3. Aslam S, Vaida F, Ritter M, Mehta RL. Systematic review and meta-analysis on management of hemodialysis catheter-related bacteremia. J Am Soc Nephrol. 2014;25(12):2927–41.
4. Blagg CR, Hickman RO, Eschbach JW, Scribner BH. Home hemodialysis: six years' experience. N Engl J Med. 1970;283:1126–31.
5. Murdoch DR, Corey GR, Hoen B, Miro JM, Fowler VG, Bayer AS, et al. Clinical presentation, etiology, and outcome of infective endocarditis in the 21st century: the International Collaboration on Endocarditis-Prospective Cohort Study. Arch Intern Med. 2009;169(5):463–73.
6. Cabell CH, Jollis JG, Peterson GE, Corey GR, Anderson DJ, Sexton DJ, et al. Changing patient characteristics and the effect on mortality in endocarditis. Arch Intern Med. 2002; 162(1):90–4.
7. Selton-Suty C, Celard M, Le Moing V, Doco-Lecompte T, Chirouze C, Iung B, et al. Preeminence of Staphylococcus aureus in infective endocarditis: a 1-year population-based survey. Clin Infect Dis. 2012;54(9):1230–9.
8. Hoen B, Alla F, Béguinot I, Bouvet A, Briancon S, Casalta JP, et al. Changing profile of infective endocarditis – results of a one-year survey in France in 1999. JAMA. 2002;288(1):75–81.
9. Abbott KC, Agodoa LY. Hospitalizations for bacterial endocarditis after initiation of chronic dialysis in the United States. Nephron. 2002;91(2):203–9.
10. Wray D, Steed L, Singleton C, Church P, Cantey JR, Gomez J. Impact of regional comorbidity on infective endocarditis in a southeastern United States medical center. Am J Med Sci. 2010;340(6):439–47.
11. Ruiz M, Sanchez MP, Dominguez JC, Pineda SO, Penas ER, Rubio MD, et al. Infective endocarditis in patients receiving chronic hemodialysis: clinical features and outcome. J Heart Valve Dis. 2005;14(1):11–4.
12. Goodkin DA, Robinson BM. Fistula versus catheter outcomes: the importance of surgical training. Kidney Int. 2013;83(3):531–2.
13. Goodkin DA, Bragg-Gresham JL, Koenig KG, Wolfe RA, Akiba T, Andreucci VE, et al. Association of comorbid conditions and mortality in hemodialysis patients in Europe, Japan, and the United States: the Dialysis Outcomes and Practice Patterns Study (DOPPS). J Am Soc Nephrol. 2003;14(12):3270–7.
14. Engemann JJ, Friedman JY, Reed SD, Griffiths RI, Szczech LA, Kaye KS, et al. Clinical outcomes and costs due to Staphylococcus aureus bacteremia among patients receiving long-term hemodialysis. Infect Control Hosp Epidemiol. 2005;26(6):534–9.
15. Le Moing V, Alla F, Doco-Lecompte T, Delahaye F, Piroth L, Chirouze C, et al. Staphylococcus aureus bloodstream infection and endocarditis – A prospective cohort study. PLoS One. 2015;10(5):e0127385.
16. Hoen B, Paul-Dauphin A, Hestin D, Kessler M. EPIBACDIAL: a multicenter prospective study of risk factors for bacteremia in chronic hemodialysis patients. J Am Soc Nephrol. 1998;9(5):869–76.
17. Powe NR, Jaar B, Furth SL, Hermann J, Briggs W. Septicemia in dialysis patients: incidence, risk factors, and prognosis. Kidney Int. 1999;55(3):1081–90.
18. Rhee CM, Leung AM, Kovesdy CP, Lynch KE, Brent GA, Kalantar-Zadeh K. Updates on the management of diabetes in dialysis patients. Semin Dial. 2014;27(2):135–45.
19. Fox CS, Larson MG, Vasan RS, Guo CY, Parise H, Levy D, et al. Cross-sectional association of kidney function with valvular and annular calcification: the Framingham heart study. J Am Soc Nephrol. 2006;17(2):521–7.
20. Choi MJ, Kim JK, Kim SG, Kim SE, Kim SJ, Kim HJ, et al. Association between cardiac valvular calcification and myocardial ischemia in asymptomatic high-risk patients with end-stage renal disease. Atherosclerosis. 2013;229(2):369–73.
21. Ikee R, Honda K, Ishioka K, Oka M, Maesato K, Moriya H, et al. Differences in associated factors between aortic and mitral valve calcification in hemodialysis. Hypertens Res. 2010; 33(6):622–6.
22. Leskinen Y, Paana T, Saha H, Groundstroem K, Lehtimaki T, Kilpinen S, et al. Valvular calcification and its relationship to atherosclerosis in chronic kidney disease. J Heart Valve Dis. 2009;18(4):429–38.

23. Sharma R, Pellerin D, Gaze DC, Mehta RL, Gregson H, Streather CP, et al. Mitral annular calcification predicts mortality and coronary artery disease in end stage renal disease. Atherosclerosis. 2007;191(2):348–54.

24. Raggi P, Boulay A, Chasan-Taber S, Amin N, Dillon M, Burke SK, et al. Cardiac calcification in adult hemodialysis patients. A link between end-stage renal disease and cardiovascular disease? J Am Coll Cardiol. 2002;39(4):695–701.

25. Ribeiro S, Ramos A, Brandao A, Rebelo JR, Guerra A, Resina C, et al. Cardiac valve calcification in haemodialysis patients: role of calcium-phosphate metabolism. Nephrol Dial Transplant. 1998;13(8):2037–40.

26. Moe SM, Drüeke TB, Block GA, Cannata-Andía JB, Elder GJ, Fukagawa M, et al. KDIGO clinical practice guideline for the diagnosis, evaluation, prevention, and treatment of Chronic Kidney Disease-Mineral and Bone Disorder (CKD-MBD). Kidney Int Suppl. 2009;113: S1–130.

27. Chang CF, Kuo BI, Chen TL, Yang WC, Lee SD, Lin CC. Infective endocarditis in maintenance hemodialysis patients: fifteen years' experience in one medical center. J Nephrol. 2004;17(2):228–35.

28. Santoro D, Benedetto F, Mondello P, Pipito N, Barilla D, Spinelli F, et al. Vascular access for hemodialysis: current perspectives. Int J Nephrol Renovasc Dis. 2014;7:281–94.

29. Taylor G, Gravel D, Johnston L, Embil J, Holton D, Paton S. Prospective surveillance for primary bloodstream infections occurring in Canadian hemodialysis units. Infect Control Hosp Epidemiol. 2002;23(12):716–20.

30. Marr KA, Kong L, Fowler VG, Gopal A, Sexton DJ, Conlon PJ, et al. Incidence and outcome of Staphylococcus aureus bacteremia in hemodialysis patients. Kidney Int. 1998;54(5):1684–9.

31. Liang SY, Marschall J. Update on emerging infections: news from the Centers for Disease Control and Prevention. Vital signs: central line-associated blood stream infections–United States, 2001, 2008, and 2009. Ann Emerg Med. 2011;58:447–51.

32. Grothe C, da Silva Belasco AG, de Cassia Bittencourt AR, Vianna LA, de Castro Cintra SR, Barbosa DA. Incidence of bloodstream infection among patients on hemodialysis by central venous catheter. Rev Lat Am Enfermagem. 2010;18(1):73–80.

33. Maraj S, Jacobs LE, Maraj R, Kotler MN. Bacteremia and infective endocarditis in patients on hemodialysis. Am J Med Sci. 2004;327(5):242–9.

34. Nielsen LH, Jensen-Fangel S, Benfield T, Skov R, Jespersen B, Larsen AR, et al. Risk and prognosis of Staphylococcus aureus bacteremia among individuals with and without end-stage renal disease: a Danish, population-based cohort study. BMC Infect Dis. 2015;15(1):6.

35. Fowler Jr VG, McIntyre LM, Yeaman MR, Peterson GE, Barth RL, Corey GR, et al. In vitro resistance to thrombin-induced platelet microbicidal protein in isolates of Staphylococcus aureus from endocarditis patients correlates with an intravascular device source. J Infect Dis. 2000;182(4):1251–4.

36. Spies C, Madison JR, Schatz IJ. Infective endocarditis in patients with end-stage renal disease: clinical presentation and outcome. Arch Intern Med. 2004;164(1):71–5.

37. Nori US, Manoharan A, Thornby JI, Yee J, Parasuraman R, Ramanathan V. Mortality risk factors in chronic haemodialysis patients with infective endocarditis. Nephrol Dial Transplant. 2006;21(8):2184–90.

38. Nguyen DB, Lessa FC, Belflower R, Mu Y, Wise M, Nadle J, et al. Invasive methicillin-resistant Staphylococcus aureus infections among patients on chronic dialysis in the United States, 2005–2011. Clin Infect Dis. 2013;57(10):1393–400.

39. Lewis SS, Sexton DJ. Metastatic complications of bloodstream infections in hemodialysis patients. Semin Dial. 2013;26(1):47–53.

40. Habib G, Hoen B, Tornos P, Thuny F, Prendergast B, Vilacosta I, et al. Guidelines on the prevention, diagnosis, and treatment of infective endocarditis (new version 2009): the Task Force on the Prevention, Diagnosis, and Treatment of Infective Endocarditis of the European Society of Cardiology (ESC). Endorsed by the European Society of Clinical Microbiology and

Infectious Diseases (ESCMID) and the International Society of Chemotherapy (ISC) for Infection and Cancer. Eur Heart J. 2009;30(19):2369–413.

41. Mermel LA, Allon M, Bouza E, Craven DE, Flynn P, O'Grady NP, et al. Clinical practice guidelines for the diagnosis and management of intravascular catheter-related infection: 2009 update by the Infectious Diseases Society of America. Clin Infect Dis. 2009;49(1):1–45.

42. Bianchi G, Solinas M, Bevilacqua S, Glauber M. Are bioprostheses associated with better outcome than mechanical valves in patients with chronic kidney disease requiring dialysis who undergo valve surgery? Interact Cardiovasc Thorac Surg. 2012;15(3):473–83.

43. Leither MD, Shroff GR, Ding S, Gilbertson DT, Herzog CA. Long-term survival of dialysis patients with bacterial endocarditis undergoing valvular replacement surgery in the United States. Circulation. 2013;128(4):344–51.

44. Kamalakannan D, Pai RM, Johnson LB, Gardin JM, Saravolatz LD. Epidemiology and clinical outcomes of infective endocarditis in hemodialysis patients. Ann Thorac Surg. 2007;83(6):2081–6.

45. Fernandez-Cean J, Alvarez A, Burguez S, Baldovinos G, Larre-Borges P, Cha M. Infective endocarditis in chronic haemodialysis: two treatment strategies. Nephrol Dial Transplant. 2002;17(12):2226–30.

46. Gallieni M, Brenna I, Brunini F, Mezzina N, Pasho S, Giordano A. Dialysis central venous catheter types and performance. J Vasc Access. 2014;15 Suppl 7:S140–6.

47. Gupta N, Cannon M, Srinivasan A. National agenda for prevention of healthcare-associated infections in dialysis centers. Semin Dial. 2013;26(4):376–83.

48. Silva TN, de Marchi D, Mendes P, Ponce D, Silva TN. Approach to prophylactic measures for central venous catheter-related infections in hemodialysis: a critical review. Hemodial Int. 2014;18(1):15–23.

49. Niyyar VD, Lok CE. Pros and cons of catheter lock solutions. Curr Opin Nephrol Hypertens. 2013;22(6):669–74.

50. Badve SV, Johnson DW. Chronic kidney disease: haemodialysis catheter care in practice. Nat Rev Nephrol. 2014;10(3):131–3.

51. Fattom A, Matalon A, Buerkert J, Taylor K, Damaso S, Boutriau D. Efficacy profile of a bivalent Staphylococcus aureus glycoconjugated vaccine in adults on hemodialysis: phase III randomized study. Hum Vaccin Immunother. 2015;11(3):632–41.

52. Shinefield H, Black S, Fattom A, Horwith G, Rasgon S, Ordonez J, et al. Use of a Staphylococcus aureus conjugate vaccine in patients receiving hemodialysis. N Engl J Med. 2002;346 (7):491–6.

53. Jansen KU, Girgenti DQ, Scully IL, Anderson AS. Vaccine review: "Staphyloccocus aureus vaccines: problems and prospects". Vaccine. 2013;31(25):2723–30.

54. Robinson DL, Fowler VG, Sexton DJ, Corey RG, Conlon PJ. Bacterial endocarditis in hemodialysis patients. Am J Kidney Dis. 1997;30(4):521–4.

55. McCarthy JT, Steckelberg JM. Infective endocarditis in patients receiving long-term hemodialysis. Mayo Clin Proc. 2000;75(10):1008–14.

56. Maraj S, Jacobs LE, Kung SC, Raja R, Krishnasamy P, Maraj R, et al. Epidemiology and outcome of infective endocarditis in hemodialysis patients. Am J Med Sci. 2002;324(5):254–60.

57. Doulton T, Sabharwal N, Cairns HS, Schelenz S, Eykyn S, O'Donnell P, et al. Infective endocarditis in dialysis patients: new challenges and old. Kidney Int. 2003;64(2):720–7.

58. Jones DA, McGill LA, Rathod KS, Matthews K, Gallagher S, Uppal R, et al. Characteristics and outcomes of dialysis patients with infective endocarditis. Nephron Clin Pract. 2013; 123(3–4):151–6.

Part VII
Treatment

Chapter 20
Antimicrobial Therapy in Infective Endocarditis

Jean-Paul Casalta, Frederique Gouriet, Gilbert Habib, and Didier Raoult

Principles and Methods

Successful treatment of infective endocarditis (IE) relies on microbial eradication by antimicrobial drugs. Surgery plays a major role in the treatment of IE [1], by removing infected material and draining abscesses. Bacteria are present in vegetations and biofilms, e.g., in prosthetic valve endocarditis (PVE), and justify the need for prolonged therapy (6 weeks) to fully sterilize infected heart valves.

In both native valve endocarditis (NVE) and PVE, the duration of treatment is based on the first day of effective antibiotic therapy, not on the day of surgery. A new full course of treatment should only start if valve cultures are positive, the choice of antibiotic being based on the susceptibility of the latest recovered bacterial isolate.

One of the most persistent problems in the failure of antibiotic therapy is the low compliance in the implementation of protocols, often related to their complexity. The goal is to implement protocols that are simple and easy to use [2].

Conflicting recommendations have been published concerning the optimal antibiotic therapy in IE.

J.-P. Casalta, MD • D. Raoult, PUPH, MD
Unité de Recherche sur les Maladies Infectieuses et Tropicales Emergentes, UMR CNRS 7278, IRD 198, Institut National de la Santé et de la Recherche Médicale (INSERM) 1095, Faculté de Médecine, Aix-Marseille Université, Marseille, France
e-mail: Jean-paul.casalta@wanadoo.fr; Didier.raoult@gmail.com

F. Gouriet, MD, PhD (✉)
Pôle de Maladies Infectieuses, Hôpital de la Timone, Marseille, France

Unité de Recherche sur les Maladies Infectieuses et Tropicales Emergentes, Aix-Marseille Université, Faculté de Médecine, Marseille, France
e-mail: Frederique.gouriet@ap-hm.fr

G. Habib, MD, FESC
Cardiology Department, HABIB Gilbert, La Timone Hospital, 13005, Marseille, France
e-mail: Gilbert.habib3@gmail.com

© Springer International Publishing Switzerland 2016
G. Habib (ed.), *Infective Endocarditis*, DOI 10.1007/978-3-319-32432-6_20

In this chapter, we present the antibiotic protocols used by our team (La Timone Hospital, Marseille, France), based on a more than 20-year endocarditis team experience. Although slightly different from current international guidelines, they are based on the simplest way to obtain maximal adherence to treatment, both from doctors and patients [2–4]

Protocols

Empirical Antimicrobial Therapy

Treatment of IE should be started promptly. Three sets of blood cultures should be drawn at 30 min intervals before initiation of antibiotics. The initial choice of empirical treatment depends on these considerations:

(i) whether the patient has received prior antibiotic therapy or not;
(ii) whether the infection affects a native valve or a prosthesis (and, if so, when surgery was performed [early vs late PVE]);

In some centers, empiric therapy and blood culture negative infective endocarditis (BCNIE) treatments are different depending on whether they are community or nosocomial acquired (increased risk of staphylococcus and Fungi).

> **Protocol**
> (a) *Community-acquired NVE and late PVE (>1 year):*
>   *Amoxicillin 12 g/day + Gentamicin 3 mg/kg/day (one shot)*
> (b) *Early PVE (<1 year), Device-related IE :*
>   *Vancomycin 30 mg/kg/j + Gentamicin 3 mg/kg/day (one shot)*

Streptococci, Escherichia Coli, HACEK, Bartonella

These microorganisms are usually susceptible to ceftriaxone. The other advantage of ceftriaxone is its use in one single injection. The patients should be treated with ceftriaxone combined with aminoglycosides.

> **Protocol**
> Ceftriaxone 2 g/day (one shot) + Gentamicin 3 mg/kg/day (one shot)
> Duration: 4 weeks of ceftriaxone IV with 2 weeks of gentamicine IV.

Enterococci

Enterococci pose two major problems. First, enterococci are highly tolerant to antibiotic-induced killing, and eradication requires prolonged administration (up to 6 weeks) of synergistic bactericidal combinations of two cell wall-inhibitors (ampicillin plus ceftriaxone, which synergise by inhibiting complementary PBPs) or one cell wall-inhibitor with aminoglycosides. The eradication on PVE requires surgery. If it is not possible, we use a treatment by amoxicillin 3 g/day orally for 1 year to decrease the incidence of recurrence [5].

Protocol
Amoxicillin 12 g/day + Ceftriaxone 2 g/day (one shot)
Duration: 6 weeks of bitherapy IV

Coagulase Negative Staphylococci (CNS), Enterococci (Amoxicillin R)

Coagulase negative staphylococci are much less aggressive but are commonly resistant and may include different clones of different sensitivities. Some authors rely on antibiotic susceptibilities of isolated strains but this may neglect slower clones resistant betalactamines.

Some authors treated all cases with a combination of vancomycin + gentamicin [2]. There is no current evidence that alternative therapies are safer or more efficient.

Protocol
Vancomycin 30 mg/kg/day + Gentamicin 3 mg/kg/day (one shot)
Duration: CNS: 6 weeks IV with 7 days of gentamicin IV.

Staphylococcus Aureus

Staphylococcus aureus is a major killer in endocarditis, with a fatality rate greater than 20% in most series. Patients may die from septic shock, multiple organ failure, or cardiac failure. Oxacillin has been used for years as the mainstream *S. aureus* treatment. Recently, we reported a dramatic reduction of the fatality rate from *S. aureus* IE by using a combination of a high dose of cotrimoxazole intravenously for 7 days, then oral + clindamycin for 7 days. Failures with this protocol were associated with positive blood cultures after 24 h of treatment and the presence of intracardiac abscesses. There is no cotrimoxazole resistance to *S. aureus* in most places [6].

S. aureus PVE carries a very high risk of mortality (>45 %) and often requires early valve replacement.

The addition of rifampin must be take place when the blood cultures are positive after 24 h of treatment and in cardiac abscesses.

Adding the gentamicin aims to quickly sterilize blood culture in the case of positive persistence.

Protocol
Clindamycin: 1.8 g IV + trimethoprim/sulfamethoxazole: 12A IV (5 g/day of sulfamethoxazole)
3 systematic blood cultures after 24 hours.
If positive, add: Rifampin IV 1800 mg/day + gentamycin IV 3 mg/kg/day
Duration: 1 week
Blood culture control at 24 h
Duration: Clindamycin 7 days, trimethoprim/sulfamethoxazole 6 weeks (1 week IV and 5 weeks orally)

Fungi (Candida, Aspergillus)

Fungi are most frequently observed in PVE and in IE affecting IVDA and immunocompromised patients and in postoperative IE [7].

Protocol
Amphothericin B: 3 mg/kg/day IV
Duration: 2 months

Coxiella Burnetii

Protocol
Doxycycline (200 mg/day) plus Hydroxychloroquine (200–400 mg/day) orally for anti-phase 1 IgG <200 and IgA and IgM <50 [8]

Trophyrema Whipplei

Protocol
Doxycycline (200 mg/day) plus Hydroxychloroquine (200–400 mg/day) orally orally for >18 months [9]

Bartonella Spp

Protocol
Doxycycline: 100 mg/12 h orally for 4 weeks and gentamycin 3 mg/kg/day IV 2 weeks [10]

References

1. Thuny F, Grisoli D, Collart F, Habib G, Raoult D. Management of infective endocarditis: challenges and perspectives. Lancet. 2012;379(9819):965–75.
2. Botelho-Nevers E, Thuny F, Casalta JP, Richet H, Gouriet F, Collart F, Riberi A, Habib G, Raoult D. Dramatic reduction in infective endocarditis-related mortality with a management-based approach. Arch Intern Med. 2009;169(14):1290–8.
3. Thuny F, Giorgi R, Habachi R, Ansaldi S, Le Dolley Y, Casalta JP, Avierinos JF, Riberi A, Renard S, Collart F, Raoult D, Habib G. Excess mortality and morbidity in patients surviving infective endocarditis. Am Heart J. 2012;164(1):94–101.
4. Thuny F, Hubert S, Tribouilloy C, Le Dolley Y, Casalta JP, Riberi A, Chevalier F, Rusinaru D, Malaquin D, Remadi JP, Ammar AB, Avierinos JF, Collart F, Raoult D, Habib G. Sudden death in patients with infective endocarditis: findings from a large cohort study. Int J Cardiol. 2013;162(2):129–32. doi:10.1016/j.ijcard.2012.06.059.
5. Casalta JP, Thuny F, Fournier PE, Lepidi H, Habib G, Grisoli D, Raoult D. DNA persistence and relapses questions on the treatment strategies of Enterococcus infections of prosthetic valves. PLoS One. 2012;7(12):e53335.
6. Casalta JP, Zaratzian C, Hubert S, Thuny F, Gouriet F, Habib G, Grisoli D, Deharo JC, Raoult D. Treatment of Staphylococcus aureus endocarditis with high doses of trimethoprim/sulfamethoxazole and clindamycin-preliminary report. Int J Antimicrob Agents. 2013;42 (2):190–1.
7. Thuny F, Fournier PE, Casalta JP, Gouriet F, Lepidi H, Riberi A, Collart F, Habib G, Raoult D. Investigation of blood culture-negative early prosthetic valve endocarditis reveals high prevalence of fungi. Heart. 2010;96(10):743–7.
8. Raoult D, Houpikian P, Tissot Dupont H, Riss JM, Arditi-Djiane J, Brouqui P. Treatment of Q fever endocarditis: comparison of 2 regimens containing doxycycline and ofloxacin or hydroxychloroquine. Arch Intern Med. 1999;159(2):167–73.
9. Fenollar F, Célard M, Lagier JC, Lepidi H, Fournier PE, Raoult D. Tropheryma whipplei endocarditis. Emerg Infect Dis. 2013;19(11):1721–30.
10. Angelakis E, Raoult D. Pathogenicity and treatment of Bartonella infections. Int J Antimicrob Agents. 2014;44(1):16–25.

Chapter 21
Surgical Techniques in Infective Endocarditis

Alberto Riberi and Fréderic Collart

Introduction

Initially always lethal [1], the prognosis of IE has been revolutionized by the introduction of antibacterial therapy and by the development of valve surgery [2]. Nevertheless, this pathology remains a severe disease, with more than 30% of patients dying within the first year after diagnosis [3, 4]. During the last decade, a trend to be surgically more aggressive and precocious has developed, with promising results [5].

Lesions and Background

The valve's infection produces inflammation of tissues, resulting initially in oedematous thickening of the valve. The persistence of infection leads to necrosis of valve tissues, which results in valve dysfunction. The tissues infection can also produce fibrin deposits at the surface of the valve, called vegetation, which can migrate, producing embolism or obstruct the valve orifice. Vegetation may be isolated but more frequently are associates with others valve involvement. The ring involvement (paravalvular infection) results in abscess. Indeed, the annular destruction produces the formation of cavities due to destruction of annular tissues and the edges of adjacent structures, the arterial or ventricular wall, depending on localisation of the lesion (Figs. 21.1 and 21.2). Under the influence of blood pressure, the weakened tissue may rupture causing a contained extravasations with formation of a false aneurysm or a fistula if the annular rupture produces a communication with another cardiac chamber or vessel (Figs. 21.3 and 21.4).

A. Riberi, MD (✉) • F. Collart, MD
Department of Cardiac Surgery, La Timone Hospital, Marseille, France
e-mail: Alberto.riberi@ap-hm.fr; Frederic.collart@ap-hm.fr

© Springer International Publishing Switzerland 2016
G. Habib (ed.), *Infective Endocarditis*, DOI 10.1007/978-3-319-32432-6_21

Fig. 21.1 Aortic IE. Surgical view of the aortic root after debridement of lesions. Resection of the aortic valve and root. Detachment of coronary arteries. *Straight dashed*: intertrigonal space; *Curve dashed*: aortic ring; *1*: Left main trunk; *2*: Kissing lesion (anterior mitral leaflet); *3*: Right main trunk; *4*: Intertrigonal abscess and involvement of the base of the anterior mitral leaflet

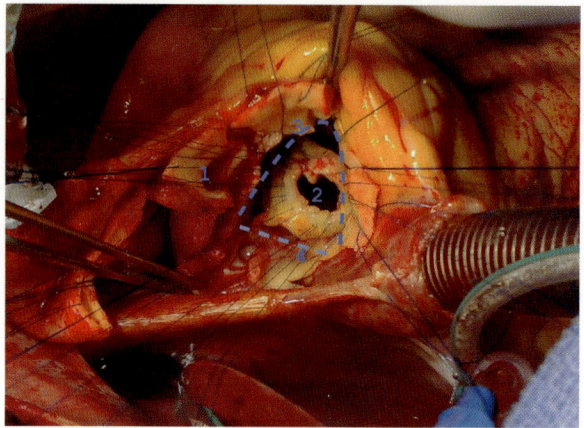

Fig. 21.2 Surgical view of the aortic root. The intertrigonal space and the mitral lesion were reconstructed with a tanned pericardial patch. *Dashed line*: aortic ring; *1*: Left main trunk; *2*: Right main trunk; *3*: Pericardial patch in the intertrigonal space; *4*: "Kissing lesion" of the mitral valve repaired. The aortic root was replaced by an aortic allograft

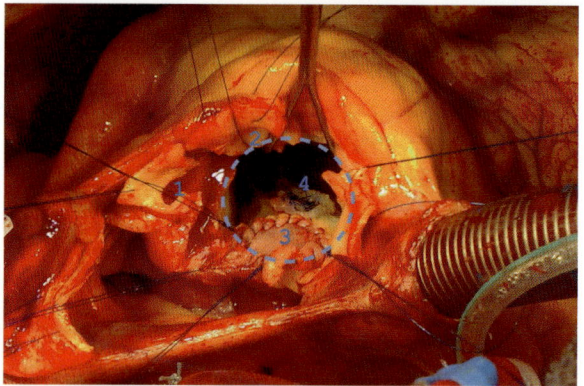

Fig. 21.3 Surgical view of the aortic valve. Aortic-atrial fistulae. Aortic valve IE with destruction of the intertrigonal space, the aortic wall of the non-coronary sinus of Valsalva and the adjacent wall of the left atrium. *AV* aortic valve, *AML* anterior mitral leaflet, *LA* left atrium

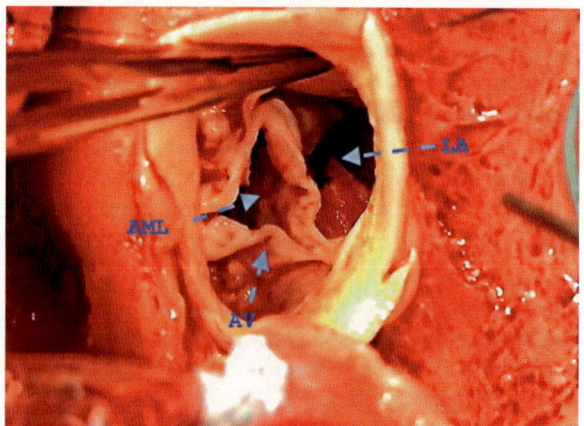

Fig. 21.4 Surgical view of the aortic root. After debridement of lesions, resection of the aortic valve, root and detachment of coronaries arteries, the reconstruction of the aortic ring is carried out with a pericardial patch, sutured at the base of the anterior mitral leaflet and the left atrium wall. The aortic root was replaced with an aortic allograft. *Dashed line*: aortic ring; *AML* anterior mitral leaflet, *LCA* left coronary artery, *RCA* right coronary artery

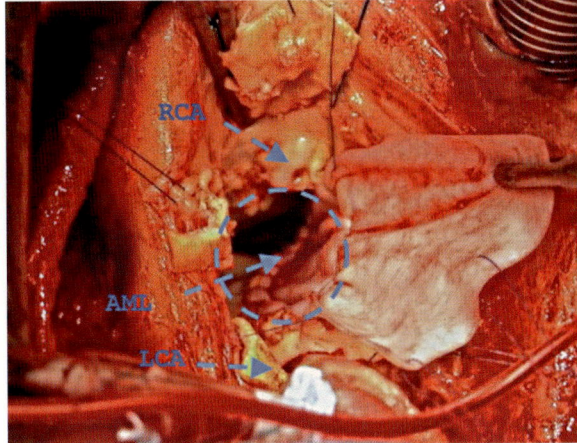

Fifty percent of patients affected by IE need surgical treatment because infection can produce valve lesions leading to valve dysfunction resulting in cardiac failure [6–8]. The cardiac insufficiency is frequently due to aortic or mitral regurgitation [8, 9]. Seldom is cardiac insufficiency secondary to valve obstruction by vegetations [10].

Infection can occur on healthy, pathological valves or prosthesis (Fig. 21.5). The aortic valve is involved in 40 % and the mitral valve in 45 %. The aortic valve required a surgical treatment more frequently, giving the false impression of being more often affected [11]. In 25 % of cases, there is a multivalvular involvement [6]. The aortic insufficiency may produce a mitral regurgitation by perforation of the anterior mitral leaflet secondary to the aortic regurgitation's flow (kissing lesion) [12] (Fig. 21.1).

In patients with valve prostheses, the regurgitation is secondary to the weakness of the valve ring by the infection and a leakage in the interface between the prosthetic and native ring that results in regurgitation.

Ring involvements are more frequently present in prosthetic IE, resulting in a higher rate of annular destruction (abscess). Sometimes the aortic or mitral insufficiency is due to the rupture of a cusp of a bioprostheses without paravalvular leakage [12].

A persistent sepsis in spite of an appropriate antibiotic treatment is due to an extravalvular extension of the infection and represents a mandatory indication for early surgery in infective endocarditis [8]. Indeed, excepting iatrogenic problems, such as inadequate antimicrobial treatment or a catheter's infection, persistent sepsis is the result of formation of an abscess, a false aneurysm, or a fistula [13, 14].

Abscess and false aneurysm are more frequently associated in aortic valve endocarditis and are often localised in the inter-trigonal space (10–40 %) [14].

Mitral abscess rarely presents in native mitral valve endocarditis, and it is localised in the inferior part of the valve ring [15, 16].

Fig. 21.5 Aortic
prosthetic IE. Surgical
view of the aortic valve.
Infective involvement
(*arrow*) of an aortic
prosthesis

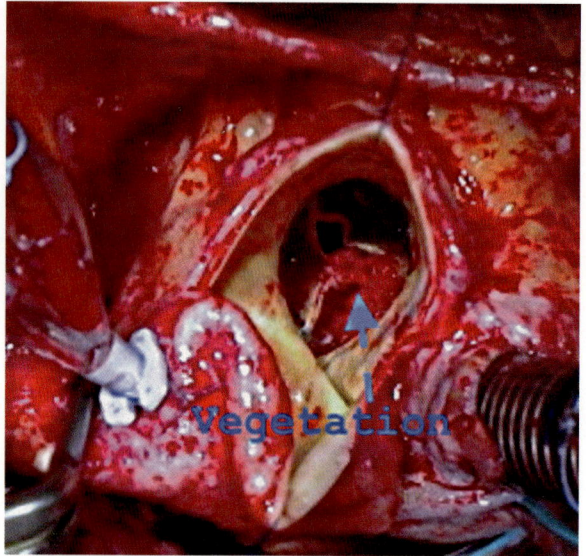

Surgical Procedures

The goals of surgical treatment in IE are to eradicate infected and necrotic tissues as well as to exclude neocavities (false aneurysm, abscess) and to restore the anatomy to preserve the valve function or to allow a prosthetic valve replacement.

Aortic Valve Endocarditis

Aortic Valve Repair

Aortic valve sparing or reconstruction is rarely possible, mostly in early surgery for IE. Patients in whom early surgery is necessary in order to avoid embolism may have had a removal of vegetation and reconstruction of the aortic cusp. Even if aortic valve repair with glutaraldhayde fixed pericardium for aortic regurgitation has been used for many decades, reported results are suboptimal [17, 18].

Aortic valve repair has been shown to be an alternative to aortic valve replacement in selected patients [19, 20]. Best results are obtained in the tricuspid aortic valve, when the free margin of the cusp is devoid of infection, and when the defect after resection can be corrected with a patch less than 10 mm. in diameter [21, 22].

Aortic Valve Replacement

When lesions are circumscribed to the native aortic valve, the aortic valve replacement is the standard treatment. In cases with ring involvement, radical debridement must be done in order to obtain healthy borders that can be directly sutured, for larger defects autologous or bovine glutaraldheyde fixed pericardium patch are needed to reinforce the ring reconstruction. The reconstruction is carried out by the suture of the aortic wall to the ventricular muscle or the intertrigonal space depending of the localisation of annular lesion. This kind of repair excludes abscess and false aneurysm of circulation and provides a strong fixation point to anchor prosthesis.

This approach of aortic IE with isolated valve involvement or with limited annular lesion provides immediately and long terms good results [11, 23].

The choice of valve prosthesis in native valve IE and prosthetic valve IE (PVE) remains controversial [16, 24–26]. Owing to the nature of the disease, it has not been possible to conduct randomized trials. Several authors have shown that the type of prosthesis used is not an important factor in achieving good early and long-term results if adequate debridement of infected tissue can be achieved and appropriate antibiotic treatment is administered. The choice of valve prosthesis (mechanical versus tissue) should be based on age, patient compliance with anticoagulation, life expectancy, and the presence of comorbidities. A bioprosthetic valve may be implanted at age more than 60 years if no other comorbidities are present [16, 24, 25, 27].

In patients in whom the risk of reinfection is high, such as in drug addict patients [28], the aortic valve replacement with aortic allograft yields better results than prosthesis [29]. Some studies have shown that the rate of reinfection is lower in patients who have undergone an aortic valve replacement with an allograft, suggesting that allograft is more resistant to infection than prosthesis [30–32]. Indeed, the risk for reinfection after an aortic valve replacement with prosthesis is higher in the first months following the surgical procedure (initial phenomenon), whereas the risk is low when allograft is utilised [30–32]. Although the reasons are not elucidated, the whole biological surface, the viability of allograft tissue, and low gradient obtained after aortic valve replacement by allograft, avoiding turbulence, seem to be the main reasons for the greater resistance to infection. In contrast, longevity (particularly in young patients), availability (mostly when surgical procedures are carried out in an emergency setting), and technical problems during a re-operation must temper the use of allograft.

Prosthetic Aortic Valve Endocarditis

When infectious involvement is limited to the aortic prosthesis with no major lesion concerning the aortic ring, the annular debridement and reconstruction should be done as described previously, followed of an aortic valve replacement. Replacement done with tissue or mechanical prosthesis yields the same immediate and long-term results [16, 25, 26, 29]. However, the STS database (Society of Thoracic Surgeons) shows a reversed trend concerning prosthetic aortic valve replacement for aortic IE, with a mechanical/biological prostheses ratio 1/2 in 2007 whereas it was 2/1 in 1994 [11].

Native or Prosthetic Aortic Valve Endocarditis with Extended Lesions of the Aortic Ring

An early surgical treatment is more frequently mandatory in patients with an aortic abscess than in isolated aortic valve involvement (87 versus 50 %) [33]. In circular destruction of the aortic ring as well as in lesions near to the coronaries ostia, in which repair can compromise the coronary circulation, is difficult to restore a strong structure in order to anchor a valve prosthesis. The aortic root replacement is the best option.

Under these conditions, the aortic root replacement is a technical challenge. The use of cryopreserved aortic allograft has some advantages. The flexibility of allograft tissue allows the achievement of suture without tension, which is important in the manipulation of weakened tissues. The allograft tissue (anterior mitral leaflet, aortic wall) can be used to reconstruct or reinforce left ventricular outflow. Moreover, allograft is more resistant to infection, as the majority of homograft series report a recurrent endocarditis rate less than 8 % [30–32]. The longevity of allograft is the same as that of bioprosthesis in aortic position.

The rate of reintervention's mortality after allograft valve or root replacement has been reported to be similar to that of bioprosthesis by some authors [34, 35]. In contrast, a significantly increased mortality has been observed in others studies [36].

Stentless bioprosthesis is an alternative to allograft in patients with aortic IE: they have the same flexibility, allowing safe suture. Moreover, large sizes are available, which is an advantage mostly for aortic rings larger than 25. In contrast, their resistance to infections is similar to bioprosthesis, and reinterventions can be as difficult [37, 38].

A recent study comparing allograft to composite tubes in IE reports similar immediate and long term results [39]. The Ross procedure may be useful in young patients where the degeneration and calcification of aortic allograft will expose the patients to a reoperative aortic root procedure [11].

In summary, when early surgery is mandatory in aortic IE, the aortic valve replacement is the standard treatment. In cases with limited annular involvement, reconstruction of the aortic ring and aortic valve replacement are safe treatments and get good immediate and long-term results. When a huge annular lesion exists aortic root replacement is the best option.

The utilisation of allograft and stentless bioprosthesis has been reported to offer advantages when compared with stented prosthesis [11].

Mitral Valve Endocarditis

The mitral valve is affected in 45 % of infective endocarditis, but only in 35 % is surgical treatment necessary [33]. The mitral valve IE is associated with an aortic valve involvement in 21 % of patients [40].

The surgical treatment of mitral valve endocarditis is primarily determined by disease severity and valvular and annular destruction. Advanced valvular and annular disease requires complete excision and mitral valve replacement (MVR) [16, 25–27, 41]. If the disease is limited to the valvular tissue, mitral valve repair is the preferred surgical option [42–44].

Mitral Valve Repair

Mitral valve repair is the optimal treatment for mitral IE. The rate for mitral reconstruction in mitral IE is reported as between 40 and 90 %, depending upon surgical experience and the rate of acute versus healed lesions [44, 45].

A North American survey including 2654 patients reported 16 % of mitral repair in patients treated in the acute phase of mitral IE and 41 % for healed lesions [41]. The STS database shows a significant increase in mitral repair for mitral IE, which went from 25 % in 1994 to 40 % in 2006 [11].

In a meta-analysis including 24 studies concerning 724 MVR and 470 mitral valve repairs, the authors reported superior event-free survival and lower in-hospital mortality for mitral valve repair compared with MVR [45]. In a French study concerning 37 patients undergoing a mitral repair in acute phase mitral IE, operative mortality was 3 % [43]. Kerchove reported an operative mortality of 4.8 % when patients were in stage I or II NYHA. The overall mortality was 17.5 %. The rate for freedom from re-intervention at 5 and 10 years was 89 % and 72 % respectively [46].

However, patients undergoing a MVR are thought to have more serious involvement of the mitral valve and mitral ring and to be more seriously ill than those undergoing a mitral repair, resulting in an increasing mortality and morbidity.

Lesions

Mitral IE may occur in previous abnormal valves with pre-existent dysfunction or in normal valves.

Anterior Mitral Leaflet

Isolated lesions of the body of the anterior mitral leaflet are prone to be repaired. Indeed, if lesions respect the free border of the leaflet, debridement and resection of the margin of the lesion followed by suture of a tanned autologous or bovine pericardial patch meet with good results. This type of lesion may be associated with an aortic regurgitation (kissing lesion) (Figs. 21.1 and 21.2) and repair can be done through the aortic orifice.

When there is no aortic dysfunction associated or when other involvements of the mitral valve--such lesion of chordae, posterior leaflet or mitral ring—exist, the atriotomy is the standard approach.

When the free margin of the anterior leaflet is involved with chordae rupture, repair is more challenging. A transfer of chordae from the posterior leaflet can be done. Repair is difficult when chordae rupture is associated with a huge destruction of the free edge of the anterior leaflet, especially on A2; under these conditions, mitral valve replacement should be considered.

Commissural Lesions

In commissural lesions of the mitral valve, debridement and resection of infected tissues followed by reconstruction by sliding plasty, or annular plicature are frequently feasible.

Sliding plasty is preferred in the anterior commisure, since annular plication may produce an obstruction of the circumflex artery.

Posterior Mitral Leaflet

When IE involves the posterior leaflet, repair can be frequently achieved. In circumscribed lesions without involvement of the free margin of the valve, repair with a patch of tanned pericardium is a safe solution. When the free margin and chordae are involved, a classical quadrangular resection with sliding plasty or annular plication can be done (Fig. 21.6). In cases of extensive destruction of the posterior mitral leaflet with huge loss of substance, reconstruction is more difficult, and large pericardial patch and neochordae are necessary. Even if immediate results are satisfactory, mid-term results are suboptimal; therefore, mitral valve replacement must be considered.

When IE involvement arises in a previously compromised mitral valve, reconstruction may be very laborious, particularly in rheumatic diseases or in advanced degenerative mitral valve disease in which mitral valve replacement is the best solution (Figs. 21.7 and 21.8).

A prosthetic annuloplasty ring may be necessary to achieve satisfactory repair during complex reconstruction [43, 47] and is well tolerated, with a low reinfection rate [43]. As an alternative, some authors have proposed using a strip of bovine or autologous glutaraldehyde- treated pericardium [46].

Mitral Valve Replacement (MVR)

Extensive involvement of the mitral valve and ring can require a mitral valve replacement; see previous discussion in this chapter.

Annular, abscesses are infrequent in native valve IE, but when they exist they are situated in the posterior part of the mitral ring. Abscesses in the intertrigonal space are almost always associated with the involvement of the aortic valve; see previous discussion in this chapter. Mitral valve replacement is carried out in the usual way.

Fig. 21.6 Surgical view
of the mitral valve.
Infective involvement of
P2.P1, P2, P3: posterior
mitral leaflet. Mitral valve
reconstruction: resection
of infective lesion (*P2*)
and sliding plasty

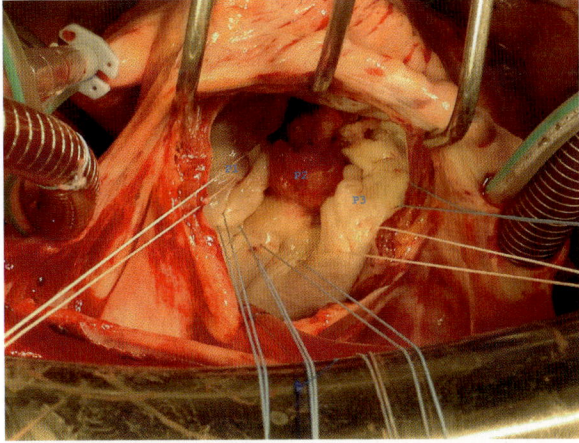

Fig. 21.7 Rheumatic
mitral valve with infective
lesion of the internal
commissure. *AL* anterior
mitral leaflet, *PL* posterior
mitral leaflet, *1*: infective
lesion

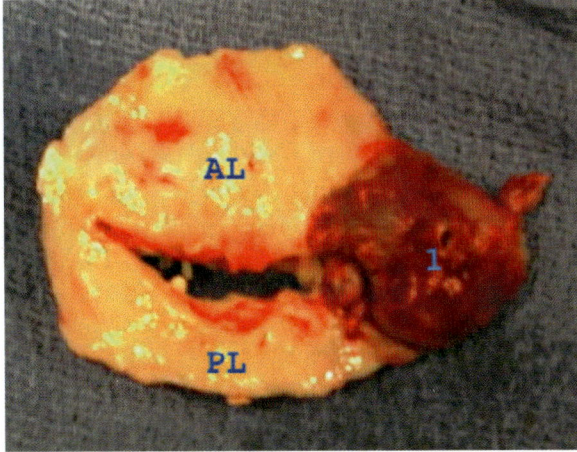

The mitral ring abscess is difficult because, even repaired, it represents a weak zone prone to desertion of the prosthesis. In mitral prosthetic IE, annular involvement is more frequently encountered and can be situated everywhere (anterior or posterior part of the mitral ring). The repair of an annular abscess is done by debridement of the lesion and reconstruction by suturing the atria to the ventricular wall. Both mechanical and bioprosthetic valves have been used in mitral valve replacement [16, 25, 41]. Although a few authors use mechanical valves almost exclusively [26, 48], the majority use both bioprosthetic and mechanical valves, with similar survival rates and freedom from reinfection [16, 25]. The risk of reoperation, however, appears to be higher among patients with tissue valve replacement [16, 24, 25]. The 5-year survival after MVR for native valve endocarditis ranges between 66 and 87 % [25, 43, 47]. Overall, valve choice should be individualized according to age, life expectancy, and presence of comorbidities.

Fig. 21.8 Surgical view of the mitral valve. Infective endocarditis of the mitral valve with degenerative disease. Extended infectious lesion of the anterior and posterior mitral leaflet. *AV* anterior mitral leaflet, *PV* posterior mitral leaflet

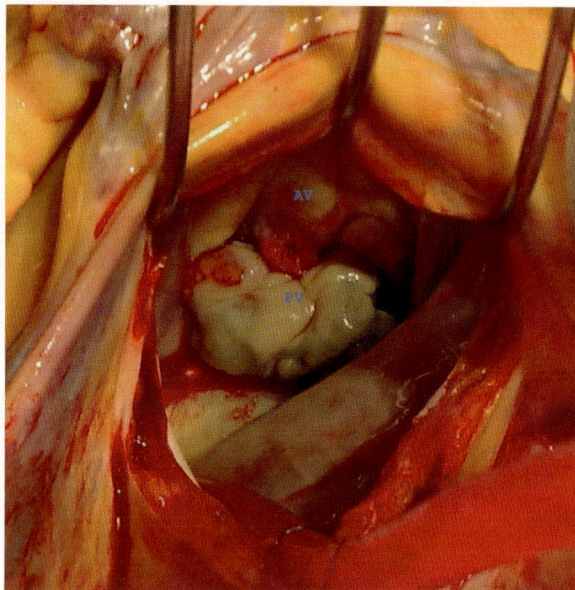

Right Sided Infective Endocarditis

Tricuspid valve IE and, rarely, pulmonary valve IE are observed in IV drug-addicts and in patients with pacemakers. The incidence varies between 5 and 10 % according to the literature [49, 50]. Surgical treatment is mandatory in patients with right cardiac failure in spite of diuretics treatment, in patients under antimicrobial treatment with persistent large vegetations (>20 mm.), and in patients with sepsis. Surgical treatment of tricuspid IE must spare the valve because a prosthetic replacement predisposes to re-infection, especially in IV drug-addict patients.

The surgical removal of the tricuspid valve [51] (Arbalu procedure) without replacement has been advocated but may be associated with severe post-operative right heart failure, particularly in patients with elevated pulmonary arterial pressure, which is often the case after multiple pulmonary emboli. It may be performed in extreme cases, but the valve should be subsequently replaced once the infection has been cured [51]. Mitral allograft has been reported as a useful alternative for tricuspid valve replacement with encouraging results [52]. Pulmonary valve IE is very infrequent. When pulmonary valve replacement is necessary, the use of pulmonary allograft is the best choice [31].

Operative mortality after treatment of right sided IE is less than 5 % [25], except in patients with uncontrolled sepsis and septic shock, in whom mortality is higher [53]. Mild and long term results are closely correlated with patient background.

Multiple Valve Endocarditis

Between 10 and 25 % of patients with infective endocarditis need repair and/or replacement of two or three valves [11]. The more frequent association is the mitro-aortic involvement. The approach in case of multiple valve involvement is the same as described previously. In case of mitro-aortic native IE, repairing the mitral valve with an aortic valve replacement whenever possible is an optimal treatment, just as in tricuspid and mitral involvement the repair of two valves must be done whenever possible. In patients with mitro-aortic prosthetic valve IE, a double valve replacement is the standard treatment. The patient's background must be considered when considering tissue or mechanical prosthesis [11]. When the mitro-aortic curtain is involved, reconstruction followed by mitro-aortic valve replacement is a difficult procedure resulting in to high morbidity and mortality [36, 54]. As an alternative to this challenging situation, reconstruction and replacement with an "in bloc mitro-aortic allograft" has been reported with promising results; however, this approach must be reserved for extreme patients [55].

Conclusion

The progress made in clinical diagnosis, imaging, antimicrobial treatment, and post- operative care has enabled the surgical treatment of patients who are more seriously ill. At present, adapted solutions can be realised in each situation. Conservative surgical treatment should take place when possible, especially for the atrioventricular valves. When a prosthetic valve replacement is necessary, the type of prosthesis (tissue or mechanical) has no influence on results and must be adapted depending on a patient's background. Despite advances, the morbidity and mortality of IE remains high, and improvements need to occur in order to optimise results.

References

1. Osler W. The gulstonian lectures, on malignant endocarditis. Br Med J. 1885;1:467–70.
2. Thuny F, Grisoli D, Collart F, Habib G, Raoult D. Management of infective endocarditis: challenges and perspectives. Lancet. 2012;379:965–75.
3. Cabell CH, Jollis JG, Peterson GE, Corey GR, et al. Changing patient characteristics and the effect on mortality in endocarditis. Arch Intern Med. 2002;162:90–4.
4. Thuny F, Di Salvo G, Belliard O, Avierinos JF, et al. Risk of embolism and death in infective endocarditis: prognostic value of echocardiography: a prospective multicenter study. Circulation. 2005;112:69–75.
5. Kang DH, Kim YJ, Kim SH, Sun BJ, et al. Early surgery versus conventional treatment for infective endocarditis. N Engl J Med. 2012;366:2466–73.
6. Revilla A, Lopez J, Vilacosta I, Villacorta E, et al. Clinical and prognostic profile of patients with infective endocarditis who need urgent surgery. Eur Heart J. 2007;28:65–71.

7. Thuny F, Beurtheret S, Mancini J, Gariboldi V, et al. The timing of surgery influences mortality and morbidity in adults with severe complicated infective endocarditis: a propensity analysis. Eur Heart J. 2011;32(16):2027–33.

8. Tornos P, Iung B, Permanyer-Miralda G, Baron G, et al. Infective endocarditis in Europe: lessons from the Euro heart survey. Heart. 2005;91:571–5.

9. Durack DT, Lukes AS, Bright DK. New criteria for diagnosis of infective endo- carditis: utilization of specific echocardiographic findings. Duke endocarditis service. Am J Med. 1994; 96:200–9.

10. Baddour LM, Wilson WR, Bayer AS, Fowler Jr VG, et al. Infective endocarditis: diagnosis, antimicrobial therapy, and management of complications: a statement for healthcare professionals from the Committee on Rheumatic Fever, Endocarditis, and Kawasaki Disease, Council on Cardiovascular Disease in the Young, and the Councils on Clinical Cardiology, Stroke, and Cardiovascular Surgery and Anesthesia, American Heart Association: endorsed by the Infectious Diseases Society of America. Circulation. 2005;111:394–434.

11. Byrne JG, Rezai K, Sanchez JA, Bernstein RA, et al. MSHA surgical management of endocarditis: the society of thoracic surgeons clinical practice guideline. Ann Thorac Surg. 2011; 91:2012–9.

12. Piper C, Hetzer R, Korfer R, Bergemann R, Horstkotte D. The importance of secondary mitral valve involvement in primary aortic valve endocarditis; the mitral kissing vegetation. Eur Heart J. 2002;23:79–86.

13. Anguera I, Miro JM, Evangelista A, Cabell CH, et al. Peri- annular complications in infective endocarditis involving native aortic valves. Am J Cardiol. 2006;98:1254–60.

14. Anguera I, Miro JM, San Roman JA, de Alarcon A, et al. Periannular complications in infective endocarditis involving prosthe- tic aortic valves. Am J Cardiol. 2006;98:1261–8.

15. Anguera I, Miro JM, Vilacosta I, Almirante B, et al. Aorto-cavitary fistulous tract formation in infective endocarditis: clinical and echocardiographic features of 76 cases and risk factors for mortality. Eur Heart J. 2005;26:288–97.

16. David TE, Gavra G, Feindel CM, Regesta T, Armstrong S, Maganti MD. Surgical treatment of active infective endocar- ditis: a continued challenge. J Thorac Cardiovasc Surg. 2007;133: 144–9.

17. Duran CM, Alonso J, Gaite L, Alonso C, Cagigas JC, Marce L, et al. Long-term results of conservative repair of rheumatic aortic valve insufficiency. Eur J Cardiothorac Surg. 1988; 2:217–23.

18. El Halees Z, Al Shahid M, Al Sanei A, Sallehuddin A, Duran C. Up to 16 years follow-up of aortic valve reconstruction with pericardium: a stent- less readily available cheap valve? Eur J Cardiothorac Surg. 2005;28:200–5.

19. Aicher D, Kunihara T, Abou Issa O, Brittner B, Gräber S, Schäfers HJ. Valve configuration determines long-term results after repair of the bi- cuspid aortic valve. Circulation. 2011;123: 178–85.

20. Boodhwani M, de Kerchove L, Glineur D, Poncelet A, Rubay J, Astarci P, et al. Repair-oriented classification of aortic insufficiency: impact on sur- gical techniques and clinical outcomes. J Thorac Cardiovasc Surg. 2009;137:286–94.

21. Chen X, Gu F, Xie D. An alternative surgical approach for aortic infective endocarditis: vegetectomy. Eur J Cardiothorac Surg. 2009;35:1096–8.

22. Mayer K, Aircher D, Feldner S, Kunihara T, Schäfers HJ. Repair versus replacement of the aortic valve in active infective endocarditis. Eur J Cardiothorac Surg. 2012;42:122–7.

23. Avierinos J, Thuny F, Chalvignac V, Giorgi R, et al. Surgical treatment of active aortic endocarditis: homografts are not the cornerstone of outcome. Ann Thorac Surg. 2007;84:1935–42.

24. Moon MR, Miller DC, Moore KA, et al. Treatment of endocarditis with valve replacement: the question of tissue versus mechanical prosthesis. Ann Thorac Surg. 2001;71:1164–71.

25. Alexiou C, Langley SM, Stafford H, Haw MP, Livesey SA, Monro JL. Surgical treatment of infective mitral valve endocarditis: predictors of early and late outcome. J Heart Valve Dis. 2000;9:327–34.

26. Guerra JM, Tornos MP, Permanyer-Miralda G, Almirante B, Murtra M, Soler-Soler J. Long-term results of mechanical prostheses for treatment of active infective endocarditis. Heart. 2001;86:63–8.
27. Delay D, Pellerin M, Carrier M, et al. Immediate and long-term results of valve replacement for native and prosthetic valve endocarditis. Ann Thorac Surg. 2000;70:1219–23.
28. Kaiser SP, Melby SJ, Zierer A, et al. Long-term outcomes in valve replacement surgery for infective endocarditis. Ann Thorac Surg. 2007;83:30–5.
29. Gulbins H, Kilian E, Roth S, Uhlig A, Kreuzer E, Reichart B. Is there an advantage in using homografts in patients with acute infective endocarditis of the aortic valve? J Heart Valve Dis. 2002;11:492–7.
30. Grinda JM, Mainardi JL, D'Attellis N, et al. Cryopreserved aortic viable homograft for active aortic endocarditis. Ann Thorac Surg. 2005;79:767–71.
31. Metras D, Angell W, Goffin Y, Gonzalez-Lanvin L, Habib G, et al. Allogreffes et autogreffes valvulaires cardiaques. Paris/Milan/Barcelona: Edition Masson; 1995.
32. Yankah AC, Klose H, Petzina R, Musci M, Siniawski H, Hetzer R. Surgical management of acute aortic root endocarditis with viable homograft: 13-year experience. Eur J Cardiothorac Surg. 2002;21:260–7.
33. Habib G, Hoen B, Tornos P, Thuny F, et al. Guidelines on the prevention, diagnosis, and treatment of infective endocarditis (new version 2009): the task force on the prevention, diagnosis, and treatment of infective endocarditis of the european society of cardiology (esc). Endorsed by the european society of clinical microbiology and infectious diseases (escmid) and the international society of chemotherapy (isc) for infection and cancer. Eur Heart J. 2009;30:2369–413.
34. Kowert A, Vogt F, Beiras-Fernandez A, Reichart B, Kilian E. Outcome after homograft redo operation in aortic position. Eur J Cardio Thoracic Surg. 2012;41(2):404–8.
35. Nowicki ER, Pettersson GB, Smedira NG, Roselli EE, Blackstone EH, Lytle BW. Aortic allograft valve reoperation: surgical challenges and patient risks. Ann Thorac Surg. 2008; 86:761–8.
36. Kaya A, Schepens MA, Morshuis WJ, Heijmen RH, De La Riviere AB, Dossche KM. Cardiovascular valve-related events after aortic root replacement with cryopreserved aortic homografts. Ann Thorac Surg. 2005;79:1491–5.
37. Heinz A, Dumfarth J, Ruttmann-Ulmer E, Grimm M, Müller LC. Freestyle root replacement for complex destructive aortic valve endocarditis. J Thorac Cardiovasc Surg. 2014;147(4): 1265–70.
38. Muller LC, Chevtchik O, Bonatti JO, Muller S, Fille M, Laufer G. Treatment of destructive aortic valve endocarditis with the freestyle aortic root bioprosthesis. Ann Thorac Surg. 2003;75:453–6.
39. Singh Jassar A, Bavaria JE, Szeto WY, Moeller PJ, et al. Graft selection for aortic root replacement in complex active endocarditis: does it matter? Ann Thorac Surg. 2012;93:480–8.
40. Horstkotte D, Follath F, Gutschik E, Lengyel M, et al. Guidelines on prevention, diagnosis and treatment of infective endocarditis executive summary; the task force on infective endocarditis of the European society of cardiology. Eur Heart J. 2004;25:267–76.
41. Gammie JS, O'Brien SM, Griffith BP, Peterson ED. Surgical treatment of mitral valve endocarditis in North America. Ann Thorac Surg. 2005;80:2199–204.
42. Iung B, Rousseau-Paziaud J, Cormier B, et al. Contemporary results of mitral valve repair for infective endocarditis. J Am Coll Cardiol. 2004;43:386–92.
43. Zegdi R, Debieche M, Latremouille C, et al. Long-term results of mitral valve repair in active endocarditis. Circulation. 2005;111:2532–6.
44. Mihaljevic T, Paul S, Leacche M, et al. Tailored surgical therapy for acute native mitral valve endocarditis. J Heart Valve Dis. 2004;13:210–6.
45. Feringa HH, Shaw LJ, Poldermans D, et al. Mitral valve repair and replacement in endocarditis: a systematic review of literature. Ann Thorac Surg. 2007;83:564–70.
46. Kerchove L, Vanoverschelde JL, Poncelet A, et al. Reconstructive surgery in active mitral valve endocarditis: feasibility, safety and durability. Eur J Cardiothorac Surg. 2007;31:592–9.

47. Ruttmann E, Legit C, Poelzl G, et al. Mitral valve repair provides improved outcome over replacement in active infective endocarditis. J Thorac Cardiovasc Surg. 2005;130:765–71.
48. Murashita T, Sugiki H, Kamikubo Y, Yasuda K. Surgical results for active endocarditis with prosthetic valve replacement: impact of culture-negative endocarditis on early and late outcomes. Eur J Cardiothorac Surg. 2004;26:1104–11.
49. Frontera JA, Gradon JD. Right-side endocarditis in injection drug users: review of proposed mechanisms of pathogenesis. Clin Infect Dis. 2000;30:374–9.
50. Wilson LE, Thomas DL, Astemborski J, Freedman TL, Vlahov D. Prospective study of infective endocarditis among injection drug users. J Infect Dis. 2002;185:1761–6.
51. Arbulu A, Holmes RJ, Asfaw I. Surgical treatment of intractable right-sided infec- tive endocarditis in drug addicts: 25 years experience. J Heart Valve Dis. 1993;2:129–37; discussion 138–139.
52. Mestres CA, Miro JM, Pare JC, Pomar JL. Six-year experience with cryopreserved mitral homografts in the treatment of tricuspid valve endocarditis in HIV-infected drug addicts. J Heart Valve Dis. 1999;8:575–7.
53. Gelsomino S, Maessen JG, van der Veen F, Livi U, et al. Emergency surgery for native mitral valve endocarditis: the impact of septic and cardiogenic shock. Ann Thorac Surg. 2012; 93:1469–76.
54. Davierwalaa PM, Binnera C, Subramaniana S, Luehra M, et al. Double valve replacement and reconstruction of the intervalvular fibrous body in patients with active infective endocarditis. Eur J Cardiothorac Surg. 2014;45(1):146–52.
55. Obadia JF, Raisky O, Sebbag L, Chocron S, Saroul C, Chassignolle JF. Monobloc aorto-mitral homograft as a treatment of complex cases of endocarditis. J Thorac Cardiovasc Surg. 2001;121:584–6.

Chapter 22
Guidelines for When to Operate in Infective Endocarditis

Gilbert Habib

Surgical treatment is used in approximately half of patients with IE because of severe complications [1]. Early surgery, i.e., performed while the patient is still receiving antibiotic treatment, aims to avoid progressive HF and irreversible structural damage caused by severe infection and to prevent systemic embolism [1–6]. The risk of early surgery is the potential risk of postoperative deterioration in unstable patients and of relapse or recurrence if surgery is performed too early, before complete action of antibiotic therapy.

For the first time, the ESC guidelines published in 2009 introduced the notion of optimal timing of surgery [7]. Recently published, the 2015 version confirmed the crucial importance of the correct selection of the optimal timing for surgery [8]. In some cases, surgery needs to be performed on an emergency (within 24 h) or urgent (within a few days) basis, irrespective of the duration of antibiotic treatment. In other cases, surgery can be postponed to allow 1 or 2 weeks of antibiotic treatment under careful clinical and echocardiographic observation before an elective surgical procedure is performed [6–9].

The three main indications for early surgery in IE are HF, uncontrolled infection, and prevention of embolic events (Table 22.1).

Heart Failure

Hemodynamic complications have been extensively described in Chap. 9. HF is the most frequent complication of IE and represents the most common indication for surgery in IE [1]. HF is observed in 42–60 % of cases of NVE and is more often present when IE affects the aortic rather than the mitral valve [3, 9, 10]. Moderate-to-severe HF is the most important predictor of in-hospital, 6-month, and 1 year

G. Habib, MD, FESC
Cardiology Department, Hôpital La Timone, Marseille, France
e-mail: Gilbert.habib3@gmail.com

© Springer International Publishing Switzerland 2016
G. Habib (ed.), *Infective Endocarditis*, DOI 10.1007/978-3-319-32432-6_22

Table 22.1 Indications and timing of surgery in left-sided valve infective endocarditis (native valve endocarditis and prosthetic valve endocarditis)

Indications for surgery	Timing	Class	Level
1. Heart Failure			
Aortic or mitral NVE or PVE with severe acute regurgitation, obstruction or fistula causing refractory pulmonary oedema or cardiogenic shock	Emergency	I	B
Aortic or mitral NVE or PVE with severe regurgitation or obstruction causing symptoms of HF or echocardiographic signs of poor haemodynamic tolerance	Urgent	I	B
2. Uncontrolled infection			
Locally uncontrolled infection (abscess, false aneurysm, fistula, enlarging vegetation)	Urgent	I	B
Infection caused by fungi or multiresistant organisms	Urgent/elective	I	C
Persisting positive blood cultures despite appropriate antibiotic therapy and adequate control of septic metastatic foci	Urgent	IIa	B
PVE caused by staphylococci or non-HACEK Gram negative bacteria	Urgent/elective	IIa	C
3. Prevention of embolism			
Aortic or mitral NVE or PVE with persistent vegetations >10 mm after one or more embolic episode despite appropriate antibiotic therapy	Urgent	I	B
Aortic or mitral NVE with vegetations >10 mm, associated with severe valve stenosis or regurgitation, and low operative risk	Urgent	IIa	B
Aortic or mitral NVE or PVE with isolated very large vegetations (>30 mm)	Urgent	IIa	B
Aortic or mitral NVE or PVE with isolated large vegetations (>15 mm) and no other indication for surgery	Urgent	IIb	C

From Habib et al. [8]. Used with permission of Oxford University Press
Emergency surgery: surgery performed within 24 h; urgent surgery: within a few days; elective surgery: after at least 1–2 weeks of antibiotic therapy
HACEK Haemophilus parainfluenzae, Haemophilus aphrophilus, Haemophilus paraphrophilus, Haemophilus influenzae, Actinobacillus actinomycetemcomitans, Cardiobacterium hominis, Eikenella corrodens, Kingella kingae and Kingella denitrificans, HF heart failure, IE infective endocarditis, NVE native valve endocarditis, PVE prosthetic valve endocarditis

mortality [3, 10–15]. Identification of surgical candidates and timing of surgery should be made by the infective endocarditis team [8]. Urgent surgery should be performed as soon as any sign of HF occurs in the setting of IE, and if there is no clear contraindication to surgery.

Surgery must be performed on an emergency basis, irrespective of the status of infection, when patients are in persistent pulmonary oedema or cardiogenic shock despite medical therapy [8]. It should be performed on an urgent basis when HF is less severe. Urgent surgery may be recommended in patients with severe aortic or mitral insufficiency without HF and large vegetations [16]. In patients with well tolerated severe valvular insufficiency and no other reasons for surgery, medical management with antibiotics under strict clinical and echocardiographic observation is a good option. Elective surgery should be considered depending on tolerance of the valve lesion and according to the recommendations of the ESC Guidelines on the Management of Valvular Heart Disease [17].

In summary, HF is the most frequent and severe complication of IE. Unless severe co-morbidity exists, the presence of HF indicates early surgery in NVE, even in patients with cardiogenic shock.

Uncontrolled Infection

Uncontrolled infection is one of the most severe complications of IE and is the second most frequent cause for surgery [1]. Uncontrolled infection is considered to be present when there is persisting infection and when there are signs of locally uncontrolled infection. Infection due to resistant or very virulent organisms often results in uncontrolled infection. The main infectious complications are described in Chap. 10.

Surgery has been indicated when fever and positive blood cultures persist for several days (7–10 days) despite an appropriate antibiotic therapy, while shorter delays (48–72 h) have been recently proposed [18].

Locally uncontrolled infection includes increasing vegetation size, abscess formation, false aneurysms or fistulae [8]. Rarely, when there are no other reasons for surgery and fever is easily controlled with antibiotics, small abscesses or false aneurysms can be treated conservatively under close clinical and echocardiographic follow-up.

Surgery is also indicated in fungal and in IE due to multiresistant organisms, e.g., MRSA or vancomycin resistant enterococci and also in the rare infections caused by Gram negative bacteria.

In summary, unless severe comorbidity exists, the presence of locally uncontrolled infection indicates early surgery in patients with IE.

Systemic Embolism

Embolic events are a frequent and life-threatening complication of IE related to the migration of cardiac vegetations. They are described in Chap. 11. The best method to reduce the risk of embolic event is the prompt institution of appropriate antibiotic therapy [19, 20]. Whilst promising [21], the addition of antiplatelet therapy did not reduce the risk of embolism in the only published randomised study [22].

The exact role of early surgery in preventing embolic events remains controversial. In the Euro Heart Survey, vegetation size was one of the reasons for surgery in

54 % of patients with NVE and in 25 % of PVE [1], but was rarely the only reason. The value of early surgery in isolated large vegetation is controversial. A recent randomized trial demonstrated that early surgery in patients with large vegetations significantly reduced the risk of death and embolic events as compared with conventional therapy [16]. However, the patients studied were at low-risk, and there was no significant difference in all-cause mortality at 6 months in the early-surgery and conventional-treatment groups.

Finally, the decision to operate early for prevention of embolism must take into account the presence of previous embolic events, other complications of IE, the size and mobility of the vegetation, the likelihood of conservative surgery, and the duration of antibiotic therapy [6]. The overall benefits of surgery should be weighed against the operative risk and must consider the clinical status and comorbidity of the patient.

The main indications and timing of surgery to prevent embolism are given in Table 22.1. The ESC guidelines [8] recommend surgical therapy in case of large (>10 mm) vegetation following one or more embolic episodes, and when the large vegetation is associated with other predictors of complicated course (heart failure, persistent infection under therapy, abscess, and prosthetic endocarditis), indicating an earlier surgical decision. The decision to operate early in isolated very large vegetation (>15 mm) is more difficult. Surgery may be preferred when a valve repair seems possible, particularly in mitral valve IE. But the most important point is that the surgery, if needed, must be performed on an urgent basis, during the first few days following initiation of antibiotic therapy, since the risk of embolism is highest at this time.

In summary, the decision to operate early to prevent embolism is always difficult and specific for the individual patient. Governing factors include size and mobility of the vegetation, previous embolism, type of microorganism, and duration of antibiotic therapy.

References

1. Tornos P, Iung B, Permanyer-Miralda G, Baron G, Delahaye F, Gohlke-Barwolf C, Butchart EG, Ravaud P, Vahanian A. Infective endocarditis in Europe: lessons from the Euro heart survey. Heart. 2005;91:571–5.
2. Baddour LM, Wilson WR, Bayer AS, Fowler Jr VG, Bolger AF, Levison ME, Ferrieri P, Gerber MA, Tani LY, Gewitz MH, Tong DC, Steckelberg JM, Baltimore RS, Shulman ST, Burns JC, Falace DA, Newburger JW, Pallasch TJ, Takahashi M, Taubert KA. Infective endocarditis: diagnosis, antimicrobial therapy, and management of complications: a statement for healthcare professionals from the Committee on Rheumatic Fever, Endocarditis, and Kawasaki Disease, Council on Cardiovascular Disease in the Young, and the Councils on Clinical Cardiology, Stroke, and Cardiovascular Surgery and Anesthesia, American Heart Association: endorsed by the Infectious Diseases Society of America. Circulation. 2005;111:e394–434.
3. Hasbun R, Vikram HR, Barakat LA, Buenconsejo J, Quagliarello VJ. Complicated left-sided native valve endocarditis in adults: risk classification for mortality. JAMA. 2003;289:1933–40.

4. Aksoy O, Sexton DJ, Wang A, Pappas PA, Kourany W, Chu V, Fowler Jr VG, Woods CW, Engemann JJ, Corey GR, Harding T, Cabell CH. Early surgery in patients with infective endocarditis: a propensity score analysis. Clin Infect Dis. 2007;44:364–72.
5. Vikram HR, Buenconsejo J, Hasbun R, Quagliarello VJ. Impact of valve surgery on 6-month mortality in adults with complicated, left-sided native valve endocarditis: a propensity analysis. JAMA. 2003;290:3207–14.
6. Thuny F, Beurtheret S, Mancini J, Gariboldi V, Casalta JP, Riberi A, Giorgi R, Gouriet F, Tafanelli L, Avierinos JF, Renard S, Collart F, Raoult D, Habib G. The timing of surgery influences mortality and morbidity in adults with severe complicated infective endocarditis: a propensity analysis. Eur Heart J. 2011;32:2027–33.
7. Habib G, Hoen B, Tornos P, et al. Guidelines on the prevention, diagnosis, and treatment of infective endocarditis (new version 2009): the Task Force on the Prevention, Diagnosis, and Treatment of Infective Endocarditis of the European Society of Cardiology (ESC). Eur Heart J. 2009;30(19):2369–413.
8. Habib G, et al. 2015 ESC Guidelines for the management of infective endocarditis: the Task Force for the Management of Infective Endocarditis of the European Society of Cardiology (ESC). Endorsed by: European Association for Cardio-Thoracic Surgery (EACTS), the European Association of Nuclear Medicine (EANM). Eur Heart J. 2015;36(44):3075–128.
9. Habib G, Avierinos JF, Thuny F. Aortic valve endocarditis: is there an optimal surgical timing? Curr Opin Cardiol. 2007;22:77–83.
10. Nadji G, Rusinaru D, Rémadi J-P, Jeu A, Sorel C, Tribouilloy C. Heart failure in left-sided native valve infective endocarditis: characteristics, prognosis, and results of surgical treatment. Eur J Heart Fail. 2009;11:668–75.
11. San Román JA, López J, Vilacosta I, Luaces M, Sarriá C, Revilla A, Ronderos R, Stoermann W, Gómez I, Fernández-Avilés F. Prognostic stratification of patients with left-sided endocarditis determined at admission. Am J Med. 2007;120:369.e1–7.
12. Revilla A, López J, Vilacosta I, Villacorta E, Rollán MJ, Echevarría JR, Carrascal Y, Di Stefano S, Fulquet E, Rodríguez E, Fiz L, San Román JA. Clinical and prognostic profile of patients with infective endocarditis who need urgent surgery. Eur Heart J. 2007;28:65–71.
13. Lopez J, Sevilla T, Vilacosta I, Garcia H, Sarria C, Pozo E, Silva J, Revilla A, Varvaro G, del Palacio M, Gomez I, San Roman JA. Clinical significance of congestive heart failure in prosthetic valve endocarditis. A multicenter study with 257 patients. Rev Esp Cardiol. 2013;66:384–90.
14. Habib G, Tribouilloy C, Thuny F, Giorgi R, Brahim A, Amazouz M, Remadi J-P, Nadji G, Casalta J-P, Coviaux F, Avierinos J-F, Lescure X, Riberi A, Weiller P-J, Metras D, Raoult D. Prosthetic valve endocarditis: who needs surgery? A multicentre study of 104 cases. Heart. 2005;91:954–9.
15. Lalani T, Chu VH, Park LP, Cecchi E, Corey GR, Durante-Mangoni E, Fowler Jr VG, Gordon D, Grossi P, Hannan M, Hoen B, Muñoz P, Rizk H, Kanj SS, Selton-Suty C, Sexton DJ, Spelman D, Ravasio V, Tripodi MF, Wang A, International Collaboration on Endocarditis–Prospective Cohort Study Investigators. In-hospital and 1-year mortality in patients undergoing early surgery for prosthetic valve endocarditis. JAMA Intern Med. 2013;173:1495–504.
16. Kang D-H, Kim Y-J, Kim S-H, Sun BJ, Kim D-H, Yun S-C, Song J-M, Choo SJ, Chung C-H, Song J-K, Lee J-W, Sohn D-W. Early surgery versus conventional treatment for infective endocarditis. N Engl J Med. 2012;366:2466–73.
17. Vahanian A, Alfieri O, Andreotti F, Antunes MJ, Barón-Esquivias G, Baumgartner H, Borger MA, Carrel TP, De Bonis M, Evangelista A, Falk V, Iung B, Lancellotti P, Pierard L, Price S, Schäfers H-J, Schuler G, Stepinska J, Swedberg K, Takkenberg J, Von Oppell UO, Windecker S, Zamorano JL, Zembala M. Guidelines on the management of valvular heart disease (version 2012). The Joint Task Force on the Management of Valvular Heart Disease of the European Society of Cardiology (ESC) and the European Association for Cardio-Thoracic Surgery (EACTS). Eur Heart J. 2012;33:2451–96.

18. Lopez J, Sevilla T, Vilacosta I, Sarria C, Revilla A, Ortiz C, Ferrera C, Olmos C, Gomez I, San Roman JA. Prognostic role of persistent positive blood cultures after initiation of antibiotic therapy in left sided infective endocarditis. Eur Heart J. 2013;34:1749–54.

19. García-Cabrera E, Fernández-Hidalgo N, Almirante B, Ivanova-Georgieva R, Noureddine M, Plata A, Lomas JM, Gálvez-Acebal J, Hidalgo-Tenorio C, Ruiz-Morales J, Martínez-Marcos FJ, Reguera JM, de la Torre-Lima J, de Alarcón González A. Neurologic complications of infective endocarditis: risk factors, outcome, and impact of cardiac surgery: a multicenter observational study. Circulation. 2013;127:2272–84.

20. Hubert S, Thuny F, Resseguier N, Giorgi R, Tribouilloy C, Le Dolley Y, Casalta JP, Riberi A, Chevalier F, Rusinaru D, Malaquin D, Remadi JP, Ammar AB, Avierinos JF, Collart F, Raoult D, Habib G. Prediction of symptomatic embolism in infective endocarditis: construction and validation of a risk calculator in a multicenter cohort. J Am Coll Cardiol. 2013;62:1384–92.

21. Anavekar NS, Tleyjeh IM, Mirzoyev Z, Steckelberg JM, Haddad C, Khandaker MH, Wilson WR, Chandrasekaran K, Baddour LM. Impact of prior antiplatelet therapy on risk of embolism in infective endocarditis. Clin Infect Dis. 2007;44:1180–6.

22. Chan KL, Dumesnil JG, Cujec B, Sanfilippo AJ, Jue J, Turek MA, Robinson TI, Moher D. A randomized trial of aspirin on the risk of embolic events in patients with infective endocarditis. J Am Coll Cardiol. 2003;42:775–80.

Part VIII
Prevention and Prophylaxis

Chapter 23
Infective Endocarditis Prophylaxis and Prevention

Xavier Duval

History of Infective Endocarditis Prophylaxis

Infective endocarditis (IE) is a rare yet severe infectious disease with an in-hospital mortality rate of around 20 % despite improvements in diagnosis and treatment [1–3]. Its overall annual incidence has not changed significantly over the last few decades. The profile of IE has recently changed. IE occurs now more frequently than before in patients without previously identified at-risk cardiac condition (PCC); IE involves prosthetic valve in 20 % of cases and intracardiac devices (pacemaker or intracardiac defibrillator) in 10 %. One patient out of two has a comorbidity, diabetes mellitus being the most frequent. *Staphylococcus aureus* is reported as the primary micro-organism in many series of IE follows by oral streptococci and enterococci. Healthcare-associated IE accounts for a quarter of IE cases [4]. Due to its high rate of mortality and morbidity, every effort should be made to reduce IE incidence. Although its efficacy has not been demonstrated in humans, antibiotic prophylaxis of IE had been recommended since 1954 for subjects with IE predisposing conditions undergoing at-risk procedures; this recommendation was maintained regularly from that date up to 2002 [5, 6]. This was based in part on the results of animal models which showed the effectiveness of antibiotics in preventing the development of IE after experimental inoculation of bacteria, and in part on force of habit.

X. Duval, MD, PhD
Department of Infectious Diseases, Bichat Claude Bernard University Hospital, Paris, France
e-mail: Xavier.duval@aphp.fr

© Springer International Publishing Switzerland 2016
G. Habib (ed.), *Infective Endocarditis*, DOI 10.1007/978-3-319-32432-6_23

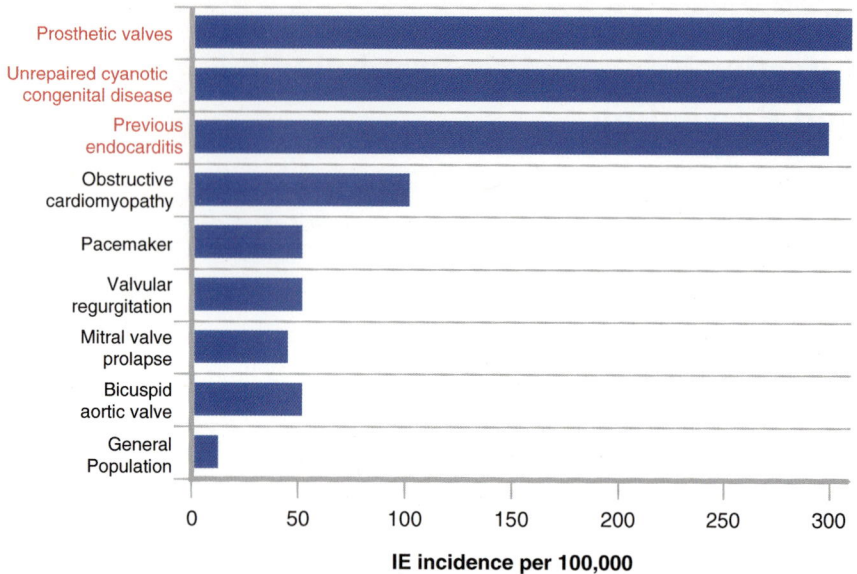

Fig. 23.1 Incidence of infective endocarditis according to different populations with predisposing underlying heart diseases and in the general population. (*Note*: Highlighted predisposing cardiac conditions are those with the highest incidences and the poorest prognosis)

Identification of IE Predisposing Conditions

The IE incidence is between three and nine cases per 100,000 individuals per year in the global population in industrialized countries [7, 8]. Some authors based on population-based studies report a stable incidence [8, 9] while others, based on inpatient databases, reported a slight but significant increase [10, 11]. This IE incidence varies markedly according to the patients' characteristics (i.e., infective endocarditis predisposing conditions) with 100-fold higher rates in certain categories of individuals, due to the existence of cardiac IE at-risk predispositions on which bacteria are grafting and/or increased incidence of bacteremia. Patients with intracardiac devices (prosthetic valves, pacemaker and defibrillator), unrepaired cyanotic congenital diseases, and history of IE, are at highest incidence of IE; HIV-infected patients, intravenous drug users, diabetic patients, individuals on hemodialysis and to a lesser extent any patients with native valve diseases, including degenerative ones are also at higher incidence than the general population (Fig. 23.1). The clustering of several of these conditions in the elderly population probably explains the higher incidence of IE in individuals older than 65 years with a rate reaching 20 cases per 100,000 males over 65 [4]. IE incidence in a given population is the complex result of the prevalence of IE predisposing cardiac conditions in this population, the susceptibility of such cardiac conditions to microorganism graft, the frequency of invasive situations (related or not to healthcare), and the prevalence of natural microorganism portals of entry (for example, the relationship between colonic tumours and group D streptococci IE in the elderly population).

Modification of the Prevalence of IE Risk Factors in the IE Population

While the overall incidence of IE has been globally stable or increasing slightly in industrialized countries, the prevalence of IE predisposing factors in the IE population has changed markedly. The number of patients with rheumatic heart disease, which represented up to 50% in the 1950' series, has decreased regularly [12] concomitantly with the decrease of rheumatic heart diseases in the general population [13], currently representing 5–12% of the IE population in industrialized countries; the prevalence of IE patients with intracardiac device infections has increased, in proportions which surpass the increase of intracardiac device use in the general population reaching a rate of 30% of the IE in recent studies [14]. The general aging of the population in industrialized countries leads to an increase of IE cases on degenerative valvulopathies. These valvulopathies are previously generally undetected explaining the progressive increase in the rate of IE occurring in patients without previously known at-risk cardiac conditions (50% of IE cases). Modifications also concern the proportion of haemodialysis patients and diabetic patients in IE series, with both proportions surpassing now 20% of IE cases in centers in North America [14] a proportion that is much higher than in the rest of the world including other industrialized countries. This could be explained by a more frequent use of central catheter for haemodialysis in the USA (a well-identified risk factor for staphylococci bacteremia) instead of arterio venous fistula, and a higher prevalence of diabetes mellitus. Considering all IE cases (on native valve and on prosthetic valve IE), the proportion of patients with previously identified heart disease has significantly decreased from 80% of IE cases in the 1970s to around 50% currently [8, 9, 15], IE must thus be evoked and prevented also in patients without known at-risk cardiac conditions.

Arguments That Led to the Modifications of IE Antibioprophylaxis Guidelines

In the context of habitual application of weakly supported guidelines, several issues had been raised before 2002 which challenged the principles underlying prophylaxis recommendations.

First, three retrospective case-control studies in three different countries were conducted in an attempt to implicate and identify dental procedures in the genesis of IE, but their findings were not homogeneous: the studies by Van der Meer et al. and by Strom et al. provided evidence that dental treatment was unlikely to be a risk factor, whereas the study by Lacassin et al. found a relationship between dental scaling and viridans streptococcal IE [16–18].

Second, the identification of procedures at risk for IE (presumptive situations of increased risk) is not based on the observation of a causal relationship but on pathophysiological considerations. Neither the number of identified IE-inducing pathogens (inoculum), colonizing the area which could enter the bloodstream in case of an invasive procedure, nor the amount of bleeding induced by the procedure, nor the rate of blood cultures isolating bacteria after a given procedure, nor the magnitude of the bacteremia following the procedure, nor the duration of the bacteremia, nor the reported cases of IE following a given procedure make possible the identification of procedures at risk for IE. Furthermore, there is wide variation in reported frequencies of these characteristics following procedures. For example, bacteremia is noted in 10–95 % of patients after tooth extraction, which probably reflects the heterogeneity of these procedures, of the host and of the experimental methodologies used [19]. Meanwhile, the rate of bacteremia following at-risk procedure has been used as a surrogate measure of the risk of IE and, as well as to identify procedures requiring antibiotic prophylaxis. However, bacteremia does not respond to the prerequisite of a pertinent (appropriate) surrogate measure. There is no evidenced-based method to decide which procedure should require prophylaxis because there are no data which show that the incidence, or the magnitude, the duration of bacteremia following a procedure increase the risk of IE. Thus any attempt at identifying procedures needing prophylaxis is artificial.

Third, transient repeated bacteremia from everyday life activities (tooth brushing, chewing, etc.) was identified as being more often responsible for bacteremia than intermittent bacteremia following occasional procedures [20, 21]. A theoretical study of cumulative bacteremia over 1 year postulated that everyday bacteremia is six million times greater than bacteremia from a single extraction [21]. These data have led, since 2002, to a drastic reduction in antibiotic indications in patients with predisposing cardiac conditions undergoing at-risk procedures [22].

Finally, the estimated risk of IE after an unprotected procedure is very low, at most 1 per 45,000 procedures [23].

Recent Modifications of IE Antibioprophylaxis Guidelines

In 2002, the French guidelines were the first to call a halt to the systematic use of antibioprophylaxis and to restrict the use of prophylaxis to patients at risk of death from IE, that is, patients with high-risk cardiac predisposing factors (in most cases: history of IE, prosthetic valves) and who had invasive dental, respiratory, gastrointestinal and/or genitourinary procedures [24]. In 2007, the American Heart Association (AHA) established new guidelines which represented a radical change from those previously published in the USA in 1997: prophylaxis was no longer recommended before dental procedures except for patients with the highest risk of adverse outcome resulting from IE and who had undergone "any dental procedure that involved manipulation of the oral mucosa" [6, 25]. The AHA advised against using prophylaxis in gastrointestinal and urogenital interventions. In 2008, the guidance from the National Institute for Health and Clinical Excellence (NICE) in the United Kingdom recommended that IE prophylaxis should be stopped for all patients and before all procedures, dental and non-dental [26]. In 2009, the European

Society of Cardiology guidelines did not follow along with this radical change but recommended, as had the 2007 US ones, the pursuit of antibiotic prophylaxis for dental procedures solely in patients at highest risk (prosthetic heart valves, congenital heart disease and history of IE). Prophylaxis was no longer recommended for patients at moderate risk or those deemed at low risk (pacemakers and/or defibrillators or who had had previous coronary artery bypass graft surgery) [27].

IE antibiotic prophylaxis had thus been then drastically modified, not because its ineffectiveness had been proven, but because the pathophysiology supporting its use was no longer convincing. There are currently two distinct IE prophylaxis positions: the radical British position based on the lack of evidence of IE efficacy and which abandoned all antibiotic prophylaxis; and the more mitigated one, adopted by the "remaining world": considering that the lack of evidence is not evidence of ineffectiveness, recommending antibiotic prophylaxis only for a limited patient population, those at very high risk of death in case of IE.

These positions have generated considerable and dramatically opposed reactions: those in favor of maintaining the antibiotic prophylaxis because there is no tangible evidence for a change; and those in favor of an abandon or a limitation because there is no tangible evidence for its continuation [28].

Current Prophylaxis Guidelines

Nowadays, antibiotic prophylaxis is restricted in most of countries to patients with prosthetic valves, history of IE, and uncorrected cyanotic diseases (patients with the highest risks of IE occurrence and of adverse outcome from IE) who will experience dental procedures that involve manipulation of gingival tissue or the periapical region of teeth or perforation of the oral mucosa (Table 23.1). The most frequent recommended regimens in adults are 2 g amoxicillin, within the hour preceding the procedure or 600 mg clindamycin in B lactams allergic individuals [25, 27]. All other cases (respiratory tract, gastro-intestinal, urogenital, skin and soft tissues procedures) no longer represent an indication for antibioprophylaxis. British guidelines adopted a more drastic attitude recommending discontinuing IE antibiotic prophylaxis altogether [26]. Prophylaxis must also focus on healthcare associated IE including early and late prosthetic valve IE and pacemaker related infection but also those occurring in cases with no previously identified heart valve diseases; this can only be conceived in a global strategy of reducing all cases of staphylococcal bacteremia and especially those secondary to all types of catheter related infections, in particular in the very elderly population.

Global oral and skin hygiene measures for everybody, including healthcare patients, to minimize the risk of community-acquired and healthcare facility-acquired bacteremia must target patients both with and without predisposing cardiac conditions [25, 27].

See Table 23.2 for an overview of recommended prophylaxis guidelines from various societies and associations for dental procedures in adults.

Table 23.1 Cardiac conditions (high risk) for which antibiotic prophylaxis is recommended in case of invasive oro-dental procedures

1. Patients with a prosthetic valve (biological, mechanical, transcatheter valves, or a prosthetic material used for cardiac valve repair)
2. Patients with previous IE
3. Patients with congenital heart disease
(a) Cyanotic congenital heart disease without surgical repair
(b) Congenital heart disease repaired with prosthetic material whether placed surgically or by percutaneous techniques, up to 6 months after the procedure
(c) Congenital heart disease with residual shunt or residual valvular regurgitation

From Habib et al. [27] (With permission of Oxford University Press)
Note: No antibiotic prophylaxis in NICE guidelines

Risk of Antibiotic Prophylaxis

Antibiotic administration carries a small risk of anaphylaxis. Considering a widespread use of prophylaxis (number of indications and of concerned individuals), this may become significant. The lethal risk of anaphylaxis is very low when using oral amoxicillin [29]. Antibiotic prophylaxis use may result in the emergence of resistant microorganisms, including oral streptococci [19]. However, to the best of our knowledge, this emergence has not been studied after a single dose of amoxicillin.

The Concept of Cumulative Exposure to Low-Grade Bacteremia

One major argument which rocked the founding principle of antibiotic prophylaxis was the concept of transient repeated bacteremia of low grade and short duration from routine daily activities (e.g., tooth- brushing, chewing, flossing, use of water irrigation devices, etc.). In fact, this repeated bacteremia might pose a greater risk for IE than intermittent bacteremia after occasional procedures [30].

The findings of two studies are very much along these lines. The first one, a double-blind, placebo-controlled study conducted by Lockhart et al., compared the incidence, duration, nature and magnitude of IE-related bacteremia from single-tooth extraction with the same information on IE-related bacteremia from tooth brushing [31]. All of the 290 individuals randomized in one of the three groups (tooth brushing, single-tooth extraction plus amoxicillin prophylaxis, and single-tooth extraction plus placebo) had had blood cultures before, during, and after the procedure. Cumulative incidence of bacteremia due to IE-related species was significantly different in the three groups: 23 % in the tooth brushing group, 33 % in the single tooth extraction+amoxicillin group, and 60 % in the extraction+placebo group. The authors concluded that, although amoxicillin has a positive impact on bacteremia after a single tooth extraction, tooth brushing may yet pose a greater risk because it is done much more often.

Table 23.2 Recommended prophylaxis guidelines for dental procedures in adults

Society	Dental prophylaxis			Predisposing cardiac conditions	
	Procedures listed	Recommended regimen			
		No allergy to B lactam	B lactam allergic patients	High risk	Moderate risk
BSAC[a] (2006)	All dental procedures involving dento-gengival manipulation or endodontics	Amoxicillin p.o. or i.v 3 g ingle dose 1 h before procedure	Clindamycin 600 mg p.o. or i.v	Recommended prophylaxis	**Prophylaxis not recommended**
AHA[b] (2007)	Any dental procedure that involves manipulation of the oral mucosa	Amoxicillin p.o. or i.v 2 g ingle dose 1 h before procedure	Clindamycin 600 mg p.o. or i.v	Recommended prophylaxis	**Prophylaxis not recommended**
NICE (2008, 2015)	All procedures	NA	NA	**Prophylaxis not recommended**	
ESC[c] (2009, 2015)	Dental procedures requiring manipulation of the gingival or periapical region of the teeth or perforation of the oral mucosa	Amoxicillin p.o. or i.v 2 g ingle dose 1 h before procedure	Clindamycin 600 mg p.o. or i.v	Recommended prophylaxis	**Prophylaxis not recommended**

Definition of High risk predisposing cardiac conditions: see Table 23.1
[a]*BSAC* British society for antimicrobial chemotherapy
[b]*AHA* American heart association
[c]*ESC* European society of cardiology

The second one, reported by Veloso et al., tried to demonstrate in animal model that IE could be caused by cumulative exposure to low-grade bacteremia occurring during daily activities [32]. This study compared the infectivity in rats of continuous low-grade bacteremia (continuous infusion of 10^3–10^6 UFC delivered at a pace of 0.0017 mL/min over 10 h) with the infectivity in rats of brief high-grade bacteremia (1 mL bolus of 10^3–10^6 UFC in 1 min). In this experiment, the number of IE induced by low-grade continuous bacteremia was not significantly different from that of IE induced by high-grade bolus bacteremia. The authors suggested that the most predictive factor of IE was the duration of the bacteremia rather than its magnitude, and that the smallest inoculum was enough to achieve a comparable infection rate.

Relationship Between Oro-Dental Status and the Risk of Endocarditis

The concept of everyday life bacteremia probably raises more questions than it answers. In fact, considering the high number of patients with cardiac conditions at risk of IE (1.7 % of the global French population and 7 % of the population 60 years old and above) and the daily repeated bacteremia capable of inducing IE, it appears surprising that IE is so rare [23]. Development of IE following everyday life bacteremia may be determined by its characteristics. It can be hypothesized that oro-dental status may interfere with the propensity to induce oral bacteremia and that poor dental condition may favor dental bacteremia originating from chewing or tooth brushing. This oro-dental status reflects the combined long-term impacts of patients' oral hygiene and of dental practitioner care, when the latter is solicited. There have been conflicting results in the literature concerning the relationship between gingival or periodontal disease and an increased risk of bacteria after tooth extraction or oral hygiene [33–35].

In the afore mentioned study conducted in "healthy" individuals by Lockhart et al. visiting a hospital-based dental service [31], the authors also looked at the association between dental status and the risk of bacteremia using a thorough clinical and radiographic examination of teeth and peridontia conducted by trained practitioners [35]. After tooth brushing, they reported a higher risk of *Streptococcal viridans* bacteremia in those individuals with high dental plaque and high calculus scores [35]; only one among five gingival inflammation measurements (generalized bleeding with tooth brushing) was also associated with *viridans Streptococci* bacteremia.

In a case-control study including IE patients, we compared oral status of patients with IE responsible microorganisms originating in the oral cavity to that of patients with IE responsible microorganisms of originating in the skin or the digestive tract. We did not find any differences concerning either calculus score or gingival inflammation between patients with oral streptococcal definite IE and patients with extra oral definite IE (mainly staphylococcal and *bovis Streptococcus* IE), signifying that the increased risk of IE-associated bacteremia noted by Lockhart et al. in patients with poor oral hygiene may not be sufficient to induce IE. Pulpal necrosis, a rare condition, was more frequently noted in case-patients, albeit only statistically significant in the bivariate analysis.

The role of dental hygiene is equally confusing. Brushing one's teeth many times a day may increase the risk of oral streptococcal IE on a short-term basis but decrease this risk on a long-term basis. In a case-control study conducted by Strom at al, which compared 287 IE patients whatever their microorganism (33.1 % of the total cohort has *viridans Streptococci* IE), authors did not find any statistical differences in the practice of scaling as compared to a control population of healthy US individuals. Case-control studies are needed to determine the risk-benefit ratio of dental hygiene and to support the current recommendations on dental hygiene.

Impact of Prophylaxis Guidelines Modification on the Epidemiology of IE

The evaluation of the impact of the drastic change in IE prophylaxis strategy on clinical and epidemiological characteristics may offer the opportunity to evaluate its efficacy a posteriori. In fact, a significant increase in the incidence of IE after scaling down prophylaxis use would be an indication of its efficacy, whereas a stable or a decreased incidence of IE would tend to support the appropriateness of prophylaxis guideline modifications. Conflicting results have been reported in the literature concerning the impact of guideline modifications in different countries.

In the USA, since 2007, a number of studies have been published that have examined the impact of the American Heart Association guidelines. Five studies did not find any impact: Rogers et al., reporting on their experience in a San Francisco medical center in 2008 [36], demonstrated no increase in the number of admissions 9 months after the guideline change. A study by Bor et al., which used National Inpatient Sample Data to assess a broad sample of patients from 1998–2009, did not show any inflection in the rise of infective endocarditis after the guideline change, nor an increase in the number of cases secondary to streptococcal infections [37]. DeSimone et al., looking at data from the start of 1999 to the end of 2010 [38], used very detailed data from the Rochester Epidemiology Project. They concluded that there was no increase in the incidence of viridans group streptococci (VGS) in their sample, but the small sample size must be considered; there were only three documented cases of VGS-IE in their sample between 2007 and 2010. Pasquali et al., looking specifically at IE in children across 37 hospitals between 2003 and 2010, found no significant change in the absolute numbers of cases before and after the guideline change [39]. Bikdeli et al. looked at admissions in patients over the age of 65 using the Medicare Inpatient Standard Analytic Files [40]. They recorded a reduction in the absolute numbers. The latest study to look at the impact of the 2007 guidelines was published in 2015; the data have been extracted from the National Inpatient Sample, as in the Bor et al. study. The authors have looked at the data between 2000 and 2011, extending the follow-up time after the change in AHA guidelines to 4 years. They have found an increase in the number of IE but there has been no acceleration of the rise since guideline modifications [41].

In the United Kingdom, the same group of authors published two successive evaluations of the UK guideline modifications (NICE), using the same methodology, the first one with a follow-up period of 2 years, the second with one of 5 years. Of note, these UK guidelines are the sole not to recommend antibiotic prophylaxis, whether or not individuals have IE predisposing cardiac conditions. Thornhill et al. used the national data on inpatient hospital activity from January 2000 to April 2010 [42]. These data were drawn from Dr Foster Intelligence, a private-public partnership health service information and intelligence organization. Before the guidelines changed, between January 2000 and March 2008, there was a trend toward an increasing number of cases of IE and deaths from IE. After the guidelines changed in March 2008, prescribing antibiotic prophylaxis (amoxicillin or clindamycin) decreased by 78.6%, especially with dentists. There was little evidence for the upward trend in cases of IE, and in particular of oral streptococci IE, and in cases of death from IE. Using a non-inferiority test, an increase in the number of cases of IE of 9.3% or more could be ruled out and in the same way, an increase in the number of deaths of 2.3% or more could also be ruled out. The authors concluded that the considerable and rapid decrease in prescriptions did not induce a large increase of IE incidence in the 2 years after the publication of the NICE guideline. When extending the follow-up period to 5 years after the modification of guidelines, the authors found contradictory results, with a small but statistically significant increase in the incidence of IE in the UK since 2008, which would account for an excess of 35 IE cases each month [43]. This increase was observed in high-risk individuals, but also in lower-risk individuals who include patients at moderate and at low risk of IE as defined in the AHA and ESC guidelines. Concomitantly, the authors observed a decrease of antibiotic prophylaxis use of almost 90%. The temporal link between these two phenomena raises the question of a causal relationship.

In France, the AEPEI study group conducted three population-based surveys over almost 20 years (the first in 1991, the second in 1999 and the last in 2008) on a population pool of 11 million inhabitants. All IE cases were validated by a centralized expert team using different case definitions (von Reyn modified by echocardiographic results, Duke classification and modified-Duke classification). Overall, IE incidence had not increased in France as of 2008, 6 years after the modification of prophylaxis guidelines. When considering IE incidence, taking into account the type of microorganisms and the IE predisposing cardiac conditions, streptococcal IE incidence, with or without a pre-existing valvulopathy, did not increase between 1999 and 2008 [44].

Even if these studies have brought us important insights into prophylaxis modification and its consequences, their results must be interpreted with caution, as all studies suffer from limitations. First, studies based on retrospective analysis of data from hospital discharge coding, did not have the IE cases validated by an expert adjudication committee. Second, in some studies, the hospital coding did not include the precise identification of the streptococcal strains in all patients, one of the major microorganisms responsible for IE originating in the mouth. Third, except for the British study which reported data on antibiotic prescription, the implementation of guidelines modification was not assessed. Fourth, in a temporal comparison analysis, multiple confounders could explain an increased IE incidence irrespective of any antibiotic prophylaxis guideline change. Finally, correlation between phenomena does not equal causation.

Should We Modify IE Prophylaxis to Target a Broader Population?

For several years, IE prophylaxis, including (or not) antibiotic prophylaxis, was targeted specifically at patients with previously identified IE predisposing cardiac conditions and focused on possible bucco dental and digestive portals of entry.

The changes in IE patient characteristics reported in the recent population-based epidemiological studies may have an impact on the population targeted by prophylaxis policy.

First, older male individuals are at the highest risk of developing IE, the annual incidence being tenfold higher in the 75–79 age range. Second, one patient out of two who develops IE is not identified as having an IE predisposing cardiac condition when he is treated by the practitioner for IE. This is concordant with the decrease in the incidence of IE reported in the French epidemiological studies in patients with previously known native heart valve disease (18.8 cases per million in 1991 to 11.4 cases per million in 1999 and 7.1 cases per million in 2008 (p = 0.007)). This applies to both the oral streptococci and *Staphylococcus aureus* IE. Third, the incidence of *Staphylococcus aureus* IE has increased since 1991, moving from 5.2 cases per million to 8.2 cases per million. It increased in patients without previously known underlying heart disease. In the 2008 French survey, *Staphylococcus aureus* is the primary micro-organism responsible for IE [4]. This could result from the increase number of patients with conditions associated with staphylococcal bacteremia, such as intracardiac implants (prosthetic valve, pacemaker), chronic hemodialysis and diabetes mellitus. Finally, and consistent with the third point, the survey conducted in France in 2008 shows that healthcare-associated IE is an emerging facet of the disease. Healthcare-associated IE were due to both *Staphylococcus aureus* and coagulase-negative staphylococci, and developed more often in older patients suffering from major debilitating conditions (hypertension, diabetes mellitus, and chronic hemodialysis) or implanted with intravascular devices. These epidemiological changes are arguments for a different approach to prophylaxis of IE not only focusing on patients with IE predisposing cardiac conditions. Many questions still remain unanswered concerning the bacterial characteristics that enable the bacteria to infect a cardiac valve, and the host factors that would enable the host to defend itself against bacterial action. To date, there is no published study that looks into the role of the factors related to the virulence of *Staphylococcus aureus* or into the role of genetic factors in host predisposition.

Benefit of Antibioprophylaxis at Cardiovascular Implantable Electronic Device Implantation

The annual pacemaker IE incidence has been estimated at 400 for 10^6 individuals with a pacemaker [45]. In most of the cases, the pacemaker is contaminated at the time of implantation. The prescription of an antibioprophylaxis when implanting a cardiovascular implantable electronic device (CIED) is now recommended. Until recently, the existing data for the use of antibioprophylaxis in this situation yielded contradictory results [46, 47]. In 1998, the meta-analysis of antibioprophylaxis for permanent pacemaker implantation by Da Costa *et al* found a significant reduction in the incidence of infection [32, 46]. However, the first major study which really demonstrated the benefit of antibioprophylaxis in the prevention of device implant infections is the trial by de Oliviera et al., a randomized, double-blind placebo-controlled trial conducted in 2009 in North America and Brazil [33, 47]. A 1000 consecutive patients who underwent the first device implantation or generator replacement were randomized in a 1:1 fashion to prophylactic antibiotics (intravenous cefazolin) or placebo. Follow-up was performed until 6 months after the procedure and the end-point was any evidence of infection (surgical site infection or systemic infection). The trial was interrupted prematurely because there was significantly less infection in the cefazolin-group *versus* the placebo-group (0.64 % *vs*. 3.28 %, RR=0.19, p=0.016). One year later, thanks to these results, the American Heart Association published a scientific statement, thus updating its 2003 statement about the prevention and the management of CIED [48, 49]. The AHA recommended, as antibioprophylaxis before CIED implantation, an antibiotic that has demonstrated in vitro effectiveness against staphylococci, that is, either a first-generation cephalosporin like cefazolin or vanco-mycin (particularly if the oxacillin resistance among staphylococci is high or if the patient is allergic to cephalosporins). Antibiotic prophylaxis is also recommended if subsequent invasive procedure of CIED is required. This antibioprophylaxis only concerns CIED implantations; the AHA does not recommend antibioprophylaxis to prevent CIED infections in patients implanted with CIED in dental or other invasive procedure which would not be directly related to a device manipulation.

Conclusion

IE co-evolved with socioeconomic changes and medical progress leading to an increase of onset age, comorbidities, intracardiac devices, and of staphylococcal IE. IE antibiotic prophylaxis has been drastically modified during the 10 last years, with currently two opposite strategies, both of them leading to a major reduction of antibiotic prophylaxis indications [50, 51]. To date, this change has not given rise to an increase in oral streptococci IE which supports a posteriori the reduction of its use. A better understanding of the physiopathology of IE and the characterization of the new valvulopathies should help better target patients not previously considered at risk of IE. Nevertheless, epidemiological surveillance is vital in order to observe rapid changes in the profile of the disease and to modify, if necessary, recommenda-tions for a better prevention.

References

1. Hoen B, Alla F, Selton-Suty C, et al. Changing profile of infective endocarditis: results of a 1-year survey in France. JAMA. 2002;288(1):75–81.
2. Hoen B, Duval X. Infective endocarditis. N Engl J Med. 2013;368:1425–33.
3. Tleyjeh IM, Steckelberg JM, Murad HS, et al. Temporal trends in infective endocarditis: a population-based study in Olmsted County, Minnesota. JAMA. 2005;293(24):3022–8.
4. Selton-Suty C, Celard M, Le Moing V, et al. Preeminence of Staphylococcus aureus in infec-tive endocarditis: a 1-year population-based survey. Clin Infect Dis. 2012;54(9):1230–9.

5. American Heart Association. Prevention of rheumatic fever and bacterial endocarditis through control of streptococcal infections. Circulation. 1955;11:317–20.
6. Dajani AS, Taubert KA, Wilson W, et al. Prevention of bacterial endocarditis. Recommendations by the American Heart Association. JAMA. 1997;277(22):1794–801.
7. Baddour LM. Prophylaxis of infective endocarditis: prevention of the perfect storm. Int J Antimicrob Agents. 2007;30 Suppl 1:S37–41.
8. Duval X, Delahaye F, Alla F, et al. Temporal trends in infective endocarditis in the context of prophylaxis guideline modifications: three successive population-based surveys. J Am Coll Cardiol. 2012;59(22):1968–76.
9. Tleyjeh IM, Abdel-Latif A, Rahbi H, et al. A systematic review of population-based studies of infective endocarditis. Chest. 2007;132(3):1025–35.
10. Fedeli U, Schievano E, Buonfrate D, et al. Increasing incidence and mortality of infective endocarditis: a population-based study through a record-linkage system. BMC Infect Dis. 2011;11:48.
11. Federspiel JJ, Stearns SC, Peppercorn AF, et al. Increasing US rates of endocarditis with Staphylococcus aureus: 1999-2008. Arch Intern Med. 2012;172(4):363–5.
12. Finland M, Barnes MW. Changing etiology of bacterial endocarditis in the antibacterial era. Experiences at Boston City Hospital 1933-1965. Ann Intern Med. 1970;72(3):341–8.
13. Seckeler MD, Hoke TR. The worldwide epidemiology of acute rheumatic fever and rheumatic heart disease. Clin Epidemiol. 2011;3:67–84.
14. Murdoch DR, Corey GR, Hoen B, et al. Clinical presentation, etiology, and outcome of infective endocarditis in the 21st century: the International Collaboration on Endocarditis-Prospective Cohort Study. Arch Intern Med. 2009;169(5):463–73.
15. Correa de Sa DD, Tleyjeh IM, Anavekar NS, et al. Epidemiological trends of infective endocarditis: a population-based study in Olmsted County, Minnesota. Mayo Clin Proc. 2010;85(5):422–6.
16. Lacassin F, Hoen B, Leport C, et al. Procedures associated with infective endocarditis in adults. A case control study. Eur Heart J. 1995;16(12):1968–74.
17. Strom BL, Abrutyn E, Berlin JA, et al. Risk factors for infective endocarditis: oral hygiene and nondental exposures. Circulation. 2000;102(23):2842–8.
18. Van der Meer JT, Van Wijk W, Thompson J, et al. Efficacy of antibiotic prophylaxis for prevention of native-valve endocarditis. Lancet. 1992;339(8786):135–9.
19. Duval X, Leport C. Prophylaxis of infective endocarditis: current tendencies, continuing controversies. Lancet Infect Dis. 2008;8(4):225–32.
20. Drangsholt MT. A new causal model of dental diseases associated with endocarditis. Ann Periodontol. 1998;3(1):184–96.
21. Roberts GJ. Dentists are innocent! "Everyday" bacteremia is the real culprit: a review and assessment of the evidence that dental surgical procedures are a principal cause of bacterial endocarditis in children. Pediatr Cardiol. 1999;20(5):317–25.
22. Durack DT. Antibiotics for prevention of endocarditis during dentistry: time to scale back? Ann Intern Med. 1998;129(10):829–31.
23. Duval X, Alla F, Hoen B, et al. Estimated risk of endocarditis in adults with predisposing cardiac conditions undergoing dental procedures with or without antibiotic prophylaxis. Clin Infect Dis. 2006;42(12):e102–7.
24. Danchin N, Duval X, Leport C. Prophylaxis of infective endocarditis: French recommendations 2002. Heart. 2005;91(6):715–8.
25. Wilson W, Taubert KA, Gewitz M, et al. Prevention of infective endocarditis: guidelines from the American Heart Association: a guideline from the American Heart Association Rheumatic Fever, Endocarditis, and Kawasaki Disease Committee, Council on Cardiovascular Disease in the Young, and the Council on Clinical Cardiology, Council on Cardiovascular Surgery and Anesthesia, and the Quality of Care and Outcomes Research Interdisciplinary Working Group. Circulation. 2007;116:1736–54.
26. Stokes T, Richey R, Wray D. Prophylaxis against infective endocarditis: summary of NICE guidance. Heart. 2008;94(7):930–1.

27. Habib G, Hoen B, Tornos P, et al. Guidelines on the prevention, diagnosis, and treatment of infective endocarditis (new version 2009): the Task Force on the Prevention, Diagnosis, and Treatment of Infective Endocarditis of the European Society of Cardiology (ESC). Eur Heart J. 2009;30(19):2369–413.
28. Shaw D, Conway DI. Pascal's Wager, infective endocarditis and the "no-lose" philosophy in medicine. Heart. 2010;96(1):15–8.
29. Lee P, Shanson D. Results of a UK survey of fatal anaphylaxis after oral amoxicillin. J Antimicrob Chemother. 2007;60(5):1172–3.
30. Moreillon P, Overholser CD, Malinverni R, et al. Predictors of endocarditis in isolates from cultures of blood following dental extractions in rats with periodontal disease. J Infect Dis. 1988;157(5):990–5.
31. Lockhart PB, Brennan MT, Sasser HC, et al. Bacteremia associated with toothbrushing and dental extraction. Circulation. 2008;117(24):3118–25.
32. Veloso TR, Amiguet M, Rousson V, et al. Induction of experimental endocarditis by continuous low-grade bacteremia mimicking spontaneous bacteremia in humans. Infect Immun. 2011;79(5):2006–11.
33. Lockhart PB. An analysis of bacteremias during dental extractions. A double-blind, placebo-controlled study of chlorhexidine. Arch Intern Med. 1996;156(5):513–20.
34. Lockhart PB, Brennan MT, Kent ML, et al. Impact of amoxicillin prophylaxis on the incidence, nature, and duration of bacteremia in children after intubation and dental procedures. Circulation. 2004;109(23):2878–84.
35. Lockhart PB, Brennan MT, Thornhill M, et al. Poor oral hygiene as a risk factor for infective endocarditis-related bacteremia. J Am Dent Assoc. 2009;140(10):1238–44.
36. Rogers AM, Schiller NB. Impact of the first nine months of revised infective endocarditis prophylaxis guidelines at a university hospital: so far so good. J Am Soc Echocardiogr. 2008;21(6):775.
37. Bor DH, Woolhandler S, Nardin R, et al. Infective endocarditis in the U.S., 1998-2009: a nationwide study. PLoS One. 2013;8(3):e60033.
38. Desimone DC, Tleyjeh IM, Correa de Sa DD, et al. Incidence of infective endocarditis caused by viridans group streptococci before and after publication of the 2007 American Heart Association's endocarditis prevention guidelines. Circulation. 2012;126(1):60–4.
39. Pasquali SK, He X, Mohamad Z, et al. Trends in endocarditis hospitalizations at US children's hospitals: impact of the 2007 American Heart Association Antibiotic Prophylaxis Guidelines. Am Heart J. 2012;163(5):894–9.
40. Bikdeli B, Wang Y, Kim N, et al. Trends in hospitalization rates and outcomes of endocarditis among Medicare beneficiaries. J Am Coll Cardiol. 2013;62(23):2217–26.
41. Pant S, Patel N, Deshmukh A. Trends in infective endocarditis incidence, microbiology and valve replacement in the United States from 2000-2011. J Am Coll Cardiol. 2015;65:2070–6.
42. Thornhill MH, Dayer MJ, Forde JM, et al. Impact of the NICE guideline recommending cessation of antibiotic prophylaxis for prevention of infective endocarditis: before and after study. BMJ. 2011;342:d2392.
43. Dayer MJ, Jones S, Prendergast B, et al. An increase in the incidence of infective endocarditis in England since 2008: a secular trend interrupted time series analysis. Lancet. 2015; 385(9974):1219–28.
44. Duval X, Alla F, Hoen B. Incidence of infective endocarditis caused by viridans group streptococci before and after publication of the 2007 American Heart Association's endocarditis prevention guidelines. Circulation. 2013;127(12):e520.
45. Duval X, Selton-Suty C, Alla F, et al. Endocarditis in patients with a permanent pacemaker: a 1-year epidemiological survey on infective endocarditis due to valvular and/or pacemaker infection. Clin Infect Dis. 2004;39(1):68–74.
46. Da Costa A, Kirkorian G, Cucherat M, et al. Antibiotic prophylaxis for permanent pacemaker implantation: a meta-analysis. Circulation. 1998;97(18):1796–801.

47. de Oliveira JC, Martinelli M, Nishioka SA, et al. Efficacy of antibiotic prophylaxis before the implantation of pacemakers and cardioverter-defibrillators: results of a large, prospective, randomized, double-blinded, placebo-controlled trial. Circ Arrhythm Electrophysiol. 2009; 2(1):29–34.
48. Baddour LM, Bettmann MA, Bolger AF, et al. Nonvalvular cardiovascular device-related infections. Circulation. 2003;108(16):2015–31.
49. Baddour LM, Epstein AE, Erickson CC, et al. Update on cardiovascular implantable electronic device infections and their management: a scientific statement from the American Heart Association. Circulation. 2010;121(3):458–77.
50. Habib G, Lancellotti P, Antunes MJ, Bongiorni MG, Casalta JP, Del Zotti F, et al. ESC Guidelines for the management of infective endocarditis: The Task Force for the Management of Infective Endocarditis of the European Society of Cardiology (ESC). Endorsed by: European Association for Cardio-Thoracic Surgery (EACTS), the European Association of Nuclear Medicine (EANM). Eur Heart J. 2015;36(44):3075–128.
51. Prophylaxis against infective endocarditis: antimicrobial prophylaxis against infective endocarditis in adults and children undergoing interventional procedures; NICE 2015; Available at: https://www.nice.org.uk/guidance/cg64/chapter/Recommendations

Part IX
Conclusion

Chapter 24
Infective Endocarditis in 2016: Main Achievements and Future Directions

Gilbert Habib

Infective endocarditis (IE) is a severe form of valve disease still associated with an unacceptably high mortality (10–30 % in-hospital mortality). The epidemiological profile of IE has changed over the last few years, with newer predisposing factors – valve prostheses, degenerative valve sclerosis, and intravenous drug abuse, associated with the increased use of invasive procedures at risk for bacteraemia. Health care-associated IE represents up to 30 % cases of IE, justifying aseptic measures during venous catheters manipulation and during any invasive procedures.

Several achievements have been accomplished in the management of infective endocarditis, but several problems are still unsolved:

1. In the field of diagnosis, the value of new imaging techniques, such as PET CT, is now clear, and these have been included in new diagnostic criteria as well as in a new diagnostic algorithm. Further investigations are needed to assess the real value of these new techniques in clinical practice.
2. The emerging role of the "endocarditis team": A multidisciplinary approach is mandatory for the treatment of patients with infective endocarditis, including cardiologists, cardiac surgeons, and specialists of infectious diseases. They must be treated in highly specialized centers with surgical facilities, and decisions should be made by the endocarditis team
3. Antibiotic prophylaxis: One of the main changes in both American and European guidelines is the reduction of antibiotic prophylaxis, because there is no real scientific proof of its efficacy and because it may be potentially dangerous.

   Despite recent publications suggesting an increasing risk of IE suspected to be in relation with the reduced antibiotic prophylaxis, prophylaxis is only recommended for patients with the highest risk of IE undergoing the highest risk dental procedures. Focus on prevention rather on prophylaxis is of utmost importance, since cases of nosocomial endocarditis are more and more frequent. However,

G. Habib, MD, FESC
Cardiology Department, Hôpital La Timone, Marseille, France
e-mail: Gilbert.habib3@gmail.com

© Springer International Publishing Switzerland 2016
G. Habib (ed.), *Infective Endocarditis*, DOI 10.1007/978-3-319-32432-6_24

prospective randomized studies are the unique way of solving the problem of prophylaxis but are still difficult to perform.

4. Antibiotic therapy: Several discrepancies still exist around the world about the optimal therapy according to the microorganism involved. New studies are needed to assess the real efficiency of several new antibiotic regimens. Simple and standardized protocols are probably better than innovative but sometimes difficult to perform new strategies. Conversely, targeted antibiotic therapy duration based on the results of imaging techniques is an interesting future objective, since giving the same duration antibiotic therapy to all patients is certainly not logical.

5. Treatment and management: The management of IE by an endocarditis team in a reference center is probably one of the most important new recommendations. The second one is the combination of early diagnosis, early antibiotic therapy, and early surgery. Endocarditis is a deadly disease if treated too late. We should think about reducing the delay in diagnosis, introducing antibiotics early, and sending the patient very early to the surgeon.

Finally, in the future, physicians should:

1. Focus on prevention rather than on prophylaxis to reduce the incidence of IE, particularly in the field of nosocomial endocarditis;
2. Understand the need for management of these patients with IE in close relationship with "endocarditis centers";
3. Send patients for an early surgical assessment as soon as possible.

Index

Printed by Printforce, the Netherlands